Chest MRI

Editor

PRACHI P. AGARWAL

MAGNETIC RESONANCE IMAGING CLINICS OF NORTH AMERICA

www.mri.theclinics.com

Consulting Editors
SURESH K. MUKHERJI
LYNNE S. STEINBACH

May 2015 • Volume 23 • Number 2

ELSEVIER

1600 John F. Kennedy Boulevard • Suite 1800 • Philadelphia, Pennsylvania, 19103-2899

http://www.mri.theclinics.com

MRI CLINICS OF NORTH AMERICA Volume 23, Number 2
May 2015 ISSN 1064-9689, ISBN 13: 978-0-323-37605-1

Editor: John Vassallo (j.vassallo@elsevier.com)
Developmental Editor: Meredith Clinton

Magnetic Resonance Imaging Clinics of North America (ISSN 1064-9689) is published quarterly by Elsevier Inc., 360 Park Avenue South, New York, NY 10010-1710. Months of issue are February, May, August, and November. Business and Editorial Offices: 1600 John F. Kennedy Blvd., Ste. 1800, Philadelphia, PA 19103-2899. Customer Service Office: 3251 Riverport Lane, Maryland Heights, MO 63043. Periodicals postage paid at New York, NY and additional mailing offices. Subscription prices are $375.00 per year (domestic individuals), $581.00 per year (domestic institutions), $190.00 per year (domestic students/residents), $420.00 per year (Canadian individuals), $755.00 per year (Canadian institutions), $545.00 per year (international individuals), $755.00 per year (international institutions), and $275.00 per year (international and Canadian students/residents). International air speed delivery is included in all *Clinics* subscription prices. All prices are subject to change without notice. **POSTMASTER:** Send address changes to *Magnetic Resonance Imaging Clinics*, Elsevier Health Sciences Division, Subscription Customer Service, 3251 Riverport Lane, Maryland Heights, MO 63043. Customer Service (orders, claims, online, change of address): Elsevier Health Sciences Division, Subscription Customer Service, 3251 Riverport Lane, Maryland Heights, MO 63043. Tel:1-800-654-2452 (U.S. and Canada); 314-447-8871 (outside U.S. and Canada). Fax: 314-447-8029. E-mail: journalscustomerservice-usa@elsevier.com (for print support); journalsonlinesupport-usa@elsevier.com (for online support).

Reprints. For copies of 100 or more of articles in this publication, please contact the Commercial Reprints Department, Elsevier Inc., 360 Park Avenue South, New York, NY 10010-1710. Tel.: 212-633-3874; Fax: 212-633-3820; E-mail: reprints@elsevier.com.

Magnetic Resonance Imaging Clinics of North America is covered in the *RSNA Index of Imaging Literature, MEDLINE/PubMed (Index Medicus), and EMBASE/Excerpta Medica.*

Contributors

CONSULTING EDITORS

SURESH K. MUKHERJI, MD, MBA, FACR
Professor and Chairman; W.F. Patenge
Endowed Chair, Department of Radiology,
Michigan State University, East Lansing,
Michigan

LYNNE S. STEINBACH, MD, FACR
Professor of Clinical Radiology and
Orthopaedic Surgery, Department of
Radiology and Biomedical Imaging, University
of California San Francisco, San Francisco,
California

EDITOR

PRACHI P. AGARWAL, MD
Co-Director, Pediatric Cardiac MR Imaging;
Associate Professor, Division of Cardiothoracic
Radiology, Department of Radiology,
University of Michigan Health System,
Ann Arbor, Michigan

AUTHORS

JEANNE B. ACKMAN, MD
Director of Thoracic MRI, Division of Thoracic
Imaging and Intervention, Department of
Radiology, Massachusetts General Hospital;
Assistant Professor, Harvard Medical School,
Boston, Massachusetts

PRACHI P. AGARWAL, MD
Co-Director, Pediatric Cardiac MR Imaging;
Associate Professor, Division of Cardiothoracic
Radiology, Department of Radiology,
University of Michigan Health System,
Ann Arbor, Michigan

AYAZ AGHAYEV, MD
Department of Radiology, Brigham and
Women's Hospital, Harvard Medical School,
Boston, Massachusetts

JUAN C. BAEZ, MD
Mid-Atlantic Permanente Medical Group,
Rockville, Maryland

MARCELO F.K. BENVENISTE, MD
Section of Thoracic Imaging, Department of
Diagnostic Radiology, The University of Texas
MD Anderson Cancer Center, Houston, Texas

BRETT W. CARTER, MD
Section of Thoracic Imaging, Department of
Diagnostic Radiology, The University of
Texas MD Anderson Cancer Center,
Houston, Texas

GI JEONG CHEON, MD, PhD
Cancer Research Institute, Seoul National
University College of Medicine; Department
of Nuclear Medicine, Seoul National University
College of Medicine, Seoul, Korea

PIERLUIGI CIET, MD, PhD
Department of Radiology and Pediatric
Pulmonology, Sophia Children's Hospital,
Erasmus Medical Center, Rotterdam, The
Netherlands; Department of Radiology, Beth
Israel Deaconess Medical Center, Harvard
Medical School, Boston, Massachusetts

ADAM L. DORFMAN, MD
Associate Professor, Pediatric Cardiology,
Departments of Pediatrics and Radiology,
University of Michigan Congenital Heart
Center, C.S. Mott Children's Hospital,
University of Michigan, Ann Arbor, Michigan

BASTIAAN DRIEHUYS, PhD
Department of Radiology, Center for In Vivo Microscopy, Duke University Medical Center, Durham, North Carolina

RITU R. GILL, MD, MPH
Assistant Professor, Department of Radiology, Brigham and Women's Hospital, Harvard Medical School, Boston, Massachusetts

GREGORY W. GLADISH, MD
Department of Diagnostic Radiology, The University of Texas MD Anderson Cancer Center, Houston, Texas

JIN MO GOO, MD, PhD
Department of Radiology, Institute of Radiation Medicine, Seoul National University Medical Research Center, Seoul National University College of Medicine; Cancer Research Institute, Seoul National University College of Medicine, Seoul, Korea

S. SIVARAM KAUSHIK, PhD
Department of Biomedical Engineering, Duke University; Department of Radiology, Center for In Vivo Microscopy, Duke University Medical Center, Durham, North Carolina

HISANOBU KOYAMA, MD, PhD
Division of Diagnostic Radiology, Department of Radiology, Kobe University Graduate School of Medicine, Kobe, Hyogo, Japan

EDWARD Y. LEE, MD, MPH
Department of Radiology, Boston Children's Hospital, Harvard Medical School, Boston, Massachusetts

SANG MIN LEE, MD
Department of Radiology, Institute of Radiation Medicine, Seoul National University Medical Research Center, Seoul National University College of Medicine, Seoul, Korea

SEBASTIAN LEY, MD
Diagnostic and Interventional Radiology, Chirurgische Klinik Dr Rinecker; Department of Clinical Radiology, Ludwig Maximilians University, Munich, Germany

JIMMY C. LU, MD
Assistant Professor, Pediatric Cardiology, Departments of Pediatrics and Radiology, University of Michigan Congenital Heart Center, C.S. Mott Children's Hospital, University of Michigan, Ann Arbor, Michigan

MARYAM GHADIMI MAHANI, MD
Assistant Professor, Department of Radiology, C.S. Mott Children's Hospital, University of Michigan, Ann Arbor, Michigan

EDITH M. MAROM, MD
Section of Thoracic Imaging, Department of Diagnostic Radiology, The University of Texas MD Anderson Cancer Center, Houston, Texas

SUMIAKI MATSUMOTO, MD, PhD
Division of Functional and Diagnostic Imaging Research, Department of Radiology; Advanced Biomedical Imaging Research Center, Kobe University Graduate School of Medicine, Kobe, Hyogo, Japan

HOLMAN P. McADAMS, MD
Department of Radiology, Duke University Medical Center, Durham, North Carolina

GISELA C. MUELLER, MD, MS
Department of Radiology, University of Michigan Health System, Ann Arbor, Michigan

ROBERT MULKERN, PhD
Department of Radiology, Boston Children's Hospital, Harvard Medical School, Boston, Massachusetts

IGA MURADYAN, PhD
Instructor, Department of Radiology, Brigham and Women's Hospital, Harvard Medical School, Boston, Massachusetts

YOSHIHARU OHNO, MD, PhD
Division of Functional and Diagnostic Imaging Research, Department of Radiology; Advanced Biomedical Imaging Research Center, Kobe University Graduate School of Medicine, Kobe, Hyogo, Japan

CHANG MIN PARK, MD, PhD
Department of Radiology, Institute of Radiation Medicine, Seoul National University Medical Research Center, Seoul National University College of Medicine; Cancer Research Institute, Seoul National University College of Medicine, Seoul, Korea

SAMUEL PATZ, PhD
Professor, Department of Radiology, Brigham and Women's Hospital, Harvard Medical School, Boston, Massachusetts

KAREN RODRIGUEZ
Department of Radiology, University of Michigan Health System, Ann Arbor, Michigan

JUSTUS E. ROOS, MD
Associate Professor, Department of Radiology, Duke University Medical Center, Durham, North Carolina

FRANK J. RYBICKI, MD, PhD
Department of Radiology, Brigham and Women's Hospital, Harvard Medical School, Boston, Massachusetts

RAVI T. SEETHAMRAJU, PhD
Magnetic Resonance, Research, and Development, Siemens Healthcare, Boston, Massachusetts

JADRANKA STOJANOVSKA, MD, MS
Assistant Professor, Department of Radiology, University of Michigan Health System, Ann Arbor, Michigan

KAZURO SUGIMURA, MD
Division of Diagnostic Radiology, Department of Radiology, Kobe University Graduate School of Medicine, Kobe, Hyogo, Japan

MYLENE T. TRUONG, MD
Section of Thoracic Imaging, Department of Diagnostic Radiology, The University of Texas MD Anderson Cancer Center, Houston, Texas

SOON HO YOON, MD
Department of Radiology, Institute of Radiation Medicine, Seoul National University Medical Research Center, Seoul National University College of Medicine, Seoul, Korea

TAKESHI YOSHIKAWA, MD, PhD
Division of Functional and Diagnostic Imaging Research, Department of Radiology; Advanced Biomedical Imaging Research Center, Kobe University Graduate School of Medicine, Kobe, Hyogo, Japan

CHANG MIN PARK, MD, PhD
Department of Radiology, Institute of Radiation
Medicine, Seoul National University Medical
Research Center, Seoul National University
College of Medicine; Cancer Research
Institute, Seoul National University College of
Medicine, Seoul, Korea

SAMUEL PATZ, PhD
Professor, Department of Radiology, Brigham
and Women's Hospital, Harvard Medical
School, Boston, Massachusetts

RAFAEL RODRIGUEZ
Department of Radiology, University of Texas

JOSHUA ROSENKRANTZ, MD

JADRANKA STOJANOVSKA, MD, MS
Assistant Professor, Department of
Radiology, University of Michigan Health
System, Ann Arbor, Michigan

KAZURO SUGIMURA, MD
Division of Diagnostic Radiology,
Department of Radiology, Kobe University
Graduate School of Medicine, Kobe,
Hyogo, Japan

MYLENE T. TRUONG, MD
Section of Thoracic Imaging, Department of
Diagnostic Radiology, The University of
Texas MD Anderson Cancer Center,
Houston, Texas

SIXIA HO, PhD, MD

FARISTH YOUSEFZADEH, MD, PhD

Contents

> The high soft tissue contrast of MR imaging enables superior tissue characterization of mediastinal masses, adding diagnostic specificity and often changing and benefiting clinical management. MR imaging can better discern cystic from solid content and can detect microscopic fat, hemorrhage, and fibrous content within lesions. In many cases, mediastinal MR imaging may prevent unnecessary diagnostic intervention. In other cases, MR imaging may indicate the optimal site for biopsy or the correct compartment for resection. Awareness of the efficacy of MR imaging with regard to mediastinal mass characterization and judicious MR imaging utilization should further improve patient care.

> Thymoma is the most common primary malignancy of the anterior mediastinum and the most common thymic epithelial neoplasm, but it is a rare tumor that constitutes less than 1% of adult malignancies. Computed tomography (CT) is currently the imaging modality of choice for distinguishing thymoma from other anterior mediastinal masses, characterizing the primary tumor, and staging the disease. However, magnetic resonance imaging is also effective in evaluating and characterizing anterior mediastinal masses and staging thymoma in patients with contraindications to contrast-material-enhanced CT such as contrast allergy and/or renal failure.

 Videos of three subjects with Mesothelioma showing dynamic perfusion in coronal plane: FLASH, TWIST and RADIAL VIBE acquisitions comparing effect of respiration accompany this article

> Computed tomography is the first-line modality for evaluation of chest diseases primarily because of its spatial resolution. Magnetic resonance (MR) imaging is used as a problem-solving tool to answer key questions that are vital to optimal patient management. MR has the potential to provide qualitative, quantitative, anatomic, and functional information without the use of ionizing radiation or nephrotoxic contrast administration. With new advances in proton MR techniques, MR

imaging can overcome some of the inherent problems associated with imaging the lung. This article describes novel MR applications for evaluation of the pleura and pleural diseases.

Tumors of the chest wall are uncommon lesions that represent approximately 5% of all thoracic malignancies. These tumors comprise a heterogeneous group of neoplasms that may arise from osseous structures or soft tissues and may be malignant or benign. Most chest wall neoplasms are malignant and include lesions that secondarily involve the chest wall via direct invasion or metastasis from intrathoracic tumors or arise as primary tumors. More than 20% of lesions may be detected on chest radiography. This review focuses on key features of malignant and benign chest wall tumors (primary and secondary) on MR imaging examinations.

Functional imaging offers information more sensitive to changes in lung structure and function. Hyperpolarized helium (^{3}He) and xenon (^{129}Xe) MR imaging of the lungs provides sensitive contrast mechanisms to probe changes in pulmonary ventilation, microstructure, and gas exchange. Gas imaging has shifted to the use of ^{129}Xe. Xenon is well-tolerated. ^{129}Xe is soluble in pulmonary tissue, which allows exploring specific lung function characteristics involved in gas exchange and alveolar oxygenation. Hyperpolarized gases and ^{129}Xe in particular stand to be an excellent probe of pulmonary structure and function, and provide sensitive and noninvasive biomarkers for pulmonary diseases.

MR imaging has emerged as a major new research and diagnostic tool for various pulmonary diseases, especially lung cancer. State-of-the art thoracic MR imaging now has the potential to be used as a substitute for traditional imaging techniques and/or to play a complementary role in patient management. This article focuses on these recent advances in MR imaging for lung cancer imaging, especially for pulmonary nodule assessment, lung cancer staging, postoperative lung function prediction, and prediction and evaluation of therapeutic response and recurrence. The potential and limitations of routine clinical application of these advances are discussed and compared with those of other modalities.

PET/MR imaging, a new hybrid modality, is thought to have great potential in oncologic imaging because it provides advantages of both PET, which allows functional imaging capability, and MR imaging, which allows high spatial resolution imaging without radiation exposure. Despite the inherent weakness of MR imaging in lung imaging, initial studies on lung cancer revealed that PET/MR imaging showed highly correlated standardized uptake values of lesions and equivalent performance in terms of lesion detection and staging compared with PET/computed tomography (CT). Thus, to affirm the actual clinical benefits of dedicated PET/MR imaging over PET/CT, prospective studies with more patients are warranted.

and complications of vascular thoracic outlet syndrome. This article reviews thoracic outlet anatomy, disorders of the vascular component, and typical imaging findings by contrast-enhanced 3D MRA.

Thoracic MR imaging in the pediatric population provides unique challenges requiring tailored protocols and a practical approach to pediatric issues, such as patient motion and sedation. Concern regarding the use of ionizing radiation in the pediatric population has continued to advance the use of MR imaging despite these challenges. This article provides a practical approach to thoracic vascular MR imaging with special attention paid to pediatric-specific issues such as sedation. Thoracic vascular anatomy and pathology are discussed with an emphasis on protocols that can facilitate accurate diagnosis.

Advances in technology coupled with optimized protocols now permit evaluation of the lungs with magnetic resonance (MR) imaging in the pediatric population. Although computed tomography remains the preferred imaging modality for this purpose, MR imaging provides a radiation-free alternative that can answer many important clinical questions and provide additional data. In addition, the use of newer techniques and equipment such as MR-imaging-compatible spirometers allows for functional assessment of the pediatric airways. This article reviews the up-to-date MR imaging techniques as well as imaging findings of selected clinically important disorders that affect the lungs and airways in the pediatric population.

MAGNETIC RESONANCE IMAGING CLINICS OF NORTH AMERICA

RELATED INTEREST

Radiologic Clinics of North America, January 2014 (Vol. 52, No. 1)
Thoracic Imaging
Jane P. Ko, *Editor*

VISIT THE CLINICS ONLINE!
Access your subscription at:
www.theclinics.com

PROGRAM OBJECTIVE

The goal of *Magnetic Resonance Imaging Clinics of North America* is to keep practicing physicians up to date with current clinical practice by providing timely articles reviewing the state of the art in patient care.

TARGET AUDIENCE

All practicing physicians and healthcare professionals who provide patient care utilizing findings from Magnetic Resonance Imaging.

LEARNING OBJECTIVES

Upon completion of this activity, participants will be able to:
1. Review the uses of MR imaging in evaluation of diseases of the chest.
2. Discuss the uses of MR imaging in cancer evaluation.
3. Recognize techniques and applications of Hyperpolarized Gas MRI.

ACCREDITATION

The Elsevier Office of Continuing Medical Education (EOCME) is accredited by the Accreditation Council for Continuing Medical Education (ACCME) to provide continuing medical education for physicians.

The EOCME designates this enduring material for a maximum of 15 *AMA PRA Category 1 Credit*(s)™. Physicians should claim only the credit commensurate with the extent of their participation in the activity.

All other health care professionals requesting continuing education credit for this enduring material will be issued a certificate of participation.

DISCLOSURE OF CONFLICTS OF INTEREST

The EOCME assesses conflict of interest with its instructors, faculty, planners, and other individuals who are in a position to control the content of CME activities. All relevant conflicts of interest that are identified are thoroughly vetted by EOCME for fair balance, scientific objectivity, and patient care recommendations. EOCME is committed to providing its learners with CME activities that promote improvements or quality in healthcare and not a specific proprietary business or a commercial interest.

The planning committee, staff, authors and editors listed below have identified no financial relationships or relationships to products or devices they or their spouse/life partner have with commercial interest related to the content of this CME activity:

Jeanne B. Ackman, MD; Prachi P. Agarwal, MD; Ayaz Aghayev, MD; Juan C. Baez, MD; Marcelo F. K. Benveniste, MD; Gi Jeong Cheon, MD, PhD; Pierluigi Ciet, MD, PhD; Adam L. Dorfman, MD; Anjali Fortna; Ritu R. Gill, MD, MPH; Gregory W. Gladish, MD; Kristen Helm; S. Sivaram Kaushik, PhD; Hisanobu Koyama, MD, PhD; Sang Min Lee, MD; Edward Y. Lee, MD, MPH; Sebastian Ley, MD; Jimmy C. Lu, MD; Maryam Ghadimi Mahani, MD; Edith M. Marom, MD; Holman P. McAdams, MD; Gisela C. Mueller, MD, MS; Suresh K. Mukherji, MD, MBA, FACR; Robert Mulkern, PhD; Iga Muradyan, PhD; Chang Min Park, MD, PhD; Samuel Patz, PhD; Karen Rodriguez; Justus E. Roos, MD; Frank J. Rybicki, MD, PhD; Lynne S. Steinbach, MD, FACR; Jadranka Stojanovska, MD, MS; Karthikeyan Subramaniam; Kazuro Sugimura, MD; Mylene T. Truong, MD; John Vassallo; Soon Ho Yoon, MD.

The planning committee, staff, authors and editors listed below have identified financial relationships or relationships to products or devices they or their spouse/life partner have with commercial interest related to the content of this CME activity:

Brett W. Carter, MD is a consultant/advisor for St. Jude Medical, Inc., has royalties/patents with Amirsys, Inc, and has research support from ACRIN.

Bastiaan Driehuys, PhD has stock ownership in Polarean.

Jin Mo Goo, MD, PhD has research support from Guerbet Korea Ltd.

Sumiaki Matsumoto, MD, PhD has research support from Toshiba Corporation.

Yoshiharu Ohno, MD, PhD has research support from Bayer AG, Daiichi Sankyo Company Limited, Eisai Co., Ltd, Guerbet LLC, Philips Electronics Japan, Ltd, and Toshiba Corporation.

Ravi Teja Seethamraju, PhD has stock ownership and an employment affiliation with Siemens AG.

Takeshi Yoshikawa, MD, PhD has research support from Eisai Co., Ltd and Toshiba Medical Systems Corporation.

UNAPPROVED/OFF-LABEL USE DISCLOSURE

The EOCME requires CME faculty to disclose to the participants:
1. When products or procedures being discussed are off-label, unlabelled, experimental, and/or investigational (not US Food and Drug Administration [FDA] approved); and
2. Any limitations on the information presented, such as data that are preliminary or that represent ongoing research, interim analyses, and/or unsupported opinions. Faculty may discuss information about pharmaceutical agents that is outside of FDA-approved labelling. This information is intended solely for CME and is not intended to promote off-label use of these

medications. If you have any questions, contact the medical affairs department of the manufacturer for the most recent prescribing information.

TO ENROLL

To enroll in the *Magnetic Resonance Imaging Clinics of North America* Continuing Medical Education program, call customer service at 1-800-654-2452 or sign up online at http://www.theclinics.com/home/cme. The CME program is available to subscribers for an additional annual fee of USD 250.

METHOD OF PARTICIPATION

In order to claim credit, participants must complete the following:
1. Complete enrolment as indicated above.
2. Read the activity.
3. Complete the CME Test and Evaluation. Participants must achieve a score of 70% on the test. All CME Tests and Evaluations must be completed online.

CME INQUIRIES/SPECIAL NEEDS

For all CME inquiries or special needs, please contact elsevierCME@elsevier.com.

Foreword
Chest MR Imaging

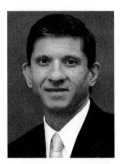

Suresh K. Mukherji, MD, MBA, FACR
Consulting Editor

Dr Prachi Agarwal is one of the brightest young minds not only in Cardiothoracic Radiology, but also in all of Radiology. She is clearly a "rising star," and I was delighted when she agreed to edit this issue of *Magnetic Resonance Imaging Clinics of North America* on the thorax. She has done an outstanding job bringing together world experts for each subject matter. The topics include MR imaging of the mediastinum, thymus, pleura, chest wall; vascular imaging (with a focus on aorta, systemic and pulmonary veins, thoracic outlet, and pulmonary arteries); and lung imaging, including lung cancer. There are also articles devoted to hyperpolarized gas imaging, PET-MR imaging, and the pediatric chest. This is a unique issue, and I thank Dr Agarwal and all of the authors for creating an outstanding issue of *Magnetic Resonance Imaging Clinics of North America*.

Suresh K. Mukherji, MD, MBA, FACR
Department of Radiology
Michigan State University
846 Service Road
East Lansing, MI 48824, USA

E-mail address:
mukherji@rad.msu.edu

Magn Reson Imaging Clin N Am 23 (2015) xv
http://dx.doi.org/10.1016/j.mric.2015.02.003
1064-9689/15/$ – see front matter © 2015 Published by Elsevier Inc.

Magn Reson Imaging Clin N Am 23 (2015) xv
http://dx.doi.org/10.1016/j.mric.2015.02.003
1064-9689/15/$ - see front matter © 2015 Published by Elsevier Inc.

Preface
Chest MR Imaging

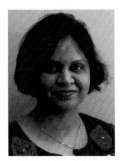

Prachi P. Agarwal, MD
Editor

There are several inherent challenges in MR imaging of the thorax. The last few decades have witnessed major strides in the field of MR imaging that have not only improved the quality of images but also widened the applicability in thoracic imaging.

Despite technological advances, thoracic MR imaging is still underutilized. A recent survey of the Society of Thoracic Radiology members[1] found that 37% (67/180) of respondents did not interpret or report a single nonvascular thoracic MR imaging, while 64% (116/182) interpreted or reported less than 10 MR images over the prior year. Importantly, 25% (41/166) of respondents felt that there was insufficient thoracic MR imaging literature and limited CME courses and lectures in this field.

It is my hope that this issue on thoracic MR imaging focusing on noncardiac applications will bridge this gap and serve as an important resource for radiologists who are interested in initiating or improving on an existing thoracic MR practice. The issue includes topics covering different facets of thoracic MR imaging, including mediastinal, thymic, and pleural assessment; vascular imaging (with a focus on aorta, systemic and pulmonary veins, thoracic outlet, and pulmonary arteries); lung imaging, including lung cancer and hyperpolarized gas imaging; novel applications such as PET MR imaging; and pediatric applications.

I express my heartfelt thanks to all the experts in the field who contributed to this issue and shared their expertise. I would also like to thank the staff at Elsevier, who has made this issue of *Magnetic Resonance Imaging Clinics of North America* possible.

Prachi P. Agarwal, MD
Division of Cardiothoracic Radiology
Department of Radiology
University of Michigan Health System
1500 East Medical Center Drive
Ann Arbor, MI 48109, USA

E-mail address:
prachia@med.umich.edu

REFERENCE

1. Ackman JB, Wu CC, Halpern EF, et al. Nonvascular thoracic magnetic resonance imaging: the current state of training, utilization, and perceived value: survey of the society of thoracic radiology membership. J Thorac Imaging 2014;29(4):252–7.

Magn Reson Imaging Clin N Am 23 (2015) xvii
http://dx.doi.org/10.1016/j.mric.2015.02.002
1064-9689/15/$ – see front matter © 2015 Published by Elsevier Inc.

Erratum

In the August 2011 issue (Volume 19, number 3), in the article on pages 429–437, "Normal Brain Anatomy on Magnetic Resonance Imaging," by Bryan Pukenas, MD, the following corrections were made to Figures 4, 7, and 11:

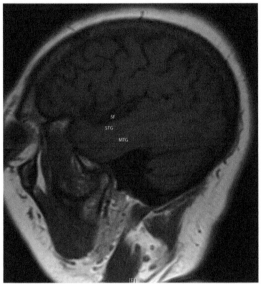

Fig. 4. Sagittal T1-weighted (TR 442, TE 9.3) far lateral image demonstrating the Sylvian fissure (SF) as well as the superior temporal (STG) and middle temporal gyri (MTG).

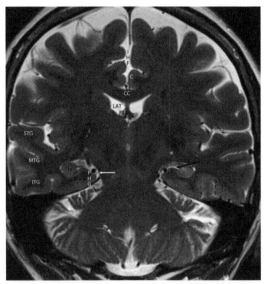

Fig. 7. Coronal T2-weighted image (repetition time, 6360 ms; echo time, 89 ms) demonstrating the inferior and medial border of the temporal lobe, the parahippocampal gyrus (PHG). The subiculum (S) and body of the hippocampus (H) are also demarcated. The hippocampal sulcus is seen on the left (black arrow), as are the collateral sulcus (cs) and the occipitotemporal sulcus (ots). Note the flow voids in the ambient cistern (white arrow) and sylvian fissure (SF). The superior, middle, and inferior temporal gyri (STG, MTG, ITG, respectively) are also seen. At this level, the bodies of the fornices (F) are present inferior to the corpus callosum (CC) and within the lateral ventricles (LAT). The cingulate gyrus (C) and interhemispheric fissure (IHF) are present in the midline.

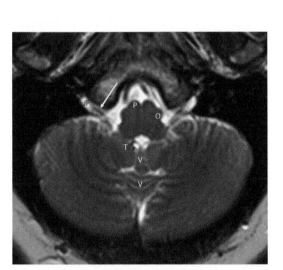

Fig. 11. Axial T2-weighted image (TR 6900 TE 96) through the medulla demonstrating the medullary pyramid (P), olive (O), cerebellar tonsil (T), and cerebellar vermis (V). The cranial nerve 9-10-11 complex (white arrow) is seen coursing through the jugular foramen (JF).

Magn Reson Imaging Clin N Am 23 (2015) xix
http://dx.doi.org/10.1016/j.mric.2015.02.001
1064-9689/15/$ – see front matter © 2015 Elsevier Inc. All rights reserved.

Magn Reson Imaging Clin N Am 23 (2015) xxx
http://dx.doi.org/10.1016/j.mric.2015.02.001

MR Imaging of Mediastinal Masses

Jeanne B. Ackman, MD

KEYWORDS

- MR imaging • Mediastinal mass • Tissue characterization • Cystic • Fibrous • Hemorrhagic
- Diagnostic specificity • Clinical management

KEY POINTS

- The high soft tissue contrast of MR imaging enables superior tissue characterization of mediastinal masses, compared with computed tomography, and often increases diagnostic specificity.
- Appropriate use of mediastinal MR imaging may prevent unnecessary diagnostic intervention.
- When intervention is needed, mediastinal MR imaging can direct interventionists toward the optimal site for biopsy or the correct compartment for resection.

INTRODUCTION

The high soft tissue contrast of MR imaging, relative to other imaging modalities including computed tomography (CT), enables superior tissue characterization of many lesions throughout the body, including those in the mediastinum. The result, in many cases, is added diagnostic specificity or virtual biopsy of the lesion. Much has been written about mediastinal masses and how their differential diagnosis can be narrowed by determination of their mediastinal compartment of origin. The premise of this method is that knowledge of the structures that normally reside in a given mediastinal compartment reduces the number of diagnostic possibilities.

This article describes how adding MR imaging to the diagnostic armamentarium yields further diagnostic precision, with potential to improve clinical management. Therefore, this article is organized not by mediastinal compartment but by MR findings that distinguish one mediastinal mass tissue type from another. The following categories are discussed in the context of their diagnostic significance, as they particularly highlight the value of MR imaging in the mediastinum:

- Discernment of cystic from solid lesions
  - Corollary: discernment of solid tissue amidst hemorrhage and necrosis; guidance for diagnostic intervention
- Detection of macroscopic and microscopic fat
- Detection of lesion T2-hypointensity
- Demonstration of a lesion's dynamic contrast enhancement pattern
- Demonstration of matching mediastinal lesions in terms of signal and enhancement in the same patient and its significance
- Detection of low apparent diffusion coefficient (ADC) values
- Determination of lesion invasiveness
- Discernment of mediastinal from paramediastinal lesions

The new International Thymic Malignancy Interest Group (ITMIG) classification of mediastinal compartments,[1] developed by a consensus of its members, is used when describing the compartment of origin of the mass under discussion in the article. Instead of basing lesion location on mediastinal compartments delineated by lines drawn on a lateral chest radiograph,[2] this more

Disclosure: The author has nothing to disclose.
Division of Thoracic Imaging and Intervention, Department of Radiology, Massachusetts General Hospital, Harvard Medical School, Founders 202, 55 Fruit Street, Boston, MA 02114, USA
E-mail address: jackman@mgh.harvard.edu

Magn Reson Imaging Clin N Am 23 (2015) 141–164
http://dx.doi.org/10.1016/j.mric.2015.01.002
1064-9689/15/$ – see front matter © 2015 Elsevier Inc. All rights reserved.

modern classification bases lesion location on its relationship to 3 compartments delineated by cross-sectional imaging that extend from the thoracic inlet to the diaphragm: a prevascular (anterior mediastinal) compartment, including all structures anterior to the pericardium and proximal ascending aorta; a visceral (middle mediastinal) compartment, including all major mediastinal visceral structures extending from anterior pericardium posteriorly to a vertical line drawn 1 cm posterior to the anterior margin of the spine (both the trachea and the esophagus are therefore included in this middle mediastinal compartment); and a paravertebral (posterior mediastinal) compartment, including all mediastinal structures posterior to this vertical line. A list of mediastinal masses typically found in each of these compartments is provided in **Table 1**.

MEDIASTINAL MAGNETIC RESONANCE PROTOCOL

High quality mediastinal MR protocols involve pulse sequences required to adequately characterize a lesion. These protocols generally include T1-weighted, T2-weighted, and T2-weighted fat-saturated pulse sequences, as well as pre-gadolinium and post-gadolinium three-dimensional (3D) ultrafast gradient echo (GRE) dynamic contrast-enhanced imaging. Ultrafast

Table 1
Mediastinal masses by compartment[a]

Anterior Mediastinum or Prevascular Compartment[a]	Middle Mediastinum or Visceral Compartment	Posterior Mediastinum or Paravertebral Compartment
Lymphadenopathy	Lymphadenopathy	Lymphadenopathy
Thyroid and parathyroid lesions	Thyroid lesions	—
—	Ascending aortic aneurysm Aortic arch aneurysm Dilated main pulmonary artery Aberrant right/left subclavian artery Descending aortic aneurysm	Descending aortic aneurysm
Thymic lesions (cyst, hyperplasia, thymic neoplasm, including lymphoma)	—	—
—	Paraganglioma and other neurogenic tumors	Neurogenic tumors including neurofibroma, schwannoma, paraganglioma
—	—	Lateral meningocele
Germ cell tumors	—	—
—	Pancreatic pseudocyst	Pancreatic pseudocyst
Pleuropericardial or mesothelial[b] cysts	Mesothelial cysts	Mesothelial cysts
—	—	Extramedullary hematopoiesis
—	Tracheal lesions	—
—	Esophageal lesions	—
Morgagni hernia	Hiatal hernia	Bochdalek hernia
Bronchogenic cysts (very rarely)	Foregut duplication cysts	Foregut duplication cysts
Abscess	Abscess	Abscess
Hematoma	Hematoma	Hematoma
Fibrosing mediastinitis	Fibrosing mediastinitis	Fibrosing mediastinitis
Hemangioma	Hemangioma	Hemangioma
Lymphangioma	Lymphangioma	Lymphangioma
Sarcoma	Sarcoma	Sarcoma

[a] Mediastinal compartments, as prescribed by the new ITMIG classification.
[b] Mesothelial cysts may be found anywhere in the body where mesothelium exists.

GRE in-phase and out-of-phase chemical shift MR imaging is recommended for T1-weighted sequences because lesion coverage for both phases can be acquired in a single 20-second breath hold and additional information is obtained regarding the presence or absence of microscopic or intravoxel fat within a lesion at no additional time cost. Supplemental diffusion-weighted and short *tau* inversion recovery imaging can be performed if the finding of low ADC values is anticipated to refine the differential diagnosis or if the detection of bone marrow edema or involvement is diagnostically or therapeutically critical, respectively.

Breath-hold imaging for all pulse sequences, including the 3-plane localizer, is strongly preferred to respiratory gating because it more reliably freezes respiratory motion and dispenses with associated respiratory motion artifact. Breath-hold imaging is almost universally successful in patients, from adolescent to elderly, provided the technologist rehearses breath-holding with the patient before the patient lies down on the table, primes the patient before each pulse sequence about the nature (length, frequency) of the breath holds, and provides MR-compatible 2-L nasal cannula oxygen[3] when breath-hold difficulty is anticipated. If a patient requires higher amounts of oxygen therapy at home or in the hospital, the volume of oxygen delivery should be suitably adjusted.

When cardiac gating is used, electrocardiogram (ECG) gating is strongly preferred to peripheral gating because ECG gating more reliably freezes cardiac motion and virtually eradicates associated pulsatility artifact.[4]

A suggested mediastinal MR imaging protocol is provided in **Table 2**. For noninvasive thymic lesion evaluation, a shortened version of this protocol can be used (**Box 1**).

TISSUE CHARACTERIZATION OF MEDIASTINAL MASSES: ITS DIAGNOSTIC AND THERAPEUTIC SIGNIFICANCE
The Diagnostic Significance of Discernment of Cystic from Solid Lesions

It is easy to misinterpret cystic lesions as solid on both noncontrast and contrast-enhanced CT.[5] Many cystic lesions in the mediastinum contain hemorrhage, proteinaceous material, and occasionally calcium oxalate (milk of calcium), all of which may increase the attenuation of a lesion and cause the lesion to appear solid on CT. Although recalling the patient for a subsequent CT scan without and with intravenous (IV) contrast could help demonstrate whether a lesion enhances, it is not practical because it substantially increases

radiation exposure and may not detect more subtly enhancing septations or small mural nodules. Dual-source CT offers some promise in this context, but it too may not show subtle lesion complexity with the same efficacy as MR imaging on account of its inferior soft tissue contrast to MR imaging, and it cannot do so without radiation exposure.

Thymic cysts are instructive in this regard. Research has shown that these benign lesions are often misinterpreted as thymomas on CT.[5] Thymic cysts may be unilocular or multilocular and may be solitary or associated with thymic hyperplasia, thymic neoplasms, and lymphoma. Congenital thymic cysts are typically unilocular and acquired thymic cysts may be unilocular or multilocular. These acquired thymic cysts, unlike their congenital counterparts, do not usually contain thymic epithelium in their walls and generally arise in the setting of inflammation and fibrosis, whether from prior surgery, trauma, infectious/inflammatory processes (human immunodeficiency virus [HIV], autoimmune), chemotherapy, or radiation. They arise from the thymopharyngeal duct remnant and may therefore occur anywhere along a line from the angle of the mandible to the thymic bed.[6,7] These lesions may be of variable attenuation on CT and of variable T1 signal on MR imaging.[8] The CT appearance of these cystic lesions can be misleading and may even prompt inappropriate intervention in some cases (**Figs. 1–3**).[5] Unilocular thymic cysts can be misinterpreted as thymomas, as was the case with the example in **Fig. 1**. It is critical to be aware that thymic cysts have been observed to measure up to 97 Hounsfield units (HU)[5] and that they can fluctuate both in size and attenuation over time and still be benign (see **Fig. 2**). A simple cyst in this context refers to a well-circumscribed, fluid-containing lesion, with a barely perceptible or thin, smooth wall and no internal lesion complexity, whether or not it contains hemorrhagic or proteinaceous material and whether or not the wall enhances. Two examples of multilocular thymic cysts are provided in **Fig. 3**.

An important caveat to the interpretation of a simple thymic cyst by MR imaging is that the malignant potential of simple cysts in the thymic bed found by MR imaging is not known. The risk of cystic thymoma arising from one of these simple cysts is apt to be low given the rarity of these tumors and the extremely low malignant potential of simple cysts found elsewhere in the body by MR imaging. Nevertheless, until future investigation reveals otherwise, these lesions warrant follow-up. The consensus reached between thoracic radiologists and thoracic surgeons at our quaternary referral institution is that these cysts be followed for up to 5 years, should they

Table 2
Mediastinal MR imaging protocol

Pulse Sequence	GE	Siemens	Philips	TR (ms)[a]	TE (ms)[b]	Flip Angle	NEX	Slice Thickness (mm)
BH axial and sagittal SSFP balanced gradient echo (GRE)	FIESTA	True FISP	BFFE	3–270	1.2–1.5 (minimum full)	45–80	1	7
BH coronal ultrafast spin echo T2	SSFSE	HASTE	UFSE	900–1000 (minimum)	80–100	NA	≤1	8
BH sagittal UFSE fat-saturated T2	SSFSE	HASTE	UFSE	900–1000 (minimum)	80–100	NA	≤1	7
BH axial in-phase and out-of-phase (chemical shift) ultrafast GRE T1 (dual echo preferable)	FSPGR	TurboFLASH	TFE	115–190	4.2–4.8/2.1–2.4	70–80	1	7
BH cardiac gated double IR T2	Double IR FSE T2	Double IR TSE T2	Double IR UFSE T2	1600–4600	110–140	NA	1	7
BH before and after 3D ultrafast GRE with automated subtraction (post-gadolinium imaging) acquired at 20 s (axial), 1 min (axial), 3 min (sagittal), and 5 min (axial)[c] upon administration of 20cc of IV gadolinium	LAVA	VIBE	THRIVE	3–5	1.5–2.5	10–12	<1	5
Optional coronal/sagittal BH STIR	Fast STIR	Turbo STIR	STIR TSE	2500	50	NA	1	7
Optional diffusion-weighted echo planar imaging	eDWI	DWI	DWI	140	1–2 (minimum)	NA	2	5–7
Optional BH cardiac gated double inversion recovery T1	Double IR prep FSE T1	Double IR prep TSE T1	Double IR prep UFSE T1	850–1100	30–40	NA	1	7
Optional BH cardiac gated sagittal double inversion recovery fat-saturated T2	Double IR FSE fat-saturated T2	Double IR TSE fat-saturated T2	Double IR UFSE fat-saturated T2	1600–4600	110–115	NA	≤1	7
Optional respiratory-triggered axial-driven equilibrium without and with fat saturation	FRFSE	RESTORE	DRIVE	4000–6000	90	NA	4	7

Abbreviations: BH, breath hold; DWI, diffusion-weighted imaging; IR, inversion recovery; NA, not applicable; NEX, number of excitations; SSFP, steady state free precession; STIR, short *tau* inversion recovery; TE, echo time; TR, recovery time; UFSE, ultrafast spin echo.

[a] Sample TR: this parameter varies as a function of MR manufacturer, body habitus, desired coverage volume, and many other factors.
[b] Sample TE: this parameter varies as a function of MR manufacturer, body habitus, desired coverage volume, and many other factors.
[c] Option to add, for example, postgadolinium axial imaging 2 minutes and 4 minutes after injection. Imaging planes can be changed to optimize lesion characterization.
Adapted from Ackman JB. A practical guide to non-vascular thoracic magnetic resonance imaging. J Thorac Imaging 2014;29(1):24; with permission.

persist, to ensure benignity. Follow-up imaging may be achieved by noncontrast MR imaging, provided the precontrast images reveal no changes of concern. The first follow-up may be performed at 6 months, with annual follow-up thereafter, provided there has been no concerning interval change.

Foregut duplication cysts are most typically found in the middle and posterior mediastinal compartments. Uncomplicated foregut duplication cysts (noninfected, and without bronchial connection) manifest as unilocular, well-circumscribed masses of variable attenuation on CT, sometimes mimicking solid lesions, and of variable T1-weighted signal on MR imaging.[9] They are almost always uniformly T2-hyperintense and may have either a barely perceptible wall or a thin, smooth, enhancing wall on MR imaging. However, this wall enhancement is seldom appreciable by CT. Mediastinal bronchogenic cysts most commonly present in the middle mediastinum (particularly the paratracheal and subcarinal spaces), less commonly in the posterior mediastinum, and rarely in the anterior mediastinum.[9] Esophageal duplication cysts closely appose the esophagus and therefore may present in the subcarinal space as well. Esophageal duplication cysts may be round or more elongated or tubular in shape and may have a slightly thicker wall than bronchogenic cysts.[6] Neurenteric cysts should show some relationship

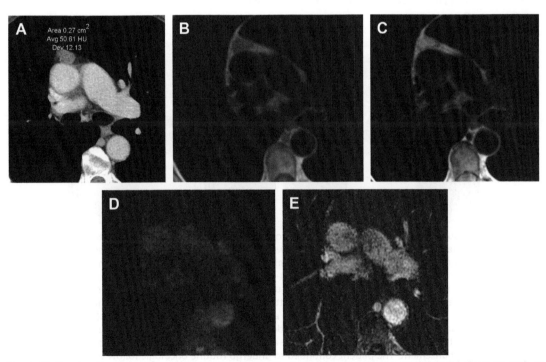

Fig. 1. Unilocular thymic cyst in a 65-year-old man with medullary thyroid cancer. (A) Axial chest CT with IV contrast revealing a lesion measuring 51 Hounsfield units (HU) in the thymic bed deemed by the reporting radiologist to be solid and likely to represent a thymic neoplasm. (B) Axial cardiac-gated double IR T1-weighted, (C) cardiac-gated double inversion recovery (IR) T2-weighted, and (D, E) pregadolinium and postgadolinium subtracted 3D ultrafast fat-saturated T1-weighted MR imaging reveal this lesion to represent a nonenhancing, unilocular cyst with intermediate T1 signal and marked T2-hyperintensity.

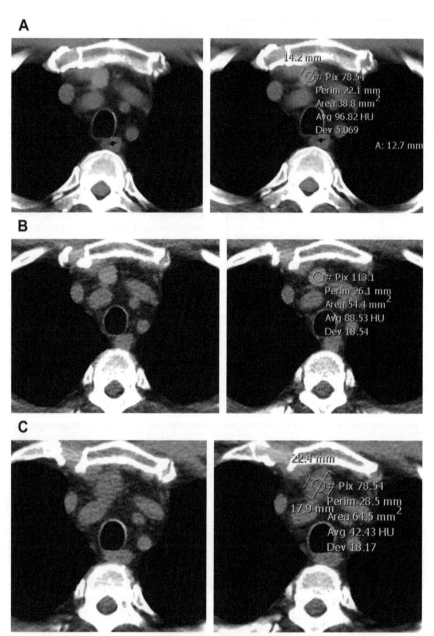

Fig. 2. Thymic nodule fluctuating in size and attenuation over time on CT in a man with a history of lung cancer undergoing routine oncologic follow-up. This lesion was proved by MR imaging and subsequent follow-up to near resolution to represent a simple, unilocular thymic cyst. At its highest attenuation, the cyst measured 97 HU. (*A*) Axial chest CT without IV contrast shows a 1.4-cm thymic nodule measuring 97 HU at baseline. (*B*) The nodule was stable in size and attenuation on follow-up noncontrast CT performed 2 years from baseline but showed an increase in size (2.2 cm) and decrease in attenuation (42 HU) on (*C*) follow-up noncontrast axial CT performed 3 years from baseline. This change in CT appearance prompted MR imaging (*D–G*). (*D*) Axial in-phase T1, (*E*) cardiac gated double IR T2, and (*F*) pregadolinium and (*G*) postgadolinium 3D ultrafast GRE MR images revealing the thymic nodule to be T1-hypointense and T2-hyperintense, with a thin, smooth enhancing wall and no internal enhancement. The patient continued to undergo routine oncologic follow-up chest CT scans for his lung cancer. (*H*) Axial chest CT with IV contrast performed 3 months after the MR imaging shows the 2.1-cm thymic nodule to measure 4 HU, revealing the difficulty in accurate attenuation measurement caused by beam hardening artifact from adjacent IV contrast in the left innominate vein. The thymic lesion almost completely disappeared on the (*I*) axial chest CT performed 4 years after the baseline study.

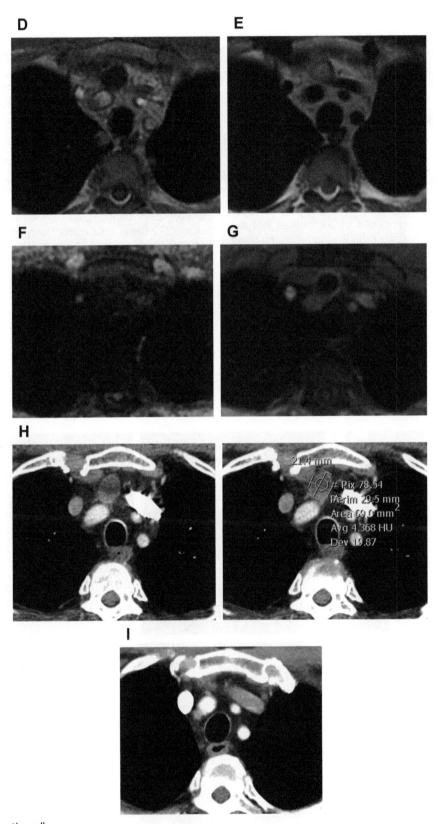

Fig. 2. (continued)

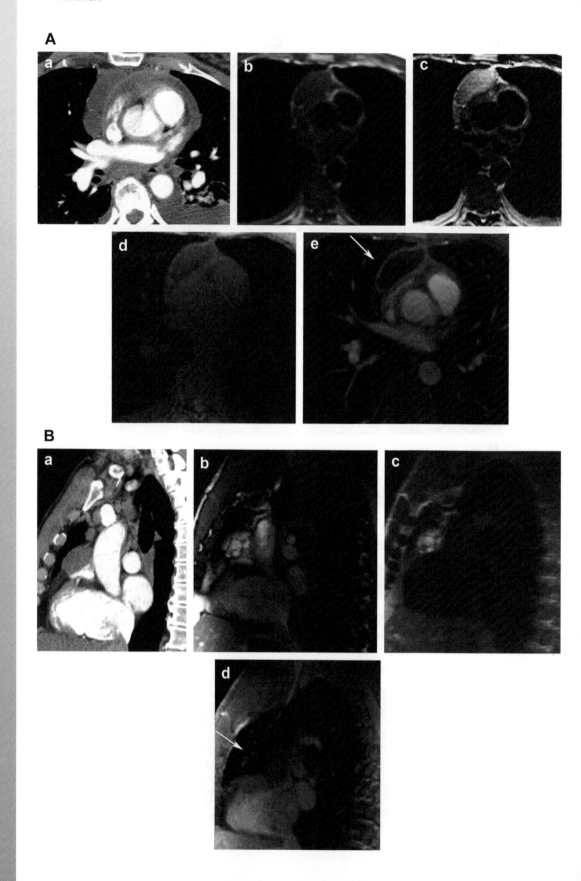

to the spine and are often associated with vertebral anomalies. Neurenteric cysts typically present early in life, unlike other foregut duplication cysts.[10]

It can be difficult to distinguish these cystic lesions from solid lesions on CT when they show high attenuation values (**Fig. 4**). It is important to be aware that CT attenuation values of up to 120 HU have been found in bronchogenic cysts,[11] whether caused by the presence of calcium oxalate or high proteinaceous or hemorrhagic content. MR imaging readily makes the distinction between cystic and solid lesions. High-attenuation cysts on CT are usually T1-isointense or T1-hyperintense to muscle on MR imaging, secondary to proteinaceous or hemorrhagic content, and uniformly T2-hyperintense, with no internal enhancement. Thin, smooth wall enhancement may be seen on MR imaging. When evaluating lesions of high T1 signal on precontrast MR imaging, postprocessed subtraction (of the precontrast from the postcontrast 3D ultrafast GRE images) is invaluable to assess for true enhancement (see **Fig. 4**).

In contrast, pericardial cysts, otherwise known as pleuropericardial cysts and mesothelial cysts, usually do not offer a diagnostic dilemma, most typically occurring in the right cardiophrenic angle, although 40% occur elsewhere in the thorax.[12] These lesions nearly always show water attenuation on CT, and T1-hypointensity, T2-hyperintensity, and no enhancement on MR imaging (**Fig. 5**).[13] Pericardial cysts may occasionally be pedunculated and wander or shift in location over time.[14]

The Diagnostic Significance of Macroscopic and/or Microscopic Fat Detection

Although macroscopic or gross fat is readily appreciated both on CT and MR imaging, microscopic or intravoxel fat is solely appreciated by chemical shift MR imaging. Chemical shift MR imaging can be used to distinguish normal thymus and thymic hyperplasia from thymic tumors because of the normal fatty involution of the thymus with age.[15] Inaoka and colleagues[16] quantified signal suppression on opposed-phase MR images with a chemical shift ratio (CSR) and found that mean CSR was significantly different ($P<.001$) between patients in the hyperplasia group (0.614 ± 0.130) and tumor group (1.026 ± 0.039). A CSR value of less than or equal to 0.7 should therefore indicate normal thymus or thymic hyperplasia, depending on the age and occasionally the sex[17,18] of the individual (**Fig. 6**). A solid thymic lesion with a CSR of 0.8 or 0.9 is considered indeterminate and warrants follow-up. A solid thymic lesion with a CSR greater than or equal to 1.0 generally indicates tumor; however, there are 3 caveats or potential pitfalls. First, awareness that not every young adult thymus suppresses on out-of-phase images is crucial to avert unnecessary thymectomy in these patients, because some thymuses involute more slowly than others.[17] A recent study revealed a sex difference in normal thymic appearance in young adults, with the thymus of young women involuting at a slower rate than that of young men.[18] If thymic hyperplasia remains possible based on otherwise suitable lesion signal and morphology, the lesion may be followed over time to ensure stability and/or eventual suppression, as age-related fatty intercalation occurs (**Fig. 7**). Second, gross fat does not suppress on out-of-phase images and can easily be discerned based on its T1/T2-hyperintensity and its decrease in signal on fat-saturated pulse sequences. Third, the CSR should not be evaluated or calculated for a thymic cyst or for a cystic component of a solid lesion. Thymic cysts, because of their fluid content, do not suppress on out-of-phase imaging and are nevertheless benign. In contradistinction, components of dermoid cysts containing intravoxel fat and water suppress on opposed-phase imaging, as expected.

Mediastinal teratomas may contain macroscopic and/or microscopic fat or no fat. Mature teratoma is the most common germ cell tumor of the mediastinum. The presence of a fat-fluid level in an anterior mediastinal mass is diagnostic of a teratoma (**Fig. 8**).[19,20]

Fig. 3. Two examples of multilocular thymic cysts (*A, B*) with CT correlation. (*A*) A multilocular thymic cyst with 2 locules (*a–e*). (*a*) Axial chest CT with IV contrast shows the thymic lesion to be of low attenuation and composed of 2 locules, with a barely perceptible wall. Small bilateral pleural effusions, a pericardial effusion, and pericardial thickening are also present. (*b*) Axial double IR T1-weighted and (*c*) T2-weighted MR images, and axial (*d*) pre-ultrafast and (*e*) post-ultrafast 3D GRE fat-saturated T1-weighted MR images reveal this thymic lesion to be T1-hypointense and T2-hyperintense, with thin smooth wall enhancement (*arrow*). (*B*) Multilocular cyst in another patient (*a–d*). (*a*) Sagittal chest CT with IV contrast, (*b*) sagittal steady state free precession (SSFP) T1-weighted/T2-weighted, (*c*) sagittal T2-weighted MR images, and (*d*) sagittal post-ultrafast 3D GRE fat-saturated T1-weighted MR image. The many locules of this multilocular thymic cyst cause this lesion to resemble a cluster of grapes on SSFP and T2-weighted MR imaging; this morphologic feature is not appreciable by CT. The enhancement of the walls and tissue between these locules is much better appreciated by MR imaging (*d, arrow*).

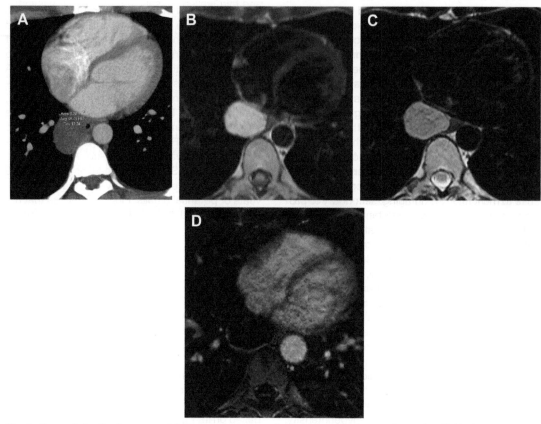

Fig. 4. Foregut duplication cyst exhibiting an intimate relationship with the esophageal wall, likely representing an esophageal duplication cyst. (*A*) Axial chest CT with IV contrast showing a 48 HU, round, well-circumscribed lesion with an imperceptible wall in the azygoesophageal recess of the middle mediastinum. (*B*, *C*) Cardiac-gated double IR T1-weighted and T2-weighted MR images (respectively), followed by a (*D*) post-contrast subtracted 3D ultrafast GRE image, showing the marked T1/T2-hyperintensity of this lesion and the lack of enhancement. The apparent enhancing material along the posterior aspect of this lesion is caused by slight misregistration of the pre-contrast and post-contrast images used for subtraction.

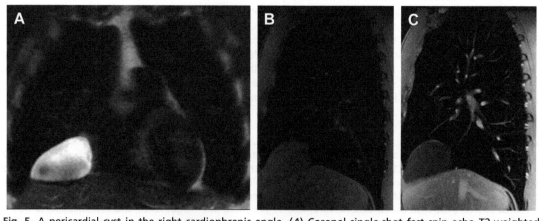

Fig. 5. A pericardial cyst in the right cardiophrenic angle. (*A*) Coronal single-shot fast spin echo T2-weighted MR image, (*B*) sagittal pre-contrast and (*C*) post-contrast 3D ultrafast GRE T1 fat-saturated MR image showing T1-hypointensity, T2-hyperintensity, and no enhancement on IV gadolinium administration. The smudgy areas of T2-hypointensity within this cyst are caused by propagated cardiac pulsation within the cyst fluid and resultant proton spin dephasing. The apparent thin, smooth, enhancing tissue (*C*) along the anterosuperior margin of this cyst likely represents mild compressive atelectasis.

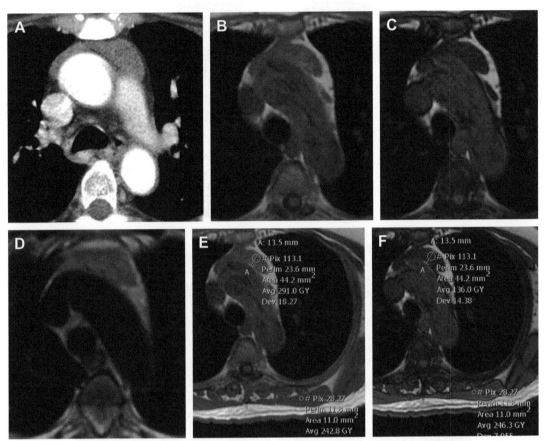

Fig. 6. Thymic hyperplasia in a 64-year-old woman with severe hyperthyroidism. (*A*) Axial chest CT with IV contrast revealing excessive, biconvex thymic soft tissue for age. (*B*) In-phase and (*C*) out-of-phase T1-weighted MR images and (*D*) cardiac-gated double IR T2-weighted MR image reveal a significant decrease in signal of this tissue on the out-of-phase image and reveal mild generalized T2-hyperintensity of this tissue. (*E*) In-phase and (*F*) out-of-phase T1-weighted MR images show region of interest (ROI) placement for the CSR calculation. CSR calculation reveals a CSR of 0.5, which is compatible with thymic hyperplasia.

$$CSR = \frac{\text{Out-of-phase signal intensity of thymic tissue/paraspinal muscle}}{\text{In-phase signal of thymic tissue/paraspinal muscle}}$$

$$CSR = \frac{136/246}{291/242}$$

$$CSR = 0.5$$

The Diagnostic Significance of Lesion T2-Hypointensity

Most cystic and solid lesions in the mediastinum are T2-hyperintense to muscle. Therefore, the finding of T2-isointensity or T2-hypointensity within a mediastinal lesion has diagnostic significance. The finding of predominantly shortened T2 relaxation time within a mediastinal lesion often confers a benign diagnosis. The typical list of T2-hypointense findings within the body includes blood products such as hemosiderin (T2-shading is not commonly found in blood-containing mediastinal lesions), hypercellular lesions, smooth muscle–containing lesions (**Fig. 9**), and fibrous or collagenous lesions.[21] It is notable that untreated mediastinal lymphoma is generally T2-hyperintense to muscle,[7] despite its hypercellular nature. Nodular sclerosing Hodgkin lymphoma is exceptional in that it may contain areas of T2-hypointensity on account of interspersed fibrosis.[7]

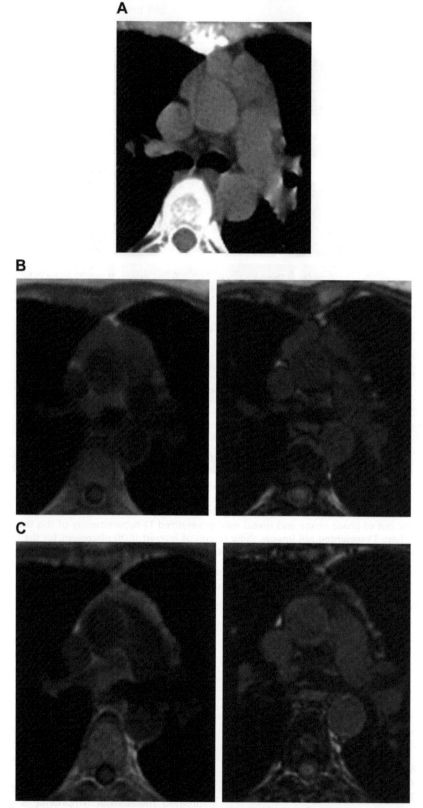

Fig. 7. Regression of thymic hyperplasia with time. (*A*) Axial chest CT without IV contrast reveals a bipyramidal, biconvex soft tissue mass in the thymic bed in a 53-year-old woman with breast cancer and subsequent aromatase therapy. (*B*) Axial in-phase and out-of-phase ultrafast GRE MR imaging 1 month later revealed partial suppression on the out-of-phase images with CSR values ranging from 0.6 to 0.8. Because of the indeterminate CSR value of 0.8 in a portion of this lesion resembling thymic hyperplasia morphologically, follow-up MR imaging was performed. (*C*) Axial in-phase and out-of-phase imaging nearly 2 years later, on discontinuation of aromatase therapy, revealed marked interval regression and suppression of the previous abundant thymic tissue, providing diagnostic proof of thymic hyperplasia at presentation.

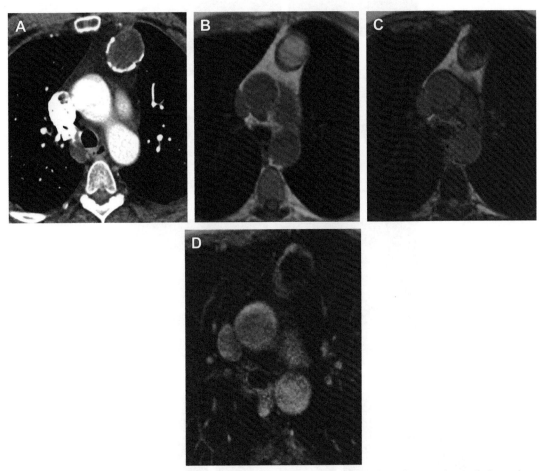

Fig. 8. Anterior mediastinal teratoma on (*A*) axial contrast-enhanced CT, (*B, C*) in-phase and out-of-phase chemical shift MR imaging, and (*D*) postcontrast subtracted 3D ultrafast GRE T1 fat-saturated MR imaging. The CT image reveals a mixed attenuation, rim-calcified, ovoid mass, without appreciable macroscopic fat. The subsequent in-phase and opposed-phase MR images (*B, C*) reveal T1-hyperintensity of internal content on the in-phase image (*B*) and suppression of the nondependent material on the opposed-phase image (*C*), findings that indicate the presence of intravoxel fat within this cyst. Postcontrast subtracted image (*D*) reveals no enhancement of internal contents of this cyst. Only the irregularly thickened wall of this lesion enhances. Note that the wall calcification of this lesion is not appreciable by MR imaging, manifesting as nonspecific low T1/T2 signal.

Mediastinal examples of fibrous or collagen-containing lesions include granulomatous lymph nodes of sarcoidosis (**Fig. 10**),[22] other calcified or noncalcified benign lymph nodes with fibrotic micronodule formation,[23] chronic fibrosing mediastinitis (**Fig. 11**), and the rare solitary fibrous tumor of the mediastinum (spindle cells amid collagenous stroma[24]).[25] T2-hypointensity may also be seen within the more central aspect of neurofibromas[26] (**Fig. 12**) and in treated lymphoma. During successful therapy for lymphoma, the T2 signal of the treated tissue decreases as water content decreases and collagen or fibrotic content increases. Enhancement of lymphomatous tissue also decreases with therapy.[27–32]

The Diagnostic Significance of Discernment of Solid Tissue Amidst Hemorrhage and Necrosis: Guidance for Diagnostic Intervention

When specific diagnosis is impossible, the high tissue contrast of MR imaging can still be helpful to guide the interventionist regarding optimal site selection and approach for biopsy. For example, by noncontrast CT, it may be unclear which components of a heterogeneous attenuation mass on CT are hemorrhagic, cystic, or solid. Thoracic MR imaging can make this distinction. By showing the solid tissue amid sites of hemorrhage and/or necrosis, the MR imaging can direct the interventionist or surgeon to the most accessible site with high diagnostic yield (**Fig. 13**).

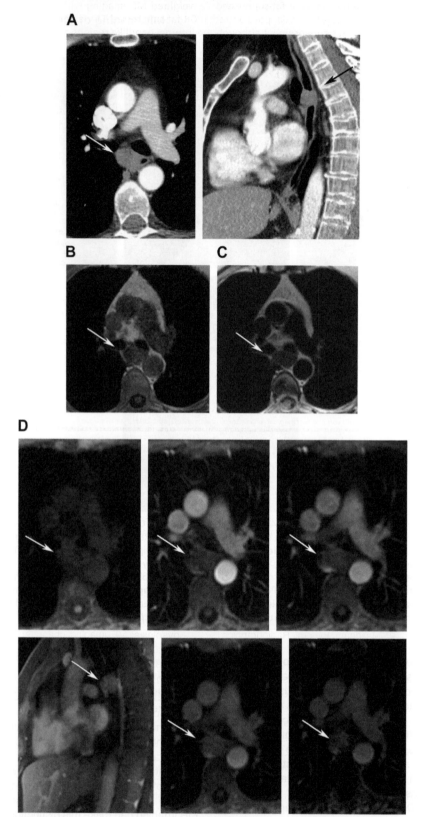

Fig. 9. Esophageal leiomyoma. (*A*) Axial and sagittal images from chest CT with IV contrast revealing a small round mass (*arrow*) isodense to muscle in the posterior subcarinal, right paraesophageal space, with no fat plane between the mass and the right lateral wall of the esophagus. (*B*) Axial in-phase T1-weighted and (*C*) cardiac gated double IR T2-weighted MR images. (*D*) From left to right, top to bottom: pre-ultrafast and post-ultrafast 3D GRE fat-saturated T1-weighted MR images at 20 seconds, 1 minute, 3 minutes (sagittal), and 5 minutes, with post-processed subtraction at 5 minutes. The MR imaging reveals this mass (*arrow*) to be of intermediate-to-low T1-weighted and T2-weighted signal and to enhance gradually and mildly.

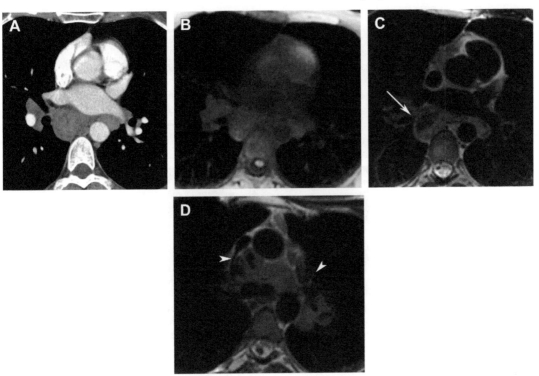

Fig. 10. Central low T2 signal in the granulomatous lymph nodes of sarcoidosis on MRI, with CT correlation. Sarcoidosis-related azygoesophageal recess and bilateral hilar lymphadenopathy on (A) chest CT with IV contrast. (B) Axial 3D ultrafast GRE fat-saturated T1-weighted image and (C, D) 2 double IR T2-weighted MR images revealing intermediate T1 signal and areas of low T2 signal within azygoesophageal recess lymphadenopathy (*white arrow*) and within the low right paratracheal and aortopulmonary (AP) window lymphadenopathy (*white arrowheads*).

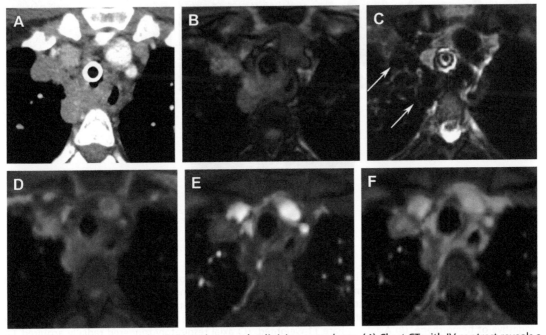

Fig. 11. Chronic fibrosing mediastinitis/pulmonary hyalinizing granuloma. (A) Chest CT with IV contrast reveals a soft tissue mass insinuating between the left posterolateral trachea and tracking directly into the right apical extrapleural space where it manifests lobulated morphology. (B) Axial 3D ultrafast GRE T1-weighted; (C) respiratory-triggered, radially acquired T2-weighted fat-saturated; and axial (D) pre-gadolinium and post-gadolinium 3D ultrafast GRE fat-saturated T1-weighted MR images, with postgadolinium images at (E) 20 seconds and (F) 5 minutes. The lesion shows intermediate T1 signal, marked T2-hypointensity (*arrows*) approaching that of air in the adjacent lung, and mild, gradual enhancement over time.

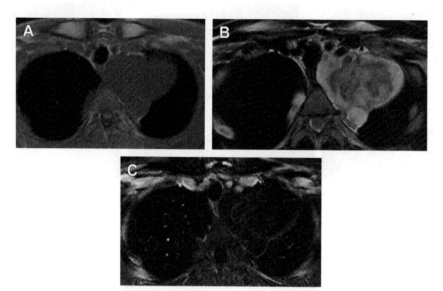

Fig. 12. Neurofibroma. (*A*) Axial in-phase T1-weighted, (*B*) cardiac-gated double IR T2-weighted, and (*C*) 3D ultrafast GRE postgadolinium subtracted MR images reveal the lobulated left mid-to-posterior mediastinal mass to show intermediate T1 signal, central T2-hypointensity with peripheral T2-hyperintensity, and minimal enhancement.

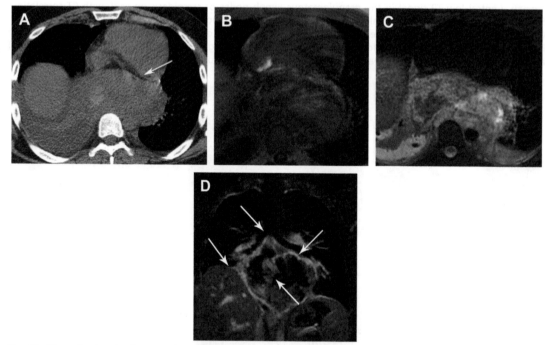

Fig. 13. Site selection for biopsy of a large, indeterminate mid-to-posterior mediastinal mass. (*A*) Non-contrast axial chest CT reveals a large, indeterminate, mixed attenuation mass in the mid-to-posterior mediastinum, displacing the esophagus anteriorly and to the left (*arrow*) and in close apposition to the descending thoracic aorta, with bilateral pleural effusions and partial right lower lobe atelectasis. The mixed attenuation of this material is suggestive of hemorrhage. (*B*) Axial in-phase T1-weighted, (*C*) axial respiratory-triggered radially acquired T2-weighted fat-saturated, and (*D*) coronal postgadolinium 3D ultrafast GRE fat-saturated T1-weighted subtracted MR images reveal the mass to exhibit heterogeneous T1-weighted and T2-weighted signal, with small areas of solid tissue centrally (*arrowhead*) and peripherally (*arrows*). The above findings are compatible with a large, hemorrhagic soft tissue mass that has ruptured into the pleural space. The aorta is intact. Subcarinal bronchoscopic biopsy yielded a high-grade, undifferentiated small round cell sarcoma.

The Diagnostic Significance of Characteristic Dynamic Contrast Enhancement Patterns

As in other parts of the body, the rate of contrast enhancement of various mediastinal lesions may prove useful. In 2002, Sakai and colleagues[33] showed that low-risk (Masaoka stage I and II) thymomas typically demonstrate more rapid time-to-peak enhancement than non-thymomas (whether advanced thymoma, thymic carcinoma, lymphoma, or germ cell tumor), with low-risk thymomas reaching peak enhancement at a mean time of 1.5 minutes. Stage III thymoma mean time-to-peak enhancement was 2.5 minutes. Non-thymomas tended to enhance more gradually over time, with a mean time of 3.2 minutes to peak enhancement. These investigators found that a cut-off value of 2 minutes to peak enhancement separated low-risk thymomas from these other lesions with 81% accuracy. This discovery offers a potential means of differentiating these anterior mediastinal masses, the most common of which (lymphoma and thymoma) warrant different management. Lymphoma warrants nonsurgical therapy, low-risk thymomas warrant surgery, and high-risk thymomas may require neoadjuvant therapy before surgery, adjuvant therapy after surgery, or no surgery if metastatic.[34] The rapid time-to-peak enhancement with partial washout over time of a low-grade thymoma is shown in **Fig. 14**.

Paragangliomas typically show intermediate T1 signal and characteristic marked T2-hyperintensity. They also tend to be hypervascular and therefore hyperenhance. Larger paragangliomas may show flow voids or a salt-and-pepper appearance. If an indeterminate mediastinal mass is found in the expected location of a mediastinal aortopulmonary paraganglion or along the para-aortic sympathetic chain on CT and is shown by MR imaging to have these signal and enhancement characteristics, a paraganglioma should be strongly considered.[35–37]

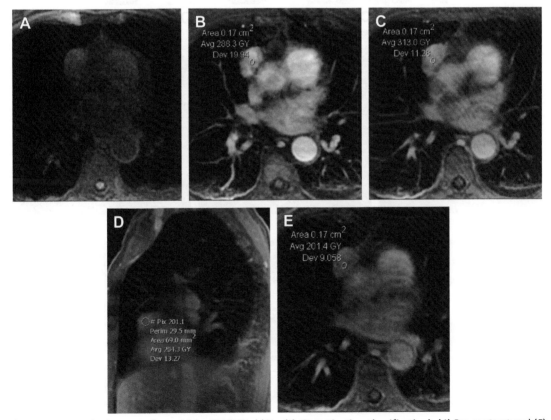

Fig. 14. Low-grade thymoma (type AB by 2004 World Health Organization classification). (*A*) Pre-contrast and (*B*) post-contrast 3D ultrafast GRE fat-saturated T1-weighted images showing rapid time-to-peak enhancement at 1 minute with washout over time; ROI signal intensity measurements on post-contrast MR images of 288, 313, 284, and 201 at 20 seconds, at (*C*) 1 minute, (*D*) 3 minutes (sagittal), and (*E*) 5 minutes respectively. Note that the 3-minute ROI was not necessarily taken at the precise location of the axial ROIs and is therefore less reliably comparative. The rapid time-to-peak enhancement at 1 minute is more typical of low-grade thymoma than high-grade thymomas or lymphoma.

Hemangiomas can occur in the mediastinum, although they are rare mediastinal masses. As in the liver, they are expected to be of low-to-intermediate T1 signal, T2-hyperintense,[38] and to show peripheral nodular enhancement with partial or complete fill-in over time.[39–41] **Fig. 15** shows a preoperatively diagnosed hemangioma, based on MR findings shared with hepatic hemangiomas.

The Diagnostic Significance of Matching Mediastinal Lesions in Terms of Signal and Enhancement Within the Same Patient

Because MR imaging offers the opportunity to characterize multiple aspects of a lesion (its anatomic location, its morphology, its T1-weighted and T2-weighted signal, its enhancement pattern, and the

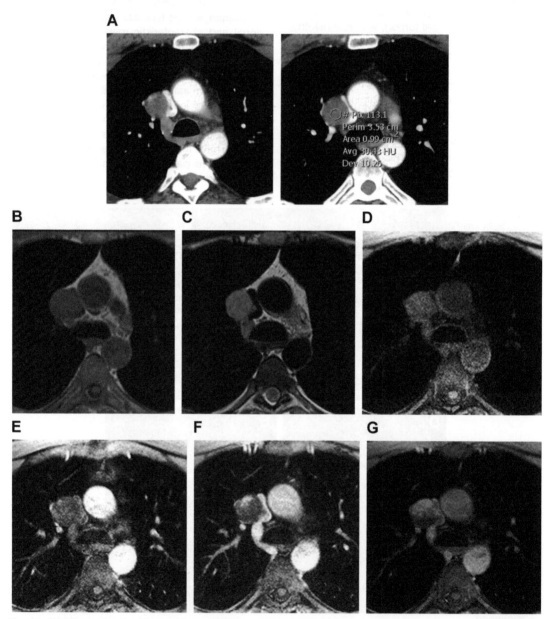

Fig. 15. Middle mediastinal hemangioma. (*A*) Two consecutive axial chest CT images with IV contrast reveal a well-defined 30 HU mass exerting mass effect on the superior vena cava (SVC), which it either indents or invades. The mass measures 30 HU centrally and contains a peripheral hyperdense focus representing early calcification or enhancement. On MR, this mass shows intermediate T1 signal on the (*B*) axial in-phase T1-weighted image, T2-hyperintensity on the (*C*) cardiac-gated double IR T2-weighted image, and peripheral nodular enhancement with fill-in over time on the (*D*) pre-contrast and (*E–G*) post-contrast 3D ultrafast GRE MR images at (*E*) 20 seconds, (*F*) 1 minute, and (*G*) 5 minutes, consistent with a hemangioma.

rate of diffusion of its water molecules), when 2 lesions in the same patient manifest similarly on every pulse sequence, the likelihood that both lesions represent the same histopathology is high. Recognition of matching lesions can help modify and, in some cases, avert intervention (**Figs. 16** and **17**).

The Diagnostic Significance of Low Apparent Diffusion Coefficient Values

Diffusion-weighted single-shot echo planar MR imaging may be helpful to distinguish benign from malignant mediastinal tumors because of the tendency of the latter to show more restricted diffusion of water. In a prospective study in 2009, Razek and

colleagues[42] showed that a threshold ADC value of 1.56×10^{-3} mm^2/s could be used to make this distinction in mediastinal tumors with 96% sensitivity, 94% specificity, and 95% accuracy. This value is similar to the threshold ADC value of 1.63 $\times 10^{-3}$ mm^2/s found by Nomori and colleagues[43] to distinguish metastatic from nonmetastatic lymph nodes with 89% accuracy. Razek and colleagues's[42] study cohort consisted of 30 malignant and 15 benign tumors. Note that noninvasive thymoma (3 in the cohort) was grouped with other benign lesions in the study cohort, including 4 neurofibromas, 4 retrosternal thyroid goiters, 3 schwannomas, and 1 thymolipoma. The malignant lesions in the study cohort included 12 lymphomas,

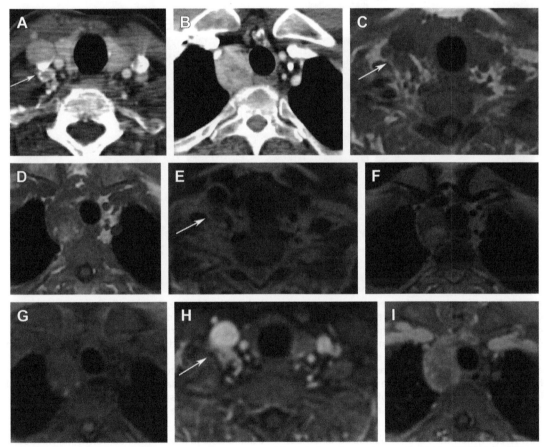

Fig. 16. Same signal and enhancement pattern, same pathology; in this case, metastatic papillary thyroid carcinoma in a 61-year-old man. (*A, B*) Chest CT with IV contrast showing (*A*) a right level IV cervical lymph node (*arrow*) lateral to the right thyroid lobe, posterior to the right internal jugular vein, and (*B*) a high right paratracheal mass. (*C, D*) Two axial in-phase T1-weighted MR images of (*C*) right level IV cervical lymph node (*arrow*) and thyroid gland, and (*D*) right paratracheal mass. (*E, F*) Axial double IR T2-weighted images of (*E*) right level IV cervical lymph node (*arrow*), thyroid gland, and (*F*) right paratracheal mass. (*G*) Axial precontrast 3D ultrafast GRE image of right paratracheal mass, and subsequent (*H, I*) postcontrast 3D ultrafast GRE images of (*H*) right level IV cervical lymph node (*arrow*), thyroid gland, and (*I*) right paratracheal mass. The MR imaging showed that the solid portion of the right paratracheal mass, the right level IV cervical lymph node, and the thyroid gland had similar signal characteristics on all pulse sequences, including all post-contrast dynamic runs, strongly suggesting all 3 lesions to be of similar histopathologic composition. A correct preoperative diagnosis of metastatic thyroid cancer was made.

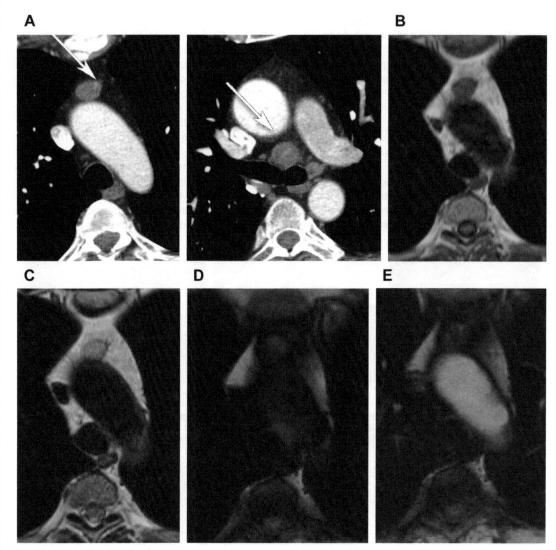

Fig. 17. Same signal and enhancement pattern, same pathology; in this case, 2 mediastinal hemangiomas. (*A*) Chest CT with IV contrast of a 56-year-old HIV-positive man revealing anterior mediastinal (*left*) and anterior sub-carinal (*right*) nodules, both of which are isodense to muscle, aside from a peripheral hyperdense focus (*arrows*). (*B*) Axial in-phase T1-weighted and (*C*) cardiac gated double IR T2-weighted MR images; (*D*) pre-contrast and postcontrast 3D ultrafast GRE fat-saturated MR images at (*E*) 20 seconds, (*F*) 1 minute, (*G*) 3 minutes (sagittal), and (*H*) 5 minutes (anterior mediastinal fat saturation is incomplete). The anterior subcarinal lesion was proved by mediastinoscopic biopsy to be a benign cavernous hemangioma. MR imaging of the anterior mediastinal lesion and that which remained of the anterior subcarinal nodule after biopsy revealed intermediate T1 signal, T2-hyperintensity, and peripheral nodular enhancement with fill-in over time characteristic of a hemangioma.

8 invasive thymomas, 8 bronchogenic carcinomas, and 2 angiosarcomas. Lymphoma showed the lowest ADC value ($1.02 \pm 0.19 \times 10^{-3}$ mm^2/s). However, the ADC values for lymphoma, invasive thymoma, and bronchogenic carcinoma in this study overlapped. These findings suggest that diffusion-weighted imaging may be helpful to differentiate lymphoma from noninvasive thymoma because of the typically lower ADC value of lymphoma. The ADC threshold values mentioned in Razek and colleagues' study are not directly

transferable to those obtained from other MR scanners and MR software, but they may be helpful as a rough guideline.

Determination of lesion invasiveness

The higher soft tissue contrast of MR, compared with CT imaging, has long been perceived to be advantageous in the detection of neurovascular and chest wall involvement, with higher sensitivity and specificity.[44] **Fig. 18** shows the utility of MR imaging in this regard, compared with

F   G   H

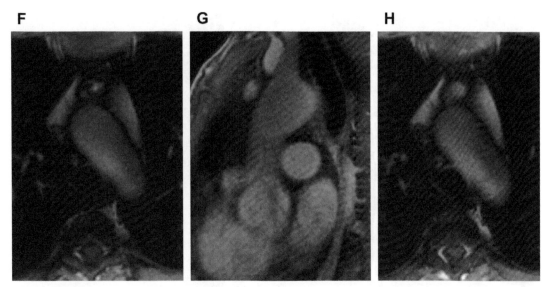

Fig. 17. (*continued*)

CT. It is important to be aware that the presence of a fat plane between a mass and adjacent structure by CT or MR does not exclude microscopic invasion. In addition, the absence of a fat plane between two structures on CT and/or MR imaging does not prove invasion.[45] Cinematic MR imaging can be of supplemental value in the detection of chest wall invasion[46] and cardiovascular involvement.[47] This cinematic technique should reveal a lack of sliding motion between the invading lesion and invaded structure. Cardiac tagging may also be useful to confirm or exclude myocardial invasion by a mediastinal mass.[48]

A   B

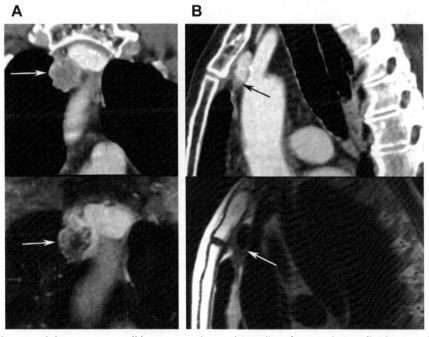

Fig. 18. Right upper lobe squamous cell lung cancer (*arrows*) invading the anterior mediastinum and, more specifically, the left innominate vein. (*A*) Matched coronal contrast-enhanced CT and post-contrast MR images and (*B*) matched sagittal contrast-enhanced CT and cardiac gated double IR T1-weighted MR images reveal solely the MR imaging to show the partial encasement and invasion of the left innominate vein by this mass; at pathology, only the innominate vein adventitia was invaded. It is difficult to appreciate the partial venous encasement or invasion by CT.

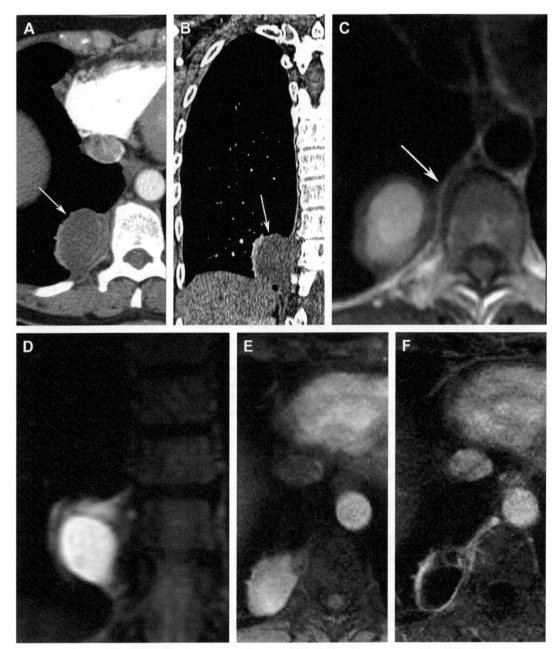

Fig. 19. Intrapleural bronchogenic cyst mistaken for a posterior mediastinal mass on CT and shown by MR imaging to reside within the right pleural space, with a resultant change in proposed differential diagnosis. (*A*) Axial and (*B*) coronal chest CT with IV contrast revealing a complex cystic mass (*arrows*) interpreted by the reporting radiologist to reside in the posterior mediastinal space and therefore to represent a neurogenic tumor. (*C*) Axial double IR T1-weighted, (*D*) coronal double IR T2-weighted, and (*E*) pre-contrast and (*F*) post-contrast T1-weighted MR images showing a preserved right paravertebral fat pad (*arrow*) and confirming the pleural location of this complex cystic lesion. Note the enhancement of its irregular wall and internal septation, as well as the T1-hyperintensity indicative of proteinaceous or hemorrhagic content. This correct compartment localization altered the preoperative diagnosis from a neurogenic tumor to an extralobar sequestration or complicated intrapleural bronchogenic cyst. Because no systemic arterial supply was demonstrated, the latter was favored. An intrapleural bronchogenic cyst was pathologically confirmed on surgical resection.

The diagnostic significance of discernment of mediastinal from paramediastinal lesions

It is occasionally difficult to distinguish a mediastinal lesion from a paramediastinal lesion on CT. The high soft tissue contrast of MR imaging can help place a lesion within an intrathoracic compartment, narrowing the differential diagnosis. For example, it can be difficult by CT to discern a posterior mediastinal lesion from a pleural lesion. MR imaging may better show preservation of paravertebral fat along the medial border of the pleural mass and absent invasion of this fat by the mass, confirming the mass to reside within the pleural space and changing the preoperative diagnosis from a neurogenic tumor to an extrapleural sequestration or intrapleural bronchogenic cyst (Fig. 19).[49]

SUMMARY

The high soft tissue contrast of MR imaging, relative to other imaging modalities including CT, enables superior tissue characterization of mediastinal masses, adding diagnostic specificity and benefiting clinical management. In many cases, mediastinal MR imaging may serve as a virtual biopsy and prevent unnecessary diagnostic intervention. In other cases, MR imaging directs the interventionist or surgeon toward the optimal site for biopsy or correct compartment for resection. Awareness of the efficacy of MR imaging with regard to mediastinal mass characterization and judicious MR utilization should further improve patient care.

REFERENCES

1. Carter BW, Tomiyama N, Bhora FY, et al. A modern definition of mediastinal compartments. J Thorac Oncol 2014;9(9):S97–101.
2. Felson B, Morgan WK, Bristol LJ, et al. Observations on the results of multiple readings of chest films in coal miners' pneumoconiosis. Radiology 1973;109(1):19–23.
3. Marks B, Mitchell DG, Simelaro JP. Breath-holding in healthy and pulmonary-compromised populations: effects of hyperventilation and oxygen inspiration. J Magn Reson Imaging 1997;7(3):595–7.
4. Ackman JB. A practical guide to nonvascular thoracic magnetic resonance imaging. J Thorac Imaging 2014;29(1):17–29.
5. Ackman JB, Verzosa S, Kovach AE, et al. High rate of unnecessary thymectomy and its cause. Can computed tomography distinguish thymoma, lymphoma, thymic hyperplasia, and thymic cysts? Eur J Radiol 2015;84(3):524–33.
6. Jeung MY, Gasser B, Gangi A, et al. Imaging of cystic masses of the mediastinum. Radiographics 2002;(22 Spec No):S79–93.
7. Takahashi K, Al-Janabi NJ. Computed tomography and magnetic resonance imaging of mediastinal tumors. J Magn Reson Imaging 2010;32(6):1325–39.
8. Murayama S, Murakami J, Watanabe H, et al. Signal intensity characteristics of mediastinal cystic masses on T1-weighted MRI. J Comput Assist Tomogr 1995;19(2):188–91.
9. McAdams HP, Kirejczyk WM, Rosado-de-Christenson ML, et al. Bronchogenic cyst: imaging features with clinical and histopathologic correlation. Radiology 2000;217(2):441–6.
10. Savage JJ, Casey JN, McNeill IT, et al. Neurenteric cysts of the spine. J Craniovertebr Junction Spine 2010;1(1):58–63.
11. Mendelson DS, Rose JS, Efremidis SC, et al. Bronchogenic cysts with high CT numbers. AJR Am J Roentgenol 1983;140(3):463–5.
12. Mouroux J, Venissac N, Leo F, et al. Usual and unusual locations of intrathoracic mesothelial cysts. Is endoscopic resection always possible? Eur J Cardiothorac Surg 2003;24(5):684–8.
13. Vinee P, Stover B, Sigmund G, et al. MR imaging of the pericardial cyst. J Magn Reson Imaging 1992;2(5):593–6.
14. Agarwal PP, Seely JM, Matzinger FR. Wandering pleuropericardial cyst. J Comput Assist Tomogr 2006;30(2):276–8.
15. Baron RL, Lee JK, Sagel SS, et al. Computed tomography of the normal thymus. Radiology 1982;142(1):121–5.
16. Inaoka T, Takahashi K, Mineta M, et al. Thymic hyperplasia and thymus gland tumors: differentiation with chemical shift MR imaging. Radiology 2007;243(3):869–76.
17. Ackman JB, Mino-Kenudson M, Morse CR. Nonsuppressing normal thymus on chemical shift magnetic resonance imaging in a young woman. J Thorac Imaging 2012;27(6):W196–8.
18. Ackman JB, Kovacina B, Carter BW, et al. Sex difference in normal thymic appearance in adults 20–30 years of age. Radiology 2013;268(1):245–53.
19. Patel IJ, Hsiao E, Ahmad AH, et al. AIRP best cases in radiologic-pathologic correlation: mediastinal mature cystic teratoma. Radiographics 2013;33(3):797–801.
20. Rosado-de-Christenson ML, Templeton PA, Moran CA. From the archives of the AFIP. Mediastinal germ cell tumors: radiologic and pathologic correlation. Radiographics 1992;12(5):1013–30.
21. Khashper A, Addley HC, Abourokbah N, et al. T2-hypointense adnexal lesions: an imaging algorithm. Radiographics 2012;32(4):1047–64.
22. Chung JH, Cox CW, Forssen AV, et al. The dark lymph node sign on magnetic resonance

imaging: a novel finding in patients with sarcoidosis. J Thorac Imaging 2014;29(2):125–9.

23. Yeh DW, Lee KS, Han J, et al. Mediastinal nodes in patients with non-small cell lung cancer: MRI findings with PET/CT and pathologic correlation. AJR Am J Roentgenol 2009;193(3):813–21.

24. Ali SZ, Hoon V, Hoda S, et al. Solitary fibrous tumor. A cytologic-histologic study with clinical, radiologic, and immunohistochemical correlations. Cancer 1997;81(2):116–21.

25. Ginat DT, Bokhari A, Bhatt S, et al. Imaging features of solitary fibrous tumors. AJR Am J Roentgenol 2011;196(3):487–95.

26. Tanaka O, Kiryu T, Hirose Y, et al. Neurogenic tumors of the mediastinum and chest wall: MR imaging appearance. J Thorac Imaging 2005;20(4):316–20.

27. Glazer HS, Levitt RG, Lee JK, et al. Differentiation of radiation fibrosis from recurrent pulmonary neoplasm by magnetic resonance imaging. AJR Am J Roentgenol 1984;143(4):729–30.

28. Rahmouni A, Luciani A, Itti E. MRI and PET in monitoring response in lymphoma. Cancer Imaging 2005;(5 Spec No A):S106–12.

29. Rahmouni A, Tempany C, Jones R, et al. Lymphoma: monitoring tumor size and signal intensity with MR imaging. Radiology 1993;188(2):445–51.

30. Nyman RS, Rehn SM, Glimelius BL, et al. Residual mediastinal masses in Hodgkin disease: prediction of size with MR imaging. Radiology 1989;170(2):435–40.

31. Gasparini MD, Balzarini L, Castellani MR, et al. Current role of gallium scan and magnetic resonance imaging in the management of mediastinal Hodgkin lymphoma. Cancer 1993;72(2):577–82.

32. Devizzi L, Maffioli L, Bonfante V, et al. Comparison of gallium scan, computed tomography, and magnetic resonance in patients with mediastinal Hodgkin's disease. Ann Oncol 1997;8(Suppl 1):53–6.

33. Sakai S, Murayama S, Soeda H, et al. Differential diagnosis between thymoma and non-thymoma by dynamic MR imaging. Acta Radiol 2002;43(3):262–8.

34. Marom EM. Advances in thymoma imaging. J Thorac Imaging 2013;28(2):69–80 [quiz: 1–3].

35. Balcombe J, Torigian DA, Kim W, et al. Cross-sectional imaging of paragangliomas of the aortic body and other thoracic branchiomeric paraganglia. AJR Am J Roentgenol 2007;188(4):1054–8.

36. Rao AB, Koeller KK, Adair CF. From the archives of the AFIP. Paragangliomas of the head and neck: radiologic-pathologic correlation. Armed Forces Institute of Pathology. Radiographics 1999;19(6):1605–32.

37. Olsen WL, Dillon WP, Kelly WM, et al. MR imaging of paragangliomas. AJR Am J Roentgenol 1987;148(1):201–4.

38. Stark DD, Felder RC, Wittenberg J, et al. Magnetic resonance imaging of cavernous hemangioma of the liver: tissue-specific characterization. AJR Am J Roentgenol 1985;145(2):213–22.

39. Cheung YC, Ng SH, Wan YL, et al. Dynamic CT features of mediastinal hemangioma: more information for evaluation. Clin Imaging 2000;24(5):276–8.

40. Semelka RC, Brown ED, Ascher SM, et al. Hepatic hemangiomas: a multi-institutional study of appearance on T2-weighted and serial gadolinium-enhanced gradient-echo MR images. Radiology 1994;192(2):401–6.

41. Yamashita Y, Ogata I, Urata J, et al. Cavernous hemangioma of the liver: pathologic correlation with dynamic CT findings. Radiology 1997;203(1):121–5.

42. Razek AA, Elmorsy A, Elshafey M, et al. Assessment of mediastinal tumors with diffusion-weighted single-shot echo-planar MRI. J Magn Reson Imaging 2009;30(3):535–40.

43. Nomori H, Mori T, Ikeda K, et al. Diffusion-weighted magnetic resonance imaging can be used in place of positron emission tomography for N staging of non-small cell lung cancer with fewer false-positive results. J Thorac Cardiovasc Surg 2008;135(4):816–22.

44. Koyama H, Ohno Y, Seki S, et al. Magnetic resonance imaging for lung cancer. J Thorac Imaging 2013;28(3):138–50.

45. Glazer HS, Duncan-Meyer J, Aronberg DJ, et al. Pleural and chest wall invasion in bronchogenic carcinoma: CT evaluation. Radiology 1985;157(1):191–4.

46. Sakai S, Murayama S, Murakami J, et al. Bronchogenic carcinoma invasion of the chest wall: evaluation with dynamic cine MRI during breathing. J Comput Assist Tomogr 1997;21(4):595–600.

47. Seo JS, Kim YJ, Choi BW, et al. Usefulness of magnetic resonance imaging for evaluation of cardiovascular invasion: evaluation of sliding motion between thoracic mass and adjacent structures on cine MR images. J Magn Reson Imaging 2005;22(2):234–41.

48. Axel L, Montillo A, Kim D. Tagged magnetic resonance imaging of the heart: a survey. Med Image Anal 2005;9(4):376–93.

49. Sugita R, Morimoto K, Yuda F. Intrapleural bronchogenic cyst. Eur J Radiol 1999;32(3):204–7.

State of the Art
MR Imaging of Thymoma

Brett W. Carter, MD*, Marcelo F.K. Benveniste, MD, Mylene T. Truong, MD,
Edith M. Marom, MD

KEYWORDS

- Thymus • Thymoma • Mediastinum • Anterior • Staging • MR imaging

KEY POINTS

- Although thymoma is a rare tumor, it is the most common primary malignancy of the anterior mediastinum.
- MR imaging is an excellent tool for characterizing anterior mediastinal masses and elegantly distinguishes normal thymus and thymic hyperplasia from malignant neoplasms involving the thymus.
- Thoracic MR imaging may be used to stage patients in whom allergy to intravenous contrast and/or renal failure precludes evaluation with contrast-enhanced chest computed tomography (CT).

INTRODUCTION

Thymoma is the most common primary malignancy of the anterior mediastinum, but it is a rare tumor that constitutes less than 1% of adult malignancies.[1] Thmyoma is the most common thymic epithelial neoplasm, a group that also includes thymic carcinoma and thymic carcinoid. Because of the rarity of thymoma, it has not been evaluated thoroughly and many of the studies regarding imaging characteristics of the tumor were single-institution studies spanning multiple decades. Increased interest in thymic malignancies and greater international collaboration over the past 5 years has ultimately resulted in the formation of the International Thymic Malignancy Interest Group (ITMIG), an organization that provides infrastructure for the study of these lesions. With the formation of an international thymic malignancy database, it is hoped that large-scale multiinstitutional studies will overcome the smaller ones of the past and advance the knowledge in the detection, staging, and treatment of this disease. CT is currently the imaging modality of choice for distinguishing thymoma from other anterior mediastinal masses, characterizing the primary tumor, and staging the disease. However, MR imaging is also effective in evaluating and characterizing anterior mediastinal masses and staging thymoma in patients with contrast allergy and/or renal failure, which preclude evaluation with contrast-material-enhanced CT. This review focuses on the characterization, classification, and staging of thymoma based on various morphologic features that may be identified on MR imaging and the impact of imaging findings on therapy and management.

EPIDEMIOLOGIC AND CLINICAL FEATURES

The incidence of thymoma is 1 to 5 cases per million individuals per year in the United States, and it is higher in African Americans and Asians. Men and women are affected equally.[2,3] The incidence of thymoma increases with age, and the condition is most common in patients older than 40 years, but decreases in incidence after 60 years of age. Children are only rarely affected.

Disclosures: B.W. Carter has received Research Support from ACRIN; he is a Consultant at St. Jude Medical, Inc; and he is a thoracic colead and an author for Amirsys, Inc. Dr M.F.K. Benveniste, Dr M.T. Truong, and Dr E.M. Marom have nothing to disclose.

Section of Thoracic Imaging, Department of Diagnostic Radiology, The University of Texas MD Anderson Cancer Center, 1515 Holcombe Boulevard, Unit 1478, Houston, TX 77030-4008, USA

* Corresponding author.

E-mail address: bcarter2@mdanderson.org

Magn Reson Imaging Clin N Am 23 (2015) 165–177
http://dx.doi.org/10.1016/j.mric.2015.01.005

The most common clinical symptoms reported at the time of diagnosis include chest pain, dyspnea, and cough.[4] These symptoms are present in up to one-third of patients and typically secondary to compression and/or invasion of mediastinal structures. Dysphagia, diaphragmatic paralysis, and superior vena cava syndrome may also be present. One-third of patients present with systemic symptoms and paraneoplastic syndromes because of the presence of hormones, antibodies, and cytokines released by the tumor. The most common paraneoplastic syndrome associated with thymoma is myasthenia gravis, which is present in 30% to 50% of patients and is more common in women than in men.[5] Other paraneoplastic syndromes include hypogammaglobulinemia and pure red cell aplasia, which are present in 10% and 5% of cases, respectively.[6] Autoimmune disorders such as systemic lupus erythematosus, polymyositis, and myocarditis may be associated with thymoma.[7] Patients may be asymptomatic, and the increased utilization of CT for the diagnosis and follow-up of benign and malignant diseases has increased the detection of incidental thymomas.[8]

HISTOLOGY AND CLASSIFICATION

Thymomas are typically solid, encapsulated tumors that are restricted to the thymus. One-third of thymomas demonstrate necrosis, hemorrhage, or cystic components, and one-third of tumors invade the capsule and adjacent structures.[9] Although thymomas are typically slow-growing malignancies, aggressive features such as invasion of surrounding structures and involvement of the pleura and pericardium may be present. However, compared with thymic carcinoma and other malignancies of the anterior mediastinum, distant metastases are rare.[9]

The histologic classification of thymoma is complex and has been the source of controversy. Histologically, thymomas are composed of neoplastic epithelial cells and nonneoplastic lymphocytes, and most tumors are heterogeneous in composition. The first histologic classification scheme developed by the World Health Organization (WHO) Consensus Committee was released in 1999 and classified thymomas into 6 separate subtypes (A, AB, B1, B2, B3, and C) based on morphologic features of the neoplastic epithelial cells and the lymphocyte:epithelial cell ratio. A revised WHO classification scheme was published in 2004 and moved type C (thymic carcinoma) to a separate category.[10] However, there are inherent limitations in this classification system. Because thymomas are typically heterogeneous tumors, many different subtypes may coexist within the

same lesion.[11] In addition, when diagnosis is made from tissue obtained via needle biopsy, the sample obtained may not be representative of the predominant subtype of the tumor.[10] For histologic classification to be useful, it should correlate with prognosis so that therapy could be selected according to the classification. The WHO classification schemes of 1999 and 2004 lacked intraobserver and interobserver reproducibility and clinical predictive value.[12] At present, the most important feature of the histologic classification of thymic epithelial malignancies is differentiation of thymic carcinoma from thymoma, because thymic carcinoma is the most distinct group histologically and clinically with worse outcomes.[13] However, worse clinical outcomes have also been shown for subtype B3 when compared with the other histologic subtypes combined.[10,14]

STAGING

Many staging systems for thymoma have been proposed.[15–18] However, the Masaoka system (Table 1) and a variant of it, the Masaoka-Koga staging system,[16,17] are the most commonly used systems. The Masaoka-Koga staging system is the one recommended by the ITMIG[19] because of its correlation with patient survival as documented in several studies (Table 2).[20] The Masaoka-Koga staging system is based on the gross and microscopic features of thymoma. Tumors are designated as stage I when completely encapsulated; stage II in the setting of microscopic invasion through the capsule (IIa) or macroscopic invasion of the surrounding fat (IIb); stage III when invasion of an adjacent structure such as the great vessels, pericardium, or lung is present; and stage IV in the setting of pleural or pericardial dissemination (IVa)

Table 1 Masaoka staging system for thymoma	
Stage	**Descriptors**
I	Complete encapsulation of tumor and no microscopic invasion of capsule
II	Macroscopic invasion into surrounding fat or mediastinal pleura Microscopic invasion into capsule
III	Invasion of pericardium, great vessels, or lung
IVa	Pleural or pericardial dissemination
IVb	Lymphatic/hematogenous metastasis

Adapted from Masaoka A, Monden Y, Nakahara K, et al. Follow-up study of thymomas with special reference to their clinical stages. Cancer 1981;48(11):2485–92; with permission.

Table 2
Masaoka-Koga staging system for thymoma

Stage	Descriptors
I	Complete encapsulation of tumor
IIa	Microscopic tumor invasion through capsule
IIb	Macroscopic tumor invasion into surrounding fat
III	Invasion of pericardium, great vessels, or lung
IVa	Pleural or pericardial dissemination
IVb	Lymphatic/hematogenous metastasis

Adapted from Koga K, Matsuno Y, Noguchi M, et al. A review of 79 thymomas: modification of staging system and reappraisal of conventional division into invasive and non-invasive thymoma. Pathol Int 1994;44(5):359–67; with permission.

or lymphatic/hematogenous metastasis (IVb). Advanced-stage disease is defined as stages III and IV. Although the Masaoka system or its variants has been the most commonly used staging mechanism, a new TNM-based staging system has been proposed and will probably replace these schemes in the future.[21]

As the Masaoka-Koga system is a postsurgical staging system, the role of the radiologist in staging thymoma is critical because neoadjuvant chemotherapy may be used for specific stages (III and IV) of disease. Therefore, good communication between the radiologist and the surgeon is necessary to determine the extent of disease and formulate appropriate treatment strategies.[22]

TREATMENT

Accurate staging and completeness of surgical resection are the 2 most important factors in formulating treatment strategies in patients with thymoma, because these factors demonstrate the strongest correlation with duration of progression-free and overall survival.[16,17,23,24] Stage I and II tumors are treated with surgical resection alone. Adjuvant chemotherapy and radiation therapy have no role in the treatment of stage I tumors and most stage II tumors because they provide no additional survival benefit.[24] However, postoperative radiation therapy is typically administered in cases of incompletely resected stage II tumors to eliminate residual disease.[20,25] When features of advanced-stage disease such as locoregional spread into adjacent structures are present, complete resection of tumor leads to prolonged survival.[26,27] In these patients, neoadjuvant chemotherapy may provide superior survival benefit when compared with adjuvant chemotherapy.[27–29] Postoperative radiation therapy is typically administered in cases of incompletely resected stage III tumors.[20,25] Chemotherapy after surgery may also be administered in this setting. The treatment of stage IVa thymomas is the same as that of stage III tumors. However, stage IVb tumor is typically treated with palliative chemotherapy only.

ROLE OF MR IMAGING

MR imaging is rarely the first imaging modality used for investigation of chest symptoms or an abnormality detected on chest radiography, because CT is generally considered to be superior to MR imaging in the evaluation and characterization of most anterior mediastinal masses. One study analyzing 127 anterior mediastinal masses of various causes, including thymic epithelial neoplasms such as thymoma and thymic carcinoma, other primary malignancies of the anterior mediastinum such as mature teratoma and malignant germ cell tumors, as well as lymphoma, demonstrated a slight advantage in the ability to correctly diagnose the lesion by CT (61%) compared with MR imaging (56%). However, this was not the case for thymic cysts, which were better visualized on MR imaging. In general, the correct diagnosis was reached in 86% using a combination of CT and MR imaging.[30] When a cystic mass is suspected or is to be investigated, MR imaging is the most useful imaging modality because it is superior to CT in distinguishing cystic from solid masses (for instance, thymic cysts from thymic neoplasms) and in identifying cystic/necrotic components within solid masses. MR imaging is also useful in differentiating thymic hyperplasia from thymic tumors and in evaluating patients with an anterior mediastinal mass suspicious for thymoma in whom iodinated contrast is contraindicated. Such patients should be imaged with MR imaging rather than an unenhanced chest CT because vessel and pericardial invasion (stage III) must be identified before surgery to enable neoadjuvant therapy in patients with thymoma. This invasion is readily demonstrated with MR imaging in such patients using black blood or white blood techniques.

The versatility of MR imaging may prove superior to that of CT in certain scenarios, which is elaborated on in the discussion of the differential diagnosis. In brief, chemical shift imaging can differentiate between normal thymus and thymic involvement with tumor, dynamic imaging can be used to distinguish thymoma from other anterior mediastinal tumors, and multishot spiral sequencing can be used for real-time imaging

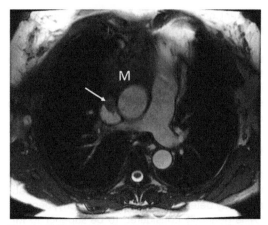

Fig. 1. Oblique true fast imaging with steady-state precession MR imaging of a 54-year-old woman with iodine allergy and thymoma demonstrates a large anterior mediastinal mass (M) that is of low signal intensity. Note the invasion of the superior vena cava (*arrow*), which would not have been identifiable on noncontrast CT. Thymoma with invasion of the superior vena cava corresponds to Masaoka-Koga stage III.

and evaluation of phrenic nerve involvement before surgery.

Imaging of Thymoma

The primary role of MR imaging in the evaluation of patients with thymoma is the staging of disease when allergy to contrast media and/or renal failure precludes the utilization of contrast-enhanced CT (Fig. 1).[31]

The typical appearance of thymoma is low to intermediate signal intensity on T1-weighted sequences and high signal intensity on T2-weighted sequences (Fig. 2).[32,33] As the signal intensity of thymoma on T2-weighted images may approach that of fat, fat-suppression techniques may be used to distinguish thymoma from adjacent mediastinal fat. Cystic changes and necrosis typically manifest as low signal intensity on T1-weighted images and high signal intensity on T2-weighted images (Fig. 3). Fibrous septa and intratumoral nodularity demonstrate low signal intensity (Fig. 4). The signal intensity of intratumoral hemorrhage is highly variable and depends on its age. For instance, hemosiderin typically manifests as low signal intensity on T1- and T2-weighted sequences, whereas acute or subacute hemorrhage may demonstrate T1 hyperintensity (Fig. 5). As the main role of clinical staging is to identify local spread (ie, pericardium, vessels, and heart) as well as pleural spread, which is often resected, the entire chest should be imaged, not limiting the field of view to the anterior mediastinum. Intravenous contrast can be helpful in the identification of small pleural metastases as tumor enhances (Fig. 6). The use of black blood or white blood techniques is helpful for evaluation of vascular invasion. Vessel distortion or tumor in the lumen of a vessel constitutes direct proof of stage III disease. Cardiac-gated black or white blood techniques are useful for better localization of tumors involving the heart, and perfusion studies are helpful when extensive cardiac muscle involvement is suspected for surgical planning.[34,35]

Phrenic nerve involvement is important to recognize, not only because it constitutes stage III disease requiring neoadjuvant therapy but also for better planning for surgical resection. With multishot spiral sequences for real-time imaging, the

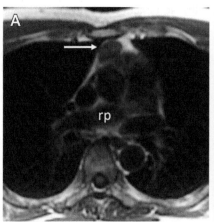
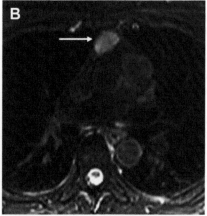

Fig. 2. MR imaging of a 55-year-old man with an anterior mediastinal mass. (*A*) Axial fast spin echo T1-weighted image at the level of the right pulmonary artery (rp) demonstrates a mass (*arrow*) that is of low signal intensity and similar to the intensity of skeletal muscle. (*B*) Axial fast spin echo fat-suppressed T2-weighted MR imaging at the same level shows that the mass (*arrow*) is of high signal intensity. Surgical resection was performed and revealed a thymoma invading the mediastinal fat, corresponding to Masaoka-Koga stage IIb.

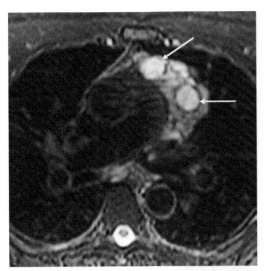

Fig. 3. Axial fast spin echo fat-suppressed T2-weighed MR imaging at the level of the right pulmonary artery demonstrates a thymoma in a 56-year-old man. The mass demonstrates lobulated regions of high signal intensity (*arrows*) that represent cystic changes and necrosis.

Fig. 5. Axial fast spin echo T1-weighted MR imaging of a 38-year-old woman with thymoma demonstrates a large mass in the anterior mediastinum that predominantly has low signal intensity. However, a focus of high signal intensity (*arrow*) within the tumor indicates acute or subacute hemorrhage.

diaphragmatic motion can be studied, obviating a separate sniff test. Paradoxic movement can be appreciated, and diaphragmatic movement span can be measured (**Fig. 7**). Although the multiplanar capabilities of MR imaging may help in identifying pericardial invasion, which represents stage III as well, its presence is often impossible to identify by imaging, and it is only identified retrospectively microscopically (**Fig. 8**). Some indirect MR imaging features of the primary tumor have been assessed

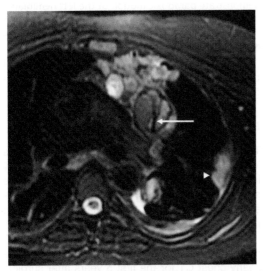

Fig. 4. Axial fast spin echo fat-suppressed T2-weighted MR imaging at the level of the pulmonary trunk bifurcation shows a large heterogeneous mass in the anterior mediastinum in a 43-year-old woman with thymoma. Note the low signal intensity fibrous septa (*arrow*) and lobulated regions of necrosis. Pleural thickening in the left hemithorax, indicates pleural metastasis (*arrowhead*), corresponding to Masaoka-Koga stage IVa.

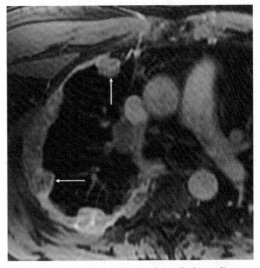

Fig. 6. Axial contrast-enhanced spoiled gradient recalled MR imaging of a 44-year-old woman with advanced-stage thymoma demonstrates extensive pleural thickening and enhancement in the right hemithorax and multiple enhancing pleural nodules (*arrows*). These findings represent pleural metastases and correspond to Masaoka-Koga stage IVa.

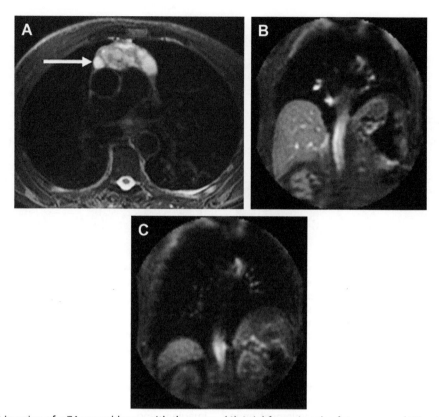

Fig. 7. MR imaging of a 74-year-old man with thymoma. (*A*) Axial fast spin echo fat-suppressed T2-weighted MR imaging at the level of the right pulmonary artery shows a large, heterogeneous mass (*arrow*) in the anterior mediastinum with multiple lobulated regions of high signal intensity. Preoperative chest radiograph (not shown) showed elevation of the left hemidiaphragm that was worrisome for phrenic nerve involvement. A multishot spiral MR imaging sequence was performed that failed to demonstrate paradoxic motion of the left hemidiaphragm. Expiratory (*B*) and inspiratory (*C*) images selected from this coronal multishot spiral MR imaging sequence show normal direction of diaphragmatic motion with a right hemidiaphragm span of 7 cm and a 3-cm span of the left hemidiaphragm. At surgery, the phrenic nerve was free of tumor.

to identify which primary tumor characteristics are less as well as more likely to be associated with local spread. A study demonstrated that 92% of stage II, III, and IV thymomas displayed heterogeneous signal intensity (**Fig. 9**) and 50% of these tumors exhibited lobulated internal features because of the presence of fibrous septa (**Fig. 10**). All stage I tumors were heterogeneous in signal, but none demonstrated lobulation.[36] Another study assessed enhancement patterns after the administration of contrast material. For instance, dynamic MR imaging has demonstrated delayed mean peak time in stage III thymomas when compared with early-stage tumors.[37] Although histologic classification of thymoma does not dictate therapy as much as staging does, some correlation of the primary tumor with MR imaging features were found. Specific findings such as visualization of the tumor capsule and fibrous septa within the tumor have been associated with less-aggressive histologies.[38] Certain findings such as heterogeneous enhancement and

predominant necrotic or cystic components suggest more aggressive histologies.

FOLLOW-UP IMAGING

The indolent nature of thymoma necessitates lengthy follow-up after initial treatment. Early identification of recurrence is crucial, because survival after complete resection of recurrent disease approaches that after initial resection, with reported 5-year survival rates of 65% to 80%.[39,40]

The current recommendations from ITMIG regarding imaging follow-up of patients include yearly chest CT for the first 5 years after surgical resection, alternating chest CT and chest radiographs through year 11, and yearly chest radiographs thereafter. For those patients with incomplete tumor resection or advanced-stage disease, follow-up chest CT every 6 months for the first 3 years is recommended. ITMIG suggests alternating between CT and MR imaging in these

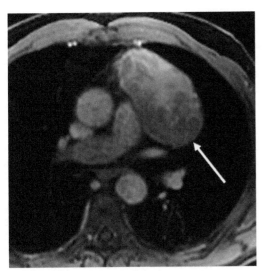

Fig. 8. Axial contrast-enhanced T1-weighted MR imaging of a 47-year-old man with thymoma demonstrates a large, enhancing mass (*arrow*) in the anterior mediastinum that is inseparable from the pulmonary trunk. At surgery, invasion of the pericardium was identified, corresponding to Masaoka-Koga stage III. Despite the multiplanar capabilities of MR imaging, it may be impossible to identify pericardial invasion.

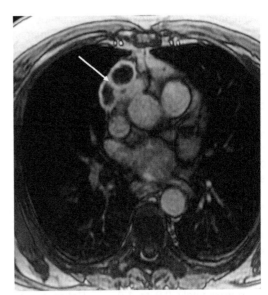

Fig. 10. Axial contrast-enhanced spoiled gradient recalled (SPGR) T1-weighted MRI of a 49-year-old woman with thymoma shows a mediastinal mass with peripheral enhancement and an enhancing internal septation (*arrow*). Invasion of the pericardium was discovered at the time of surgical resection, corresponding to Masaoka-Koga stage III. Advanced-stage thymomas are more likely to demonstrate lobulated internal features because of fibrous septa than early-stage thymomas.

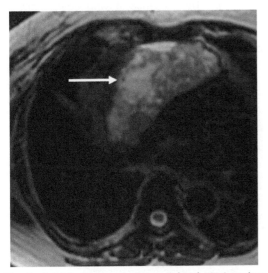

Fig. 9. Axial fast spin echo T2-weighted MR imaging of a 51-year-old woman shows a large mass (*arrow*) in the anterior mediastinum that is heterogeneous in signal intensity. Invasion of the pericardium, corresponding to Masaoka-Koga stage III, was present at the time of surgery. Advanced-stage thymomas are more likely to demonstrate signal heterogeneity than early-stage thymomas.

patients to decrease the cumulative radiation dose.[19] However, there are currently no studies in the literature comparing the accuracies of these modalities for detecting tumor recurrence.

DIFFERENTIAL DIAGNOSIS

The differential diagnosis for malignancies of the anterior mediastinum includes additional primary thymic epithelial neoplasms such as thymic carcinoma and thymic carcinoid, nonthymic malignancies such as lymphoma and germ cell tumors, metastatic disease from nonmediastinal primary neoplasms, and benign lesions such as thymic cysts or thymic hyperplasia. Patient demographics such as gender, age, tumor characteristics on imaging studies such as tissue composition and invasiveness, and associated abnormalities such as lymphadenopathy, pleural and/or pericardial effusions, and metastatic disease may help narrow the differential diagnosis when an anterior mediastinal mass is identified.

Thymic Hyperplasia

Thymic hyperplasia typically manifests as diffuse thickening and enlargement of the thymus with maintenance of the normal thymiform shape. The appearance of thymic hyperplasia on MR imaging is similar to that of normal thymus. However, occasionally, the appearance of thymic hyperplasia may be confused with thymic malignancy. In- and out-of-phase gradient echo sequences may be useful to differentiate thymic hyperplasia and normal thymus from other masses of the anterior mediastinum, because thymic hyperplasia and the normal thymus demonstrate loss of signal on out-of-phase images secondary to the suppression of microscopic fat interspersed between non-neoplastic thymic tissue (**Fig. 11**).[41,42] Thymic malignancies and lymphoma do not suppress on out-of-phase images. The signal loss expected with the normal thymus and with thymic hyperplasia can be measured by demonstrating chemical shift ratios (CSRs) of 0.5 to 0.6, whereas thymic malignancies and lymphoma exhibit higher CSRs of approximately 0.9 to 1.0.[41,42] Ratios greater than 0.6 and less than 0.9 are indeterminate. The CSR is calculated as follows: CSR = (thymus SI OP/paraspinal muscle SI OP)/(thymus SI IP/paraspinal muscle SI IP), where SI is the signal intensity, IP denotes in-phase sequences, and OP denotes out-of-phase sequences. The chemical shift MR imaging depicts intravoxel fat and water, and thus a sufficient amount of fat should exist within the voxel for this chemical shift to occur. As the thymus involutes with age, fat gradually replaces it. It has been found that normal thymus in patients younger than 10 years does not show signal loss with chemical shift imaging, whereas signal loss is present in up to 50% of patients aged 11 to 15 years.[43] Although signal loss is expected to occur in patients older than 16 years with a normal or hyperplastic thymus,[43] occasionally, young adults may lack this signal loss because of lack of sufficient fat within the thymus, as was described in a recent case report of a 21-year-old woman.[44]

Other Anterior Mediastinal Masses

Dynamic MR imaging has been assessed for differentiating anterior mediastinal masses in 59 patients using sequential imaging at 30 seconds for 5 minutes after the administration of gadopentetate dimeglumine. The mean peak of the time-intensity curve was significantly shorter for thymomas (1.5 minutes; 31 tumors) than nonthymomas, which included thymic carcinoma, lymphoma, malignant germ cell tumor, and thymic carcinoid (3.2 minutes; 28 tumors).[36]

Thymic Carcinoma

Thymic carcinoma is the second most common thymic epithelial neoplasm after thymoma. Although the appearance of thymic carcinoma on MR imaging is similar to that of thymoma and thymic carcinoid, thymic carcinomas may demonstrate hyperintensity relative to muscle on both T1- and T2-weighted sequences. Heterogeneous signal intensity secondary to cystic changes, necrosis, and hemorrhage may be present (**Fig. 12**).[45] The presence of lymphadenopathy or a pleural effusion suggests a thymic epithelial neoplasm such as thymic carcinoid or thymic carcinoma other than thymoma.[46]

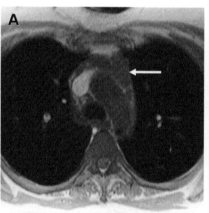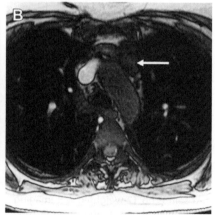

Fig. 11. MR imaging of a 38-year-old woman with thymic hyperplasia. (*A*) Axial in-phase T1-weighted imaging at the level of the transverse thoracic aorta demonstrates soft tissue in the anterior mediastinum (*arrow*) that is similar in signal intensity to muscle. (*B*) Axial out-of-phase T1-weighted imaging at the same level shows complete loss of signal intensity in this region (*arrow*). Thymic hyperplasia and normal thymus demonstrate loss of signal on out-of-phase imaging secondary to the suppression of microscopic fat interspersed between normal thymic tissue.

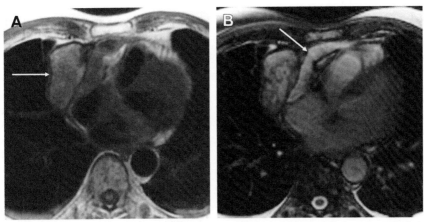

Fig. 12. MR imaging of a 39-year-old woman with thymic carcinoma. (*A*) Axial fast spin echo T1-weighted imaging at the level of the atria demonstrates a heterogeneous mass in the right anterior mediastinum (*arrow*). (*B*) Axial fast spin echo T2-weighted imaging at the same level shows a high-signal-intensity pericardial effusion (*arrow*) adjacent to the mass. Thymic carcinoma was discovered at surgery. Features such as lymphadenopathy, pericardial effusion, or pleural effusion are much more likely to be present in thymic carcinoma than thymoma.

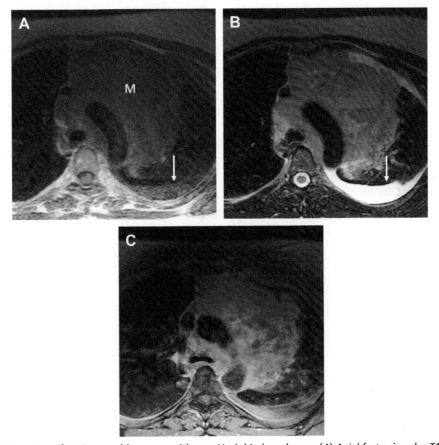

Fig. 13. MR imaging of a 49-year-old woman with non-Hodgkin lymphoma. (*A*) Axial fast spin echo T1-weighted imaging at the level of the transverse thoracic aorta demonstrates a large, heterogeneous, and infiltrative mass (M) in the mediastinum, and a small left pleural effusion (*arrow*). (*B*) Axial fast spin echo fat-suppressed T2-weighted imaging at the same level shows heterogeneous signal intensity of the mass and high-signal-intensity left pleural effusion (*arrow*). (*C*) Axial contrast-enhanced fast spin echo fat-suppressed T1-weighted imaging at a slightly more caudal level shows enhancement of most part of the mediastinal mass. The diffuse nature of the tumor in the mediastinum and the left pleural effusion are much more common in lymphoma than thymoma.

Thymic Carcinoid

Thymic carcinoid is the least common thymic epithelial neoplasm after thymoma and thymic carcinoma and originates from thymic cells of neural crest origin. Although the appearance of thymic carcinoid on MR imaging may be similar to that of thymoma and thymic carcinoma, carcinoid tumors may demonstrate hyperenhancement.[39] The presence of lymphadenopathy suggests a thymic epithelial neoplasm such as thymic carcinoid or thymic carcinoma other than thymoma.[46]

Lymphoma

Primary lymphoma of the thymus is a rare malignancy that is typically primary mediastinal B-cell lymphoma, a type of non-Hodgkin lymphoma.[47] This neoplasm typically manifests as homogeneous hypointensity on T1- and T2-weighted images. Enhancement is usually homogeneous after the administration of intravenous contrast material, although heterogeneity secondary to necrosis may be present (**Fig. 13**).[48] The thymus may also become secondarily involved by primary lymphomas from intrathoracic and extrathoracic locations.

Germ Cell Tumors

The most common germ cell tumors of the anterior mediastinum include teratomas and seminomas. Benign teratomas, which may be mature or immature depending on the differentiation of the tissues, typically manifest as multilocular cystic masses containing various amounts of fluid, fat, soft tissue, and calcification. The fluid component is typically hypointense on T1-weighted images and hyperintense on T2-weighted images (**Fig. 14**). Hemorrhagic and proteinaceous components may result in T1 hyperintensity. The fat component is typically hyperintense on T1-weighted images. The utilization of fat saturation technique may enable the identification of fat within these lesions. Seminomas are primary malignant germ cell tumors of the mediastinum that occur almost exclusively in younger men. The most common appearance of this tumor on MR imaging is a homogeneous mass with internal septations that are T2 hypointense but enhance after the administration of intravenous contrast.[48]

Thymic Cysts

Thymic cysts are typically asymptomatic mediastinal masses that may be congenital or acquired. Thymic cysts manifest as well-circumscribed anterior mediastinal masses with low signal intensity on T1-weighted sequences and high signal intensity on T2-weighted sequences (**Fig. 15**). T1 hyperintensity may be seen in cysts complicated by hemorrhage or infection. The cyst wall is typically visible as a low-signal-intensity rim on T2-weighted images. The absence of intracystic mural nodules allows differentiation of thymic cysts from cystic thymomas.[49] Minimal enhancement along the peripheral aspect of the cyst may be visualized, although no enhancing internal components should be identified.

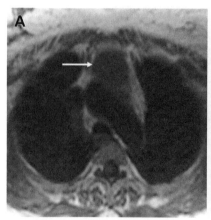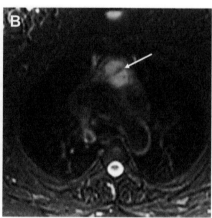

Fig. 14. Mature teratoma in a 33-year-old woman with elevated levels of α-fetoprotein (AFP). (*A*) Axial fast spin echo T1-weighted MR imaging at the level of the transverse thoracic aorta shows a well-circumscribed mass (*arrow*) in the anterior mediastinum that is of low signal intensity. (*B*) Axial fast spin echo fat-suppressed T2-weighted imaging at the same level demonstrates the mass to be of high signal intensity with an internal septation (*arrow*) of low signal intensity. Mature teratoma was revealed at surgery. Unlike patients with thymoma, those with germ cell tumors may demonstrate elevated levels of specific markers such as AFP or β-human chorionic gonadotropin.

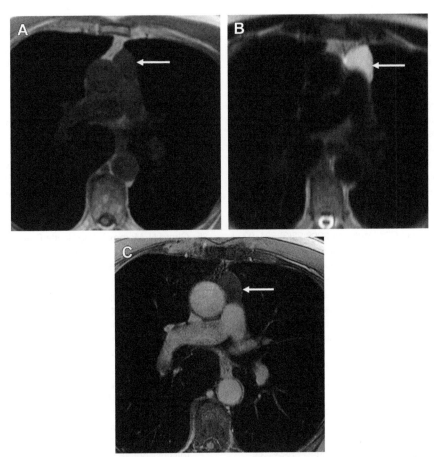

Fig. 15. Thymic cyst in a 32-year-old woman. (*A*) Axial precontrast spoiled gradient recalled (SPGR) MR imaging at the level of the pulmonary trunk bifurcation demonstrates a well-circumscribed anterior mediastinal mass (*arrow*) of low signal intensity. (*B*) Axial single-shot fast spin echo T2-weighted imaging at the same level shows high signal intensity within the mass (*arrow*) with absence of any nodular soft tissue component. (*C*) Axial contrast-enhanced (SPGR) fat-suppressed MR imaging at the same level demonstrates minimal enhancement along the peripheral aspect of the cyst (*arrow*) but no enhancing internal components.

SUMMARY

Thymoma is a rare tumor that represents the most common primary malignancy of the anterior mediastinum. Accurate imaging of the tumor is crucial to the diagnosis, staging, and treatment of thymoma. CT is generally superior to MR imaging in the evaluation of most anterior mediastinal masses, and surgeons are more familiar with the appearance of CT for the staging of patients with thymoma. However, MR imaging plays a critical role in the differentiation of benign lesions such as thymic hyperplasia and thymic cysts from other anterior mediastinal lesions, staging of thymoma in those individuals unable to undergo CT scanning secondary to contrast allergy and/or renal failure, and as a component of routine follow-up imaging in an effort to reduce the cumulative radiation dose. The excellent contrast resolution of MR imaging can be used in difficult cases when CT is inconclusive.

REFERENCES

1. Morgenthaler TI, Brown LR, Colby TV, et al. Thymoma. Mayo Clin Proc 1993;68(11):1110–23.
2. Engels EA. Epidemiology of thymoma and associated malignancies. J Thorac Oncol 2010;5: S260–5.
3. Travis WD, Brambilla E, Müller-Hermelink HK, et al, editors. Pathology & genetics: tumours of the lung, pleura, thymus and heart. World Health Organization classification of tumours, vol. 10. Lyon (France): IARC; 2004.
4. Lewis JE, Wick MR, Scheithauer BW, et al. Thymoma: a clinicopathologic review. Cancer 1987; 60(11):2727–43.
5. Osserman KE, Genkins G. Studies in myasthenia gravis: review of a twenty-year experience in over 1200 patients. Mt Sinai J Med 1971;38(6):497–537.
6. Cameron RB, Loehrer PJS, Thomas CRJ. Neoplasms of the mediastinum. In: DeVita VTJ, Hellman S, Rosenberg SA, editors. Cancer: principles and

practice of oncology. Philadelphia: Lippincott Williams & Wilkins; 2005. p. 845–58.

7. Levy Y, Afek A, Sherer Y, et al. Malignant thymoma associated with autoimmune diseases: a retrospective study and review of the literature. Semin Arthritis Rheum 1998;28(2):73–9.

8. Henschke CI, Lee IJ, Wu N, et al. CT screening for lung cancer: prevalence and incidence of mediastinal masses. Radiology 2006;239(2):586–90.

9. Regnard JF, Magdeleinat P, Dromer C, et al. Prognostic factors and long-term results after thymoma resection: a series of 307 patients. J Thorac Cardiovasc Surg 1996;112(2):376–84.

10. Suster S, Moran CA. Histologic classification of thymoma: the World Health Organization and beyond. Hematol Oncol Clin North Am 2008;22(3):381–92.

11. Moran CA, Weissferdt A, Kalhor N, et al. Thymomas I: a clinicopathologic correlation of 250 cases with emphasis on the World Health Organization schema. Am J Clin Pathol 2012;137:444–50.

12. Rieker RJ, Hoegel J, Morresi-Hauf A, et al. Histologic classification of thymic epithelial tumors: comparison of established classification schemes. Int J Cancer 2002;98(6):900–6.

13. Detterbeck FC. Clinical value of the WHO classification system of thymoma. Ann Thorac Surg 2006; 81(6):2328–34.

14. Suster S, Moran CA. Thymoma, atypical thymoma, and thymic carcinoma. A novel conceptual approach to the classification of thymic epithelial neoplasms. Am J Clin Pathol 1999;111:826–33.

15. Gamondès JP, Balawi A, Greenland T, et al. Seventeen years of surgical treatment of thymoma: factors influencing survival. Eur J Cardiothorac Surg 1991; 5(3):124–31.

16. Masaoka A, Monden Y, Nakahara K, et al. Follow-up study of thymomas with special reference to their clinical stages. Cancer 1981;48(11):2485–92.

17. Koga K, Matsuno Y, Noguchi M, et al. A review of 79 thymomas: modification of staging system and reappraisal of conventional division into invasive and non-invasive thymoma. Pathol Int 1994;44(5): 359–67.

18. Yamakawa Y, Masaoka A, Hashimoto T, et al. A tentative tumor-node-metastasis classification of thymoma. Cancer 1991;68(9):1984–7.

19. Huang J, Detterbeck FC, Wang Z, et al. Standard outcome measures for thymic malignancies. J Thorac Oncol 2010;5(12):2017–23.

20. Falkson CB, Bezjak A, Darling G, et al. The management of thymoma: a systematic review and practice guideline. J Thorac Oncol 2009;4(7):911–9.

21. Detterbeck FC, Stratton K, Giroux D, et al. The IASLC/ITMIG thymic epithelial tumors staging project: proposal for an evidence-based stage classification system for the forthcoming (8th) edition of the TNM classification of malignant tumors. J Thorac Oncol 2014;9(9 Suppl 2):S65–72.

22. Detterbeck FC, Moran C, Huang J, et al. Which way is up? policies and procedures for surgeons and pathologists of resection specimens of thymic malignancy. J Thorac Oncol 2011;6(7 Suppl 3): S1730–8.

23. Casey EM, Kiel PJ, Loehrer PJ Sr. Clinical management of thymoma patients. Hematol Oncol Clin North Am 2008;22:457–73.

24. Moran CA, Walsh G, Suster S, et al. Thymomas II: a clinicopathologic correlation of 250 cases with a proposed staging system with emphasis on pathologic assessment. Am J Clin Pathol 2012; 137:451–61.

25. Girard N, Mornex F, Van Houtte P, et al. Thymoma: a focus on current therapeutic management. J Thorac Oncol 2009;4:119–26.

26. Kim ES, Putnam JB, Komaki R, et al. Phase II study of a multidisciplinary approach with induction chemotherapy, followed by surgical resection, radiation therapy, and consolidation chemotherapy for unresectable malignant thymomas: final report. Lung Cancer 2004;44:369–79.

27. Rea F, Sartori F, Loy M, et al. Chemotherapy and operation for invasive thymoma. J Thorac Cardiovasc Surg 1993;106:543–9.

28. Venuta F, Rendina EA, Longo F, et al. Long-term outcome after multimodality treatment for stage III thymic tumors. Ann Thorac Surg 2003;76:1866–72 [discussion: 1872].

29. Venuta F, Rendina EA, Pescarmona EO, et al. Multimodality treatment of thymoma: a prospective study. Ann Thorac Surg 1997;64:1585–91 [discussion: 1591–2].

30. Tomiyama N, Honda O, Tsubamoto M, et al. Anterior mediastinal tumors: diagnostic accuracy of CT and MRI. Eur J Radiol 2009;69(2):280–8.

31. Marom EM. Advances in thymoma imaging. J Thorac Imaging 2013;28(2):69–83.

32. Restrepo CS, Pandit M, Rojas IC, et al. Imaging findings of expansile lesions of the thymus. Curr Probl Diagn Radiol 2005;34:22–34.

33. Maher MM, Shepard JA. Imaging of thymoma. Semin Thorac Cardiovasc Surg 2005;17:12–9.

34. Thomas A, Shanbhag S, Haglund K, et al. Characterization and management of cardiac involvement of thymic epithelial tumors. J Thorac Oncol 2013; 8(2):246–9.

35. Goldman M, Matthews R, Meng H, et al. Evaluation of cardiac involvement with mediastinal lymphoma: the role of innovative integrated cardiovascular imaging. Echocardiography 2012;29(8):E189–92.

36. Sakai S, Murayama S, Soeda H, et al. Differential diagnosis between thymoma and non-thymoma by dynamic MR imaging. Acta Radiol 2002;43:262–8.

37. Reubi JC, Waser B, Horisberger U, et al. In vitro autoradiographic and in vivo scintigraphic localization of somatostatin receptors in human lymphatic tissue. Blood 1993;82:2143–51.

38. Sadohara J, Fujimoto K, Muller NL, et al. Thymic epithelial tumors: comparison of CT and MR imaging findings of low-risk thymomas, high-risk thymomas, and thymic carcinomas. Eur J Radiol 2006;60:70–9.

39. Regnard JF, Zinzindohoue F, Magdeleinat P, et al. Results of re-resection for recurrent thymomas. Ann Thorac Surg 1997;64(6):1593–8.

40. Ströbel P, Bauer A, Puppe B, et al. Tumor recurrence and survival in patients treated for thymomas and thymic squamous cell carcinomas: a retrospective analysis. J Clin Oncol 2004;22(8):1501–9.

41. Inaoka T, Takahashi K, Mineta M, et al. Thymic hyperplasia and thymus gland tumors: differentiation with chemical shift MR imaging. Radiology 2007; 243:869–76.

42. Takahashi K, Inaoka T, Murakami N, et al. Characterization of the normal and hyperplastic thymus on chemical-shift MR imaging. Am J Roentgenol 2003; 180:1265–9.

43. Inaoka T, Takahashi K, Iwata K, et al. Evaluation of normal fatty replacement of the thymus with chemical-shift MR imaging for identification of the normal thymus. J Magn Reson Imaging 2005; 22(3):341–6.

44. Ackman JB, Mino-Kenudson M, Morse CR. Nonsuppressing normal thymus on chemical shift magnetic resonance imaging in a young woman. J Thorac Imaging 2012;27:W196–8.

45. Rosado-de-Christenson ML, Strollo DC, Marom EM. Imaging of thymic epithelial neoplasms. Hematol Oncol Clin North Am 2008;22(3):409–31.

46. Nishino M, Ashiku SK, Kocher ON, et al. The thymus: a comprehensive review. Radiographics 2006;26(2): 335–48.

47. Johnson PW, Davies AJ. Primary mediastinal B-cell lymphoma. Hematology Am Soc Hematol Educ Program 2008;349–58.

48. Takahashi K, Al-Janabi NJ. Computed tomography and magnetic resonance imaging of mediastinal tumors. J Magn Reson Imaging 2010;32(6):1325–39.

49. Nasseri F, Eftekhari F. Clinical and radiologic review of the normal and abnormal thymus: pearls and pitfalls. Radiographics 2010;30(2):413–28.

Novel MR Imaging Applications for Pleural evaluation

Ritu R. Gill, MD, MPH[a],*, Samuel Patz, PhD[a],
Iga Muradyan, PhD[a], Ravi T. Seethamraju, PhD[b]

KEYWORDS

- MR imaging • MR imaging technique • Novel applications • Pleura • Pleural tumors
- Mesothelioma

KEY POINTS

- Optimizing current magnetic resonance (MR) protocols provide more efficient and valuable MR applications and potentially help identify imaging biomarkers that can be predictive and prognostic.
- Diffusion-weighted (DW) and perfusion imaging are emerging techniques and can provide complementary information, which can be used in evaluation and management of pleural diseases.
- MR imaging continues to play a vital role is assessing suitability for surgical resection and continues to be superior to other cross-sectional modalities.

 Videos of three subjects with Mesothelioma showing dynamic perfusion in coronal plane: FLASH, TWIST and RADIAL VIBE acquisitions comparing effect of respiration accompany this article at http://www.mri.theclinics.com/

INTRODUCTION

MR imaging is an excellent modality for differentiating benign from malignant pleural diseases. Owing to better soft-tissue contrast and higher intrinsic flow sensitivity, it is superior to computed tomography (CT) and fluorodeoxyglucose (FDG) PET-CT.[1–4] MR imaging plays a vital role in determining resectability of primary and secondary pleural tumors, especially malignant pleural mesothelioma (MPM),[5] and is superior to other cross-sectional imaging modalities in evaluating invasion of the chest wall, diaphragm, heart, vessels, airways, and other critical structures.[6–9] Optimizing standard MR imaging sequences to reduce susceptibility and improve spatial and temporal resolution can improve the sensitivity and specificity of imaging findings and help in surgical planning and response assessment.

Even though the differential diagnosis of pleural diseases is limited and the lesions are easy to biopsy, the diagnostic yield of biopsies is low and more invasive procedures are often needed to make a diagnosis.[10–13] A variety of MR imaging techniques can help differentiate benign from malignant diseases and guide biopsy, thus improving the yield and diagnostic accuracy.[14] Although CT is the mainstay of chest imaging and has good sensitivity and specificity, MR imaging and PET seem to have higher accuracy. MR imaging has the added benefit of being an excellent aid in

Disclosures: no relevant disclosures (R.R. Gill, S. Patz, and I. Muradyan); Dr Seethamraju has stock ownership and an employment affiliation with Siemens AG.
[a] Department of Radiology, Brigham and Women's Hospital, Harvard Medical School, 75 Francis Street, Boston, MA 02120, USA; [b] Magnetic Resonance, Research and Development, Siemens Healthcare, 1620 tremont st., Boston, MA 02120, USA
* Corresponding author. Department of Radiology, Brigham and Women's Hospital, Harvard Medical School, 15 Francis Street, Boston, MA.
E-mail address: rgill@partners.org

Magn Reson Imaging Clin N Am 23 (2015) 179–195
http://dx.doi.org/10.1016/j.mric.2015.01.006
1064-9689/15/$ – see front matter © 2015 Elsevier Inc. All rights reserved.

determining surgical resectability of tumors[6] without irradiation.

Pathologic pleural involvement ranges from pleural effusions to pleural thickening and masses, both due to primary chest processes or secondary to a disease outside the thorax.[15] CT remains the gold standard imaging modality in chest, as it provides exquisite resolution of the anatomic structures of the lungs and airways, has fast acquisition times, and does not require complex planning or postprocessing to extract the desired information. MR imaging has been advocated as a powerful adjunctive tool and can provide complementary information when assessing pleural pathology.[16]

In the past, the proton-poor environment in the chest, rapid signal dephasing, and respiratory and cardiac motion presented significant obstacles for widespread adoption and clinical use of MR imaging in evaluation of noncardiac chest diseases. Advances in pulmonary MR imaging methods, optimization of MR protocols, and individualization of pulse sequences for the clinical question at hand have increased the utilization of MR in evaluation of the pleural abnormalities in recent times.[17] The future of chest MR imaging will include a greater emphasis on quantitative imaging. This article provides comprehensive information regarding the utility and applicability of novel MR imaging techniques for evaluation of pleural diseases.

MR IMAGING PLEURAL PROTOCOLS

MR protocols comprise sequences designed for both anatomic and functional imaging, thus allowing a comprehensive evaluation of chest tumors and pathologies in a single examination.[18–20] Pulse sequences, imaging planes, and parameters such as slice thickness and interslice gap are specified according to the anatomic range being imaged and the study objectives. T1-weighted (T1W) images are known for their excellent anatomic resolution and ability to resolve and differentiate between the pleural space and extrapleural fat. T2-weighted (T2W) images allow differentiation of pleural thickening and nodularity from pleural fluid and help delineate tumor from adjacent muscle. Gadolinium administration further enhances tissue contrast and increases the conspicuity of the borders between lesions and adjacent normal structures on T1W images with fat saturation. Short tau inversion recovery (STIR) images are particularly sensitive for bone involvement by tumor or infection, denoted by fluid signal in place of normal dark to intermediate marrow signal and breach of the normal dark cortical line.[21]

Parallel MR imaging used with sequences that allow for high temporal resolution cine imaging, such as steady state free precession, may reveal subtle invasion of mediastinal structures and the chest wall.[22] Additional sequences that have utility in selected cases of tumor assessment include diffusion-weighted imaging (DWI) and dynamic contrast-enhanced (DCE) or perfusion MR imaging.[19]

The authors' clinical MR protocol for pleural tumor evaluation is performed on a 3-T whole-body system (Magnetom TIM Trio, Siemens AG, Erlangen, Germany) using the manufacturer's body array coil for signal reception and body coil for transmission. Initial anatomic-based imaging consists of coronal and transverse T2W single-shot acquisition (half Fourier acquisition single-shot turbo spin echo [HASTE]; repetition time, 1200 milliseconds; echo time, 101 milliseconds; section thickness, 5.0 mm; interslice gap, 1.5 mm; signal averages 1; field of view [FOV],400 mm; matrix size, 320 × 224; parallel imaging factor 2) and 3-dimensional (3D) T1W volume interpolated gradient echo acquisitions (volume interpolated breath-hold examination [VIBE]; repetition time, 3.34 milliseconds; echo time, 1.26 milliseconds; section thickness, 4.0 mm; interslice gap, 0 mm; signal averages 1; FOV, 400 mm; matrix size, 320 × 256; parallel imaging factor 2) to cover the entire thoracic cavity and diaphragm using a breath-hold technique.

Diffusion-Weighted Imaging

Axial DWI scans in the authors' institution are acquired with fat suppression using a free-breathing single-shot spin echo- echo planar imaging sequence (repetition time 5000 milliseconds, echo time 82 milliseconds, section thickness 8.0 mm, interslice gap 1.5 mm, signal averages 6, FOV 400 mm, matrix size 160 × 96, parallel imaging factor 2).

The number and range of b-values used are chosen to optimize apparent diffusion coefficient ADC calculation by providing 4 data points for calculating each ADC value while reducing intravascular water perfusion effects on b-value DW images. The total imaging time for DWI is approximately 6.5 minutes.[23] The ADC value is calculated by a logarithmic linear fit of signal intensity versus the b values; this yields a monocompartmental fit for the raw signal intensity data. The major limitation is the lack of consensus on standardization of region of interest analysis and utilization of mean and minimal ADC values (Table 1).[24]

Perfusion MR Imaging

Perfusion imaging is performed using a 3D GRE based sequence (repetition time/echo time

Table 1 ADC calculation	
Methods of ADC Calculation	**Evaluation**
Parametric ADC	Graphical representation of changes in ADC on a voxel-by-voxel basis
ADC histogram	Depiction of each voxel in multiple ROIs as a histogram

Abbreviation: ROI, region of interest.

Table 2 Common parameters generated using Toft model	
MR Pharmacokinetic Parameter	**Units**
Transfer constant (K^{trans})	min^{-1}
Rate constant (Kep)	min^{-1}
Elimination constant (Ve)	None

[TR/TE], 2.02/0.84 ms; flip angle, 10°; acquisition matrix, 256 × 135; slab thickness, 168–200 mm; 42–56 slice encoding; pixel spacing, 1.76–1.88 mm; scan time, 2.84–3.96 s/image). Follow-up chest radiograph obtained after treatment demonstrated internal resolution. Postprocessing and calculation of perfusion indices is performed using the Toft model (**Fig. 1**). The area under the curve (AUC) represents the area under the plot of plasma concentration of gadolinium (not logarithm of the concentration) against time and can be used to calculate the apparent volume of distribution of gadolinium in the tissues or tumors. The AUC is often used in addition to or as an alternative to parameters derived from pharmacokinetic modeling of T1W DCE MR imaging data. AUC has been shown to be a mixed parameter that can display correlation with transfer constant (K^{trans}), elimination constant (v_e), and rate constant (K_{ep}) and can have a relationship with all three (**Table 2**). Furthermore, it has been demonstrated that AUC is not affected by vascular input function.

CLINICAL APPLICATIONS IN PLEURAL DISEASES
Characterization of Pleural Pathologies

Various pleural pathologies have different imaging features as summarized in (**Table 3**).

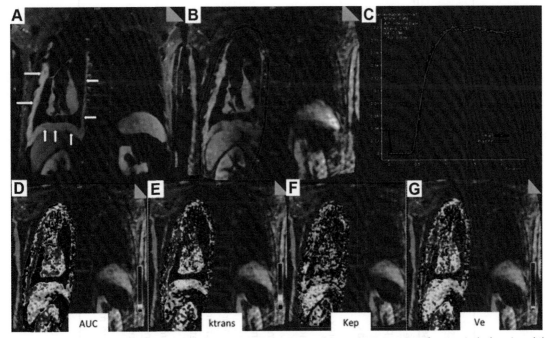

Fig. 1. A 48-year-old man with epithelial mesothelioma who underwent MR imaging for surgical planning. (*A*) Coronal postcontrast VIBE image demonstrates right pleural mesothelioma (*arrows*) and associated effusion. (*B*) Region of interest drawn to demarcate the area for calculation of perfusion parameters. (*C*) The enhancement curve showing goodness of fit. Multiparametric maps depicting the perfusion parameters of the tumor: area under the curve (AUC) (*D*), transfer constant (ktrans) (*E*), rate constant (Kep) (*F*), and elimination constant (Ve) (*G*).

Table 3
MR characteristics of pleural diseases

Pleural Disease/Abnormality	T1W	T2W	Postcontrast	ADC Value (mm²/s)	Other Features and Associations
Transudate pleural effusion	Low	High	−	$3.42 \pm 0.76 \times 10^{-3}$	Absence of loculations
Exudative pleural effusion	Low	High	+++	$3.18 \pm 1.82 \times 10^{-3}$	Pleural thickening, split pleura sign, loculations, modularity, internal septations
Chylothorax	High	Low	−	—	Signal comparable to fat, associated with lymphoma, lymphangioleiomyomatosis, and postsurgical
Hemothrorax	High	High	−	—	Concentric rim sign due to T1 shortening on T1W and T2W imaging
Pleural plaques	Low	Low	−/+	$2.6 \pm 1.82 \times 10^{-3}$	Extrapleural fat, round atelectasis, and pleural effusion
Lipoma	High	Moderate to high	−	—	Fat suppression sequences are helpful
Liposarcoma	Low	High	+/+ +/+ + +	—	Heterogeneous, calcifications may be present
Fibrous tumor of the pleura	Low	Low	+++	—	Myxoid degeneration and calcifications can be present, pedunculated
Malignant fibrous tumor	Low	High	+++	—	Lower ADC than benign fibrous tumor of the pleura
Synovial sarcoma	Low	Mixed	+++	—	Triple sign, bunch of grapes appearance on T2W image
Pleural metastases	Low	Low/high	++/+ + +		Enhancement and morphologic characteristics similar to primary tumor
Lymphoma	Low	Low	++	$1.23 \pm 0.3 \times 10^{-3}$	Multistation adenopathy, marrow involvement
Lung cancer	Low	Mixed	+++	$2.12 \pm 0.6 \times 10^{-3}$	Pleural effusion, lung masses and adenopathy
Epithelial mesothelioma	Low	Low	+++	$1.31 \pm 0.15 \times 10^{-3}$	Asbestos exposure, circumferential tumor, pleural effusion
Sarcomatoid mesothelioma	Low	Mixed	+++	$0.99 \pm 0.07 \times 10^{-3}$	Circumferential tumor, pleural effusion, pleural masses, chest wall invasion

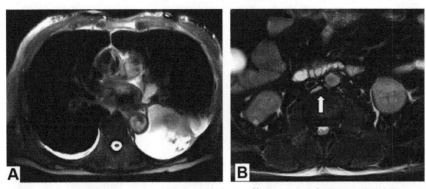

Fig. 2. An 87-year-old man presenting with bilateral chylous effusions. Axial T2W HASTE image at the level of T12/L1 (*A*) vertebral bodies showing bilateral chylous effusions, left greater than right. (*B*) Enlarged thoracic duct (*arrow*). The patient underwent subsequent thoracic duct embolization.

Pleural effusions

Differentiation between transudative and exudative pleural effusions often requires combination of clinical, biochemical, and pathologic findings. Hounsfield unit measurements on CT scans can be unreliable. Conventional MR imaging techniques based on the degree of enhancement on T1W spin echo images after the administration of gadolinium-DTPA (0.1 mmol/kg) have been used to distinguish exudative effusions from transudative effusions, but they are not reliable.[25] The cause of pleural effusions is based on the presence or absence of specific morphologic features (pleural thickening, split pleura sign, loculations, nodularity, internal septations, and enhancement postgadolinium administration).[26] Transudative

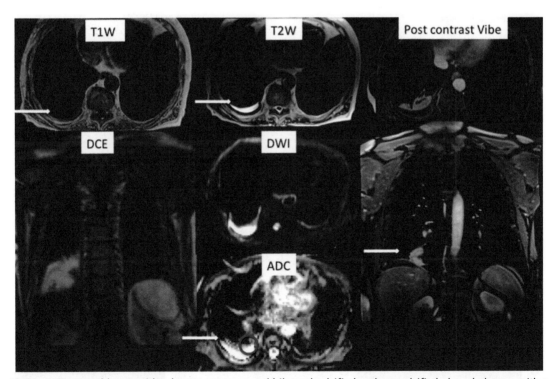

Fig. 3. A 57-year-old man with asbestos exposure and bilateral calcified and noncalcified pleural plaques with a masslike opacity in the right lower lobe. The consolidation in the right lower lobe is isointense to hypointense on T1W and T2W (*white arrows*) images, shows moderate enhancement, and has a comet tail appearance on postcontrast images (*white arrow*). The DCE coronal image shows uniform enhancement of the right lower lobe consolidation. The effusion does not show restriction on DW image and ADC image (*white arrow*). The ADC value of the effusion is 3.40×10^{-3} mm^2/s (*red region of interest*).

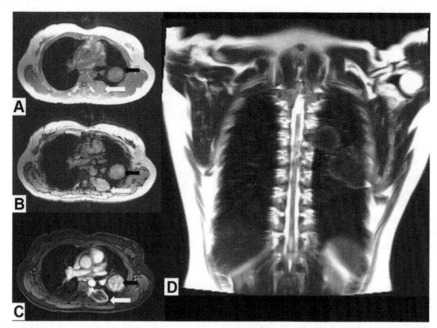

Fig. 4. A 49-year-old women with chest pain underwent MR imaging to characterize 2 left-sided tumors. The left paraspinal pleural-based lesion (*white arrow*) and the fissural pleural-based lesion (*black arrow*) are isointense on T1W (*A, B*) and hypointense on T2W images (*D*). The fissural lesion (*black arrow*) shows homogenous intense enhancement and the paraspinal lesion (*white arrow*) shows peripheral enhancement post gadolinium administration (*C*). The patient underwent surgical resection, and the final pathology was consistent with fibrous tumor of the pleura.

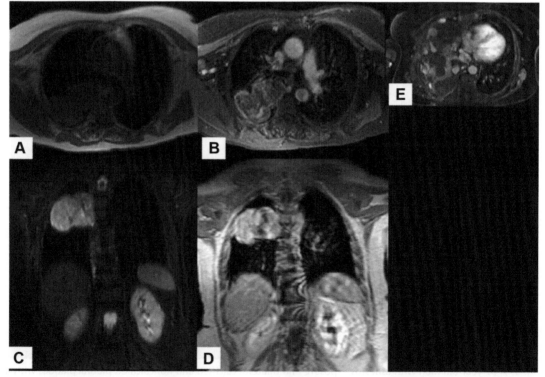

Fig. 5. A 67-year-old women with biopsy-proven malignant fibrous tumor of the pleura. The mass is isointense on axial T1W images (*A*) but is hyperintense to muscles on coronal T2W images (*C*) and shows heterogeneous enhancement (*B, D*) after contrast administration. The mass was successfully resected but recurred in 6 months (*E*). Heterogeneously enhancing mass within the right hemithorax consistent with recurrent malignant fibrous tumor (*E*).

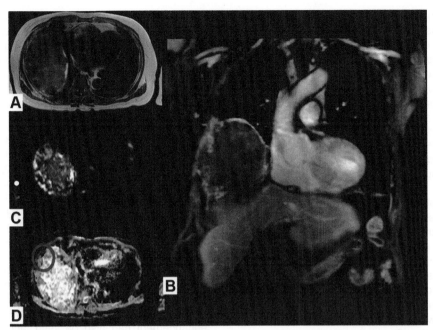

Fig. 6. A 70-year-old man with a known right-sided pleural tumor showing growth over 6 months. The large right pleural-based lesion is hypointense on T1W images (*A*) and shows peripheral enhancement after contrast (*B*). The lesion shows heterogeneity and some areas of restricted diffusion (*C*) within it. The mean ADC value of the lesion is 2.40×10^{-3} mm^2/s and ranged between 3.40×10^{-3} mm^2/s and 1.7×10^{-3} mm^2/s (*D*). The biopsy of the restricted areas showed no evidence of malignant transformation (*red circle*).

effusions have a mean ADC value of $3.42 \pm 0.76 \times 10^{-3}$ mm^2/s compared with exudative effusions, which have a slightly lower mean ADC value of $3.18 \pm 1.82 \times 10^{-3}$ mm^2/s.[27] Inan and colleagues[27] were able to differentiate pleural effusions using a cutoff value of 3.6×10^{-3} mm^2/s with a sensitivity of 71% and specificity of 63%. MR evaluation also plays a key role in the management of chylous effusions. Localization of the thoracic duct before embolization procedures by MR imaging is standard of care (**Fig. 2**).[28] Subacute or chronic hemothrorax has high signal

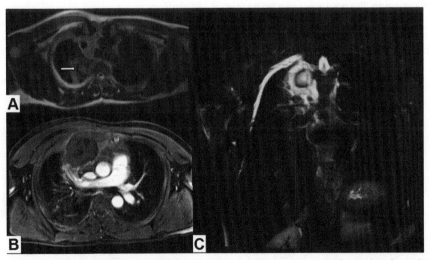

Fig. 7. A 38-year-old women after bone marrow transplant and known Mucor infection in the right upper lobe with evidence of mediastinitis and chest wall invasion. Note the dark rim surrounding the lesion on axial T1W (*arrow*) (*A*) and peripheral contrast enhancement on postcontrast VIBE image (*B*). There is also a small right pleural effusion. The coronal STIR image (*C*) is useful in delineating the overall extent and distribution of the disease process.

intensity on T1W and T2W images. Chronic pleural hematomas can be identified on MR imaging by the presence of the concentric ring sign caused by the bright central signal intensity (methemoglobin) related to the T1 shortening effects, surrounded by the dark outer ring representing hemosiderin on T1W and T2W images.

Round atelectasis

Chronic pleural effusions and pleural thickening are associated with round atelectasis, a rounded area of lung collapse, which can remain stable or even grow over a period. Even though it has a characteristic comet tail appearance on CT scans, anxiety over an underlying malignancy can lead to unnecessary invasive procedures. DCE MR imaging can be used to characterize round atelectasis. Signal intensity curves from round atelectasis are similar in shape to the pulmonary artery blood flow and normal lung with a steeper slope during wash-in and washout and higher relative signal increase when compared with tumors,[29] thus increasing the diagnostic yield when combined with morphologic assessment (**Fig. 3**).

Pleural plaques and thickening

Bilateral pleural plaques are related to asbestos exposure and tend to have low signal intensity on T1W and T2W sequences and show minimal to no enhancement after gadolinium administration. MR imaging can also help identify associated anatomic features such as extrapleural fat hypertrophy, diffuse pleural thickening, and pleural effusions. DWI can be used to differentiate benign plaques from malignant degeneration, and when combined with DCE MR imaging, the accuracy can be further improved.[30] Diffuse pleural thickening can be secondary to several causes such as mycobacterial tuberculosis infection, empyema, trauma, drug exposure, and collagen vascular disease apart from asbestos exposure. It is preceded by pleural effusion, leading to fibrosis and subsequently sheetlike pleural thickening involving the visceral pleura measuring at least 5 cm in length and 3 mm in thickness.[31]

Fibrous tumor of the pleura

The MR imaging features of fibrous tumors of the pleura depend on the lesion size. The intratumoral heterogeneity increases with increasing size due to necrosis, myxoid degeneration, and development of dystrophic calcification. It may be possible to visualize a vascular pedicle in approximately 40% of small tumors, accounting for their mobility.[31] The MR appearance of these tumors is similar to fibrous tissue; they tend to appear hypointense on T1W and T2W sequences in most cases and tend to have intense inhomogeneous enhancement in most cases after gadolinium administration.[30] Nodular and homogeneous enhancement can also be seen, and the lesion may have a rim of low signal on T2W images. Approximately 10% tumors are isointense to muscle and 10% are hyperintense on T1W and T2W sequences. Areas of necrosis and myxoid degeneration appearing as high signal on T1W and T2W images can also be seen (**Fig. 4**).[30]

The malignant fibrous tumors tend to be hyperintense on both T2W and STIR images and show intense enhancement. ADC values can potentially be used to identify malignant degeneration and also the malignant counterparts (**Figs. 5 and 6**).[32]

Miscellaneous benign pleural abnormalities

Sometimes, focal liver herniation through a diaphragmatic defect can mimic a solitary fibrous tumor, in which case liver-specific contrast agents

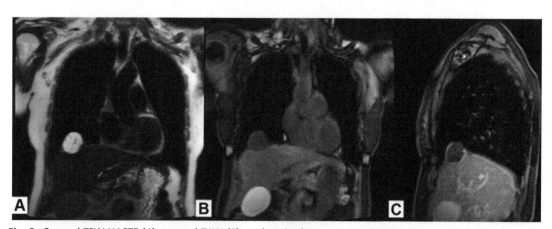

Fig. 8. Coronal T2W HASTE (*A*), coronal T1W (*B*), and sagittal postcontrast 3D GRE images (*C*) showing a multiloculated cyst (T1 hypointense and T2 hyperintense) within the diaphragm, with capsular enhancement. The differential diagnosis includes a congenital cyst and hydatid cyst.

such as Gadoextate sodium (Eovist, Bayer) can easily differentiate the two.

Infectious processes involving the pleura are well assessed on coronal STIR images, which help delineate the overall extent and distribution of the disease process. Other rare benign diaphragmatic pathologies can also sometimes mimic pleural pathology on CT images. T2W and postcontrast 3D gradient recalled echo (GRE) images in multiple planes can help resolve the dilemma (**Figs. 7 and 8**).

Metastatic pleural disease

Malignant involvement of the pleura is most commonly related to metastatic disease and presents as malignant effusions with pleural thickening and pleural nodularity. Primary bronchogenic carcinoma is the most common tumor metastatic to the pleura followed by breast (20%) and lymphoma (10%).

Thymic epithelial neoplasms can involve the pleura either contiguously or by drop metastases. The MR characteristics of malignant pleural involvement are similar to the primary tumor; the ADC values can be used potentially as an imaging biomarker to identify pleural and nodal metastases if the ADC value of the original tumor is known.[31] STIR images can help delineate the extent and help plan resection margins.

Sarcomas involving the pleura

Primary sarcomas that involve the pleura are rare and include liposarcoma, synovial sarcoma, and undifferentiated pleomorphic sarcoma (previously known as malignant fibrous histiocytoma).

Pleural liposarcoma is often asymptomatic and on MR imaging appears hyperintense on T2W sequences due to myxoid degeneration and hypointense on T1W sequences, with variable enhancement after administration of contrast.[31] Thoracic synovial sarcoma is less common than its extrathoracic counterpart and may arise in the chest wall, pleura, mediastinum, heart, or lung and can be associated with ipsilateral pleural effusions. The triple sign is pathognomic of synovial sarcomas and describes the presence of hyperintense, isointense, and hypointense areas on T2W MR imaging.[33] On MR imaging, nodular soft tissue with multiloculated fluid-filled components is typical and rim enhancement is seen after administration of intravenous contrast.

Epithelioid hemangioendothelioma is a low- to intermediate-grade aggressive neoplasm that rarely arises in the pleura. It is more common in the bone, liver, soft tissue, and lung. The pleural form more commonly affects men than women. Presenting symptoms are somewhat nonspecific and include chest pain, dyspnea, fever, and cough. Imaging findings include pleural effusion and volume loss in the affected hemithorax and are similar to those of MPM and pleural carcinomatosis (**Figs. 9 and 10**).[34]

Malignant pleural mesothelioma

MPM is a rare and aggressive primary pleural neoplasm related to asbestos exposure. MR imaging plays an important role in evaluation and assessment for treatment and is superior to CT in both anatomic delineation (because of superior contrast)

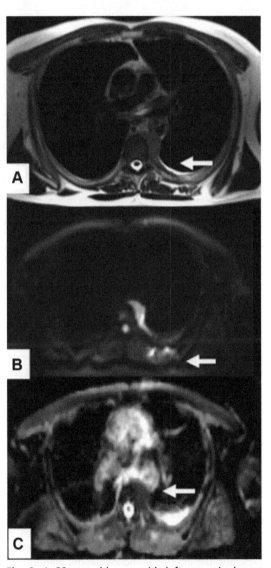

Fig. 9. A 66-year-old man with left paraspinal mass (*arrow*) that is low in signal on T2W image (*A*); note increased signal (*arrow*) in the chest wall muscles similar to the left paraspinal mass depicting subtle chest wall involvement on the DW image (*B*) and demonstrating restricted diffusion on the ADC map (*C*). Pathology: B-cell lymphoma.

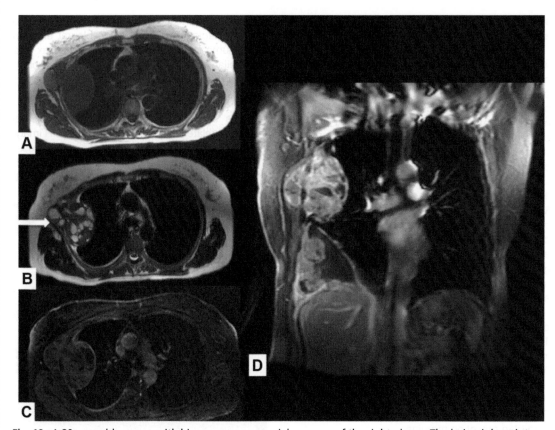

Fig. 10. A 39-year-old women with biopsy-proven synovial sarcoma of the right pleura. The lesion is hypointense on T1W images (*A*) and depicts the triple sign on T2W images (*arrow, B*). The mass shows intense enhancement after contrast (*C, D*).

and correlation with histopathology.[5,30,31,33] MPM tends to have intermediate to slightly high signal intensity on T1W images and moderately high signal intensity onT2W images (compared with adjacent musculature and chest wall) and shows moderate enhancement after contrast administration. MR imaging has higher sensitivity than CT in detecting early chest wall invasion, diaphragmatic involvement, and vascular invasion. Additional techniques such as fat suppression and subtraction images further help identify chest wall invasion and fissural involvement. DWI and DCE MR imaging can further help characterize the histologic cell types of mesothelioma. The epithelial subtype tends to have higher ADC value than the sarcomatoid subtype and an ADC value of 1.31×10^{-3} mm^2/s can be used as a cutoff to differentiate the 2 histologic cell types.[23] Giesel and colleagues[35] were able to correlate perfusion parameters in mesothelioma with angiogenesis in these tumors (**Figs. 11–15**).

Determining Resectability

Metastatic involvement of the pleura is not considered as resectable disease; surgical options are reserved for localized disease and for primary malignant pleural tumors localized to the ipsilateral hemithroax.[34] Two types of surgical resections can be considered: (1) pleurectomy or pleural decortication, in which both the visceral and parietal pleura are resected, and (2) extrapleural pneumonectomy, in which the whole lung is resected with resection of the pleura with or without the diaphragm. MR imaging is superior to CT in evaluating a patient for resectability, when evaluating the chest wall, diaphragm, endothoracic fascia, mediastinal fat, and vascular invasion (**Figs. 16** and **17**).[5] Parallel MR imaging techniques in conjunction with generalized auto calibrating partially parallel acquisition, true fast imaging with steady state precession, and FLASH can help in delineating subtle invasion of the mediastinal structures such as myocardium and chest wall.[34] Fat suppression and subtraction images especially coronal images are helpful in looking for subtle endothoracic fascial involvement. Coolen and colleagues[36] described the sign of pointillism on high–b-value images. These images highlight areas of chest wall invasion, look similar to FDG PET-CT images, and are helpful for surgical planning (see **Figs. 15–17; Figs. 18–20**).[35]

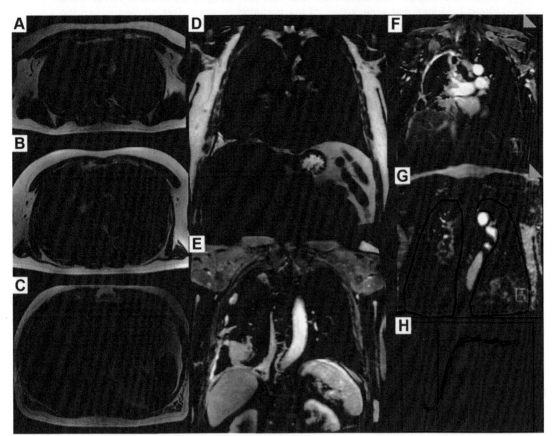

Fig. 11. A 57-year-old man with right malignant pleural mesothelioma. Axial T1W (*A–C*), T2W (*D*), and postcontrast images (*E, F*) show a circumferential right-sided pleural tumor with no evidence of chest wall involvement, transdiaphragmatic extent, or contralateral disease. The patient underwent a radical pleurectomy. (*G*) Placement of region of interest for calculation of perfusion parameters; (*H*) enhancement curve.

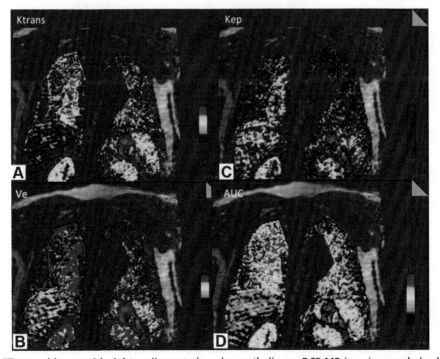

Fig. 12. A 57-year-old man with right malignant pleural mesothelioma. DCE MR imaging can help characterize the perfusion parameters (*A*) Ktrans, (*B*) Ve, (*C*) Kep, and (*D*) AUC of the tumor and can be used for assessing treatment response.

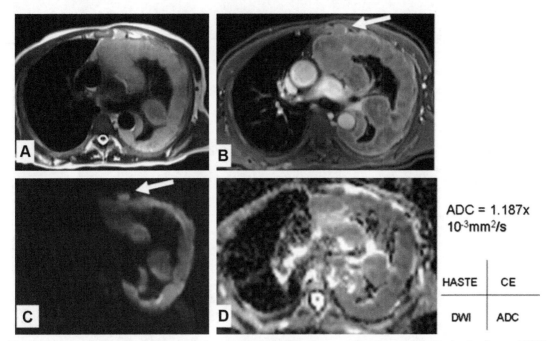

Fig. 13. A 71-year-old man with a circumferential left pleural tumor on T2W image (*A*). Contrast-enhanced VIBE shows enhancement and anterior chest wall invasion (*arrow*) (*B*). DWI demonstrates higher intensity than skeletal muscle and confirms chest wall invasion (*arrow*) (*C*). (*D*) ADC map. Pathology: Epithelioid mesothelioma.

ADC = 1.187x 10⁻³mm²/s

| HASTE | CE |
| DWI | ADC |

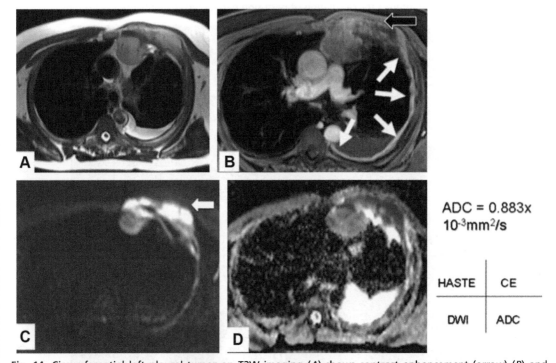

ADC = 0.883x 10⁻³mm²/s

| HASTE | CE |
| DWI | ADC |

Fig. 14. Circumferential left pleural tumor on T2W imaging (*A*) shows contrast enhancement (*arrow*) (*B*) and anterior chest wall invasion (*black arrow*) (*C*). Pointillism sign (*white arrow*) showing chest wall involvement on DW images. (*D*) ADC map showing restricted diffusion in the tumor. The ADC value is consistent with sarcomatoid subtype of mesothelioma. A small left pleural effusion is present as well.

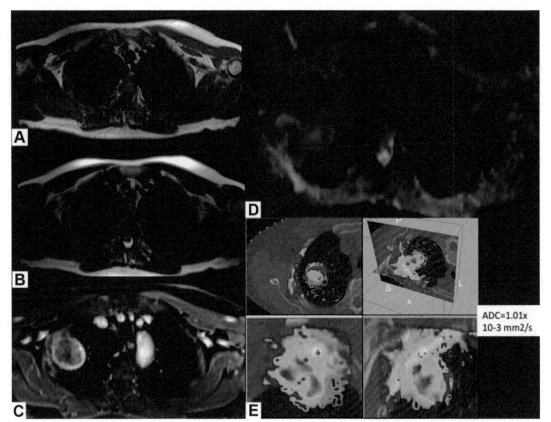

Fig. 15. A 67-year-old man presenting a right upper pleural-based mass causing focal chest wall invasion seen on T1W (*A*), T2W (*B*), and contrast-enhanced axial images (*C*). The ADC value is suggestive of a biphasic mesothelioma with an epithelial predominant component (*D*). Multiparametric map superimposed over CT images shows intratumoral heterogeneity and distribution of the sarcomatoid component in the periphery depicted in red and the predominant epithelial component in green (*E*).

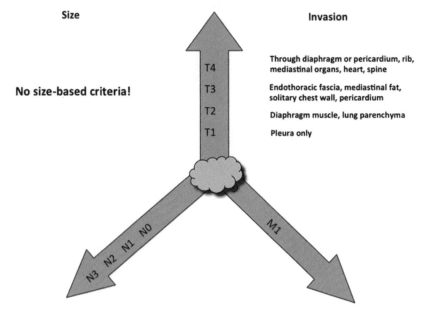

Fig. 16. *T* classification of malignant pleural mesothelioma and criteria for determining resectability.

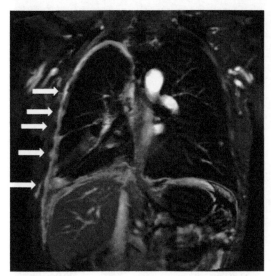

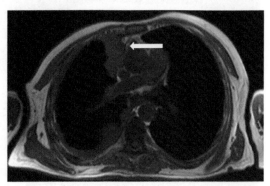

Fig. 18. Axial T1W image showing mediastinal fat invasion by tumor (*arrow*).

Fig. 17. Coronal 3D GRE subtraction images can help identify subtle multifocal endothoracic fascial involvement. Note the irregular outline of the outer pleural margin representing fingerlike invasion into the fascial plane (*arrows*) thus making complete macroscopic resection difficult.

Assessment of Treatment Response

DCE MR imaging after the administration of gadolinium contrast material can be used to assess perfusion and vascularity of tumors by mapping the pharmacokinetics of the contrast through the tumor. Signal intensity curves can be plotted by tracking wash-in and washout of contrast in 3D volume of the tumor. Multiparametric maps can be derived and used to predict the probability of response to chemotherapy and can also be used longitudinally to assess response to therapy. Giesel and colleagues[35] studied the feasibility of DCE to monitor response to chemotherapy in patients with mesothelioma. Their study showed that patients who had lower permeability coefficient (kep <2.6 min) were less likely to respond to chemotherapy than those with a higher kep (>3.6 min) and enjoyed a survival advantage (460 vs 780 days).[35,37]

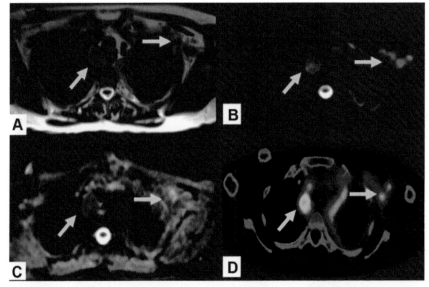

Fig. 19. A 63-year-old man with mesothelioma. Enlarged right upper mediastinal and left axillary lymph nodes (*arrow*) on T2W image (*A*) demonstrate restricted diffusion (*B, C*). These correspond to avid uptake on ¹⁸F FDG PET-CT (*D*). Pathology: Metastatic mesothelioma.

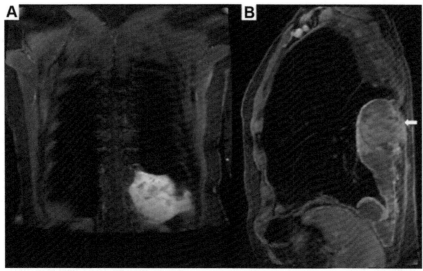

Fig. 20. (*A*) Coronal T2W and (*B*) sagittal postcontrast VIBE image showing that the diaphragm is not involved by the tumor but there is contiguous focal chest wall invasion (*arrow*).

FUTURE DIRECTIONS

MR imaging in the lung suffers from 2 key problems: (1) short T2* due to air that causes dephasing and loss of signal and (2) motion artifacts due to the beating heart and respiratory motion. Shortening echo times can reduce susceptibility issues; however, it is difficult to achieve optimal motion compensation when simultaneously using high temporal resolution as required for reasonable pharmacokinetic analysis. By optimizing a radial stack of stars VIBE sequence for DCE imaging, it is possible to overcome both difficulties.[38] This sequence is robust to motion and aliasing and therefore ideal for dynamic acquisitions, because the center of k-space is updated for every excitation (Videos 1–3).

RESOLVE (readout segmented spin echo diffusion) is a revolutionary new approach for obtaining high-quality, high-resolution DW images even in body regions strongly affected by susceptibility artifacts such as the lung. It is largely free of distortions and delivers sharper imaging at higher spatial resolution. RESOLVE is especially

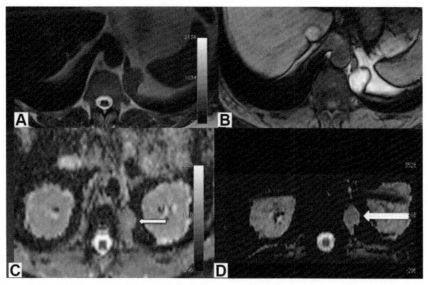

Fig. 21. Left diaphragmatic cyst. It is hypointense on T2W image (*A*) and hyperintense on T1W image (*B*) and shows no restriction on zoomed DW images (*arrows, C* and *D*). Findings are consistent with a protienaceous cyst.

attractive for the evaluation of smaller lesions in a wide range of DWI and diffusion tensor imaging examinations.[35,39–41] Zoomed (reduced FOV) diffusion can also generate improved diffusion images and allow for more accurate ADC measurements (**Fig. 21**).

SUPPLEMENTARY DATA

Supplementary data related to this article can be found online at http://dx.doi.org/10.1016/j.mric. 2015.01.006.

REFERENCES

1. Knuuttila A, Kivisaari L, Kivisaari A, et al. Evaluation of pleural disease using MR and CT. With special reference to malignant pleural mesothelioma. Acta Radiol 2001;42:502–7.
2. Low RN, Sigeti JS, Song SY, et al. Dynamic contrast-enhanced breath-hold MR imaging of thoracic malignancy using cardiac compensation. J Magn Reson Imaging 1996;6:625–31.
3. Mayo JR. Magnetic resonance imaging of the chest. Where we stand. Radiol Clin North Am 1994;32(4): 795–809.
4. Helm EJ, Matin TN, Gleeson FV. Imaging of the pleura. J Magn Reson Imaging 2010;32(6):1275–86.
5. Gill RR. Imaging of mesothelioma. Malignant mesothelioma. Berlin; Heidelberg (Germany): Springer; 2011. p. 27–43.
6. Gill RR, Gerbaudo VH, Sugarbaker DJ, et al. Current trends in radiologic management of malignant pleural mesothelioma. Semin Thorac Cardiovasc Surg 2009;21(2):111–20.
7. McLoud TC, Woods BO, Carrington CB, et al. Diffuse pleural thickening in an asbestos-exposed population: prevalence and causes. AJR Am J Roentgenol 1985;144(1):9–18.
8. Light RW. Pleural diseases. Lippincott Williams & Wilkins; 2007.
9. Sahn SA. Pleural diseases related to metastatic malignancies. Eur Respir J 1997;10(8):1907–13.
10. Benamore RE, Scott K, Richards CJ, et al. Image-guided pleural biopsy: diagnostic yield and complications. Clin Radiol 2006;61(8):700–5.
11. Maskell NA, Gleeson FV, Davies RJ. Standard pleural biopsy versus CT-guided cutting-needle biopsy for diagnosis of malignant disease in pleural effusions: a randomised controlled trial. Lancet 2003;361(9366):1326–30.
12. Agarwal P, Seely JM, Matzinger FR, et al. Pleural mesothelioma: sensitivity and incidence of needle track seeding after image-guided biopsy versus surgical biopsy. Radiology 2006;241(2):589–94.
13. Bueno R, Reblando J, Glickman J, et al. Pleural biopsy: a reliable method for determining the diagnosis but not subtype in mesothelioma. Ann Thorac Surg 2004;78(5):1774–6.
14. Falaschi F, Battolla L, Mascalchi M, et al. Usefulness of MR signal intensity in distinguishing benign from malignant pleural disease. AJR Am J Roentgenol 1996;166(4):963–8.
15. Hierholzer J, Luo L, Bittner R, et al. MRI and CT in the differential diagnosis of pleural disease. Chest 2000;118(3):604–9.
16. Yamamuro M, Gerbaudo VH, Gill RR, et al. Morphologic and functional imaging of malignant pleural mesothelioma. Eur J Radiol 2007;64(3):356–66.
17. Dietrich O, Reiser MF, Schoenberg SO. Artifacts in 3-T MRI: physical background and reduction strategies. Eur J Radiol 2008;65(1):29–35.
18. Bellomi M. Non-conventional imaging of lung cancer. Cancer Imaging 2010;10(1A):S161.
19. Weinreb JC, Naidich DP. Thoracic magnetic resonance imaging. Clin Chest Med 1991;12(1):33–54.
20. Kwee TC, Takahara T, Ochiai R, et al. Whole-body diffusion-weighted magnetic resonance imaging. Eur J Radiol 2009;70:409–17.
21. Schmidt GP, Reiser MF, Baur-Melnyk A. Whole-body MRI for the staging and follow-up of patients with metastasis. Eur J Radiol 2009;70(3):393–400.
22. Schoenberg SO, Baert AL, Dietrich O, et al. Parallel imaging in clinical MR applications. Springer; 2007.
23. Gill RR, Umeoka S, Mamata H, et al. Diffusion-weighted MRI of malignant pleural mesothelioma: preliminary assessment of apparent diffusion coefficient in histologic subtypes. Am J Roentgenol 2010; 195(2):W125–30.
24. Luna A, Martín T, Sánchez González J. Diffusion-weighted imaging in the evaluation of lung, mediastinum, heart, and chest wall. Diffusion MRI outside the brain. Berlin; Heidelberg (Germany): Springer; 2012. p. 279–306.
25. Frola C, Cantoni S, Turtulici I, et al. Transudative vs exudative pleural effusions: differentiation using Gd-DTPA-enhanced MRI. Eur Radiol 1997;7(6): 860–4.
26. Baysal T, Bulut T, Gökirmak M, et al. Diffusion-weighted MR imaging of pleural fluid: differentiation of transudative vs exudative pleural effusions. Eur Radiol 2004;14(5):890–6.
27. Inan N, Arslan A, Akansel G, et al. Diffusion-weighted MRI in the characterization of pleural effusions. Diagn Interv Radiol 2009;15(1):13–8.
28. Campisi C, Bellini C, Eretta C, et al. Diagnosis and management of primary chylous ascites. J Vasc Surg 2006;43(6):1244–8.
29. Horn M, Oechsner M, Gardarsdottir M, et al. Dynamic contrast-enhanced MR imaging for differentiation of rounded atelectasis from neoplasm. J Magn Reson Imaging 2010;31(6):1364–70.
30. Tateishi U, Nishihara H, Morikawa T, et al. Solitary fibrous tumor of the pleura: MR appearance and

enhancement pattern. J Comput Assist Tomogr 2002;26(2):174–9.

31. Gill RR, Gerbaudo VH, Jacobson FL, et al. MR imaging of benign and malignant pleural disease. Magn Reson Imaging Clin N Am 2008;16(2):319–39.

32. Inaoka T, Takahashi K, Miyokawa N, et al. Solitary fibrous tumor of the pleura: apparent diffusion coefficient (ADC) value and ADC map to predict malignant transformation. J Magn Reson Imaging 2007; 26(1):155–8.

33. Mirzoyan M, Muslimani A, Setrakian S, et al. Primary pleuropulmonary synovial sarcoma. Clin Lung Cancer 2008;9(5):257–61.

34. Crotty EJ, McAdams HP, Erasmus JJ, et al. Epithelioid hemangioendothelioma of the pleura: clinical and radiologic features. AJR Am J Roentgenol 2000;175(6):1545–9.

35. Giesel FL, Bischoff H, von Tengg-Kobligk H, et al. Dynamic contrast-enhanced MRI of malignant pleural mesothelioma feasibility study of noninvasive assessment, therapeutic follow-up, and possible predictor of improved outcome. Chest 2006;129(6):1570–6.

36. Coolen J, De Keyzer F, Nafteux P, et al. Malignant pleural disease: diagnosis by using diffusion-weighted and dynamic contrast-enhanced MR imaging—initial experience. Radiology 2012; 263(3):884–92.

37. Giesel FL, Choyke PL, Mehndiratta A, et al. Pharmacokinetic analysis of malignant pleural mesothelioma—initial results of tumor microcirculation and its correlation to microvessel density (CD-34). Acad Radiol 2008;15(5):563–70.

38. Plathow C, Ley S, Fink C, et al. Analysis of intrathoracic tumor mobility during whole breathing cycle by dynamic MRI. Int J Radiat Oncol Biol Phys 2004; 59(4):952–9.

39. Armato SG III, Labby ZE, Coolen J, et al. Imaging in pleural mesothelioma: a review of the 11th International Conference of the International Mesothelioma Interest Group. Lung Cancer 2013;82(2):190–6.

40. Block KT, Chandarana H, Fatterpekar G, et al. Improving the Robustness of Clinical T1-Weighted MRI Using Radial VIBE, MAGNETOM Flash 5/2013: 6–11 Clinical NeurologyJulien.

41. Cohen-Adad High-Resolution DWI in Brain and Spinal Cord with syngo RESOLVE; MAGNETOM Flash 2/2012.

MR Imaging of Chest Wall Tumors

Brett W. Carter, MD*, Gregory W. Gladish, MD

KEYWORDS

- Chest wall • Neoplasm • Tumor • Benign • Malignant • MRI

KEY POINTS

- Tumors of the chest wall account for only 5% of all thoracic neoplasms and represent a heterogeneous group of lesions that may arise from osseous structures or soft tissues.
- A majority of chest wall tumors are malignant lesions that result from direct invasion or metastasis from intrathoracic primary malignancies or arise as primary tumors.
- Cross-sectional imaging with MR imaging allows for lesion characterization, differentiation from non-neoplastic diseases, and delineation of disease extent.
- Because imaging findings may be nonspecific, a combination of clinical, radiologic, and histopathologic information is often necessary to establish the correct diagnosis.

INTRODUCTION

Chest wall tumors are uncommon lesions that represent approximately 5% of all thoracic malignancies[1] and are less common than osseous and soft tissue tumors that occur elsewhere in the body.[2,3] Thus, radiologists may be unfamiliar with the typical clinical presentation and imaging features of these rare neoplasms. Because chest wall tumors represent a heterogeneous group of lesions, several different classification schemes have been developed and may be used in clinical practice. These tumors are typically divided into categories based on the site of origin and tissue composition (osseous or soft tissue) as well as whether they are malignant or benign. Greater than 20% of chest wall tumors may be detected on chest radiography.[4] Full characterization of these lesions is limited, however, on radiography, and cross-sectional techniques, such as multidetector CT (MDCT) and MR imaging, are the imaging modalities of choice. Although radiologic findings may be nonspecific for many of these tumors, a combination of clinical features, imaging characteristics, and histopathologic findings usually enables a definitive diagnosis, subsequently guiding further patient management.[5,6] This article reviews the most common malignant and benign chest wall tumors of osseous and soft tissue origin, with emphasis placed on clinical presentation and characteristic features on MR imaging.

CLASSIFICATION OF CHEST WALL TUMORS

Because neoplasms of the chest wall represent a heterogeneous group of lesions, no specific classification scheme is universally accepted for use in clinical practice. Most systems divide these neoplasms into several groups, however, based on site of origin, tissue composition, and whether tumors are malignant or benign. A majority of osseous tumors arise from cartilage or bone. The 2002 World Health Organization (WHO) classification system for soft tissue tumors recognizes 9 specific categories: adipocytic, vascular, fibroblastic-myofibroblastic, fibrohistiocytic, smooth muscle, pericytic, skeletal muscle, chondro-osseous, and tumors of uncertain differentiation.[7] A classification system for soft tissue

Disclosures: Dr B.W. Carter has received research support from ACRIN; he is a Consultant at St. Jude Medical, Inc; and he is a Thoracic co-lead and author for Amirsys, Inc. Dr G.W. Gladish has nothing to disclose.
Department of Diagnostic Radiology, The University of Texas MD Anderson Cancer Center, 1515 Holcombe Boulevard, Unit 1478, Houston, TX 77030-4008, USA
* Corresponding author.
E-mail address: bcarter2@mdanderson.org

mri.theclinics.com

tumors suggested by Nam and colleagues[6] includes adipocytic, vascular, fibroblastic-myofibroblastic, and fibrohistiocytic categories and adds peripheral nerve sheath and cutaneous categories; this scheme is used in this review. Additional causes of chest wall tumors, such as metastatic disease, direct invasion by lung cancer, and lymphoma, also are discussed.

APPROACH TO CHEST WALL TUMORS

When a chest wall mass is identified, a multidisciplinary approach using multiple sources of information and evaluation techniques is key to distinguishing between different tumor types, narrowing the differential diagnosis, and guiding further management. To this extent, several important features have been identified that are useful in formulating an approach: (1) patient demographics and clinical features; (2) site of chest wall involvement; (3) presence and pattern of mineralization on radiologic studies; and (4) correlation between imaging features and histopathologic findings.[6]

CLINICAL PRESENTATION

Patients with chest wall tumors may be symptomatic or asymptomatic at the time of presentation. In contrast to patients with benign chest wall tumors, a majority of patients with malignant chest wall tumors are symptomatic.[8–10] The most common overall clinical symptom is chest pain. In the setting of malignant tumors, the presence of chest wall pain is suggestive of osseous involvement and should raise concern for invasion. In general, malignant tumors tend to manifest as larger lesions, grow more quickly, and result in specific symptoms, such as pain, compared with benign lesions.[8,11] Older patients tend to present with larger, aggressive malignant tumors, whereas younger patients tend to present with smaller benign lesions.[4] Extrathoracic neoplasms are more likely to manifest as a growing mass than intrathoracic lesions.[12]

IMAGING EVALUATION

Chest radiography may be the first imaging study to suggest the presence of a chest wall mass given its widespread availability and utilization. More than 20% of lesions are visible on chest radiography.[4] Chest radiographs are most beneficial in demonstrating the location, size, and growth rate of chest wall masses.[10] Although mineralization, such as calcification or ossification, may be present, the high-kilovoltage technique used for radiography is not optimal for evaluation of small deposits. Such small deposits, however, may be detected on the low-kilovoltage technique used for bone radiography, which also better delineates soft tissue planes.[5] Many benign chest wall tumors exhibit slow growth over time; therefore, these tumors may result in well-defined soft tissue planes with erosion of adjacent osseous structures.

Cross-sectional imaging techniques are more accurate in identifying and characterizing chest wall tumors. MDCT elegantly demonstrates the size and extent of local tumor as well as additional features, such as the tissue of origin, lesion morphology, and composition.[8,9] Administration of intravenous (IV) contrast can be used to illustrate tumor vascularity.[5] 2-[fluorine-18] fluoro-2-deoxy-d-glucose (FDG) positron emission tomography (PET)/CT is not routinely performed to evaluate chest wall tumors, because many primary and secondary malignancies may demonstrate increased FDG uptake. PET/CT may be used, however, to determine the presence and extent of metastatic disease and assess response to therapy.

MR imaging is the optimal modality for evaluating and characterizing neoplasms of the chest wall, because the superior soft tissue contrast and spatial resolution enable differentiation of tumor from the normal chest wall and infectious and inflammatory processes.[5] The administration of IV gadolinium contrast is helpful in this regard. The most common sequences used to evaluate chest wall tumors include standard spin-echo and fast spin-echo sequences.[5] In cases complicated by excessive motion, either due to proximity to the heart or from breathing, cardiac gating and respiratory compensation, respectively, can be used.[5] Different coils can be used to optimally evaluate tumors depending on their location. For instance, surface coils are beneficial in evaluating superficial chest wall lesions, and torso coils are used to characterize tumors that have more prominent intrathoracic components.

MALIGNANT OSSEOUS TUMORS

Malignant osseous tumors of the chest wall account for approximately 55% of all chest wall masses.[4] The most common primary malignancies include sarcomas, such as chondrosarcoma, osteosarcoma, and the Ewing sarcoma family of tumors (ESFT) as well as multiple myeloma (MM) whereas metastatic disease and direct invasion from intrathoracic malignancies are the most frequent secondary causes.[3] The overall 5-year survival of malignant osseous neoplasms is 60%.[4]

Chondrosarcoma

Chondrosarcoma is the most common primary osseous malignancy of the chest wall and accounts for 30% of all primary malignant osseous lesions and 33% of all primary rib tumors.[13] In addition to arising as primary tumors, these lesions have also been associated with malignant degeneration of benign chondromas,[14] trauma,[4] and radiation therapy.[3] Approximately 10% of chondrosarcomas occur in the chest wall. Most tumors are identified in the anterior chest wall, in the superior 5 ribs, adjacent to costochondral junctions, or in the paravertebral regions.[11] Origin within the soft tissues is uncommon.[15] Although chondrosarcomas may be encountered in individuals of any age, they are typically diagnosed in the fourth to seventh decades of life and are more common in men than in women.[4] The most common symptom reported at the time of diagnosis is a palpable and painful anterior chest wall mass.

On MR imaging, the cartilage background of osteosarcomas is heterogeneous but typically iso- to hypointense to muscle on T1-weighted images and hyperintense to muscle on T2-weighted images. Regions of mineralization, such as the highly characteristic rings and arcs configuration that may be present on MDCT, are hypointense to muscle on both T1- and T2-weighted images.[6] After the administration of IV contrast, enhancement is heterogeneous, especially at the peripheral aspect of tumors (**Fig. 1**).[16–18] Myxoid chondrosarcomas do not contain mineralization and may demonstrate markedly high signal intensity on T2-weighted images.[11]

Osteosarcoma

Osteosarcomas are high-grade malignant mesenchymal tumors that account for 10% to 15% of malignant chest wall tumors[4,11] and are most frequently diagnosed in children and

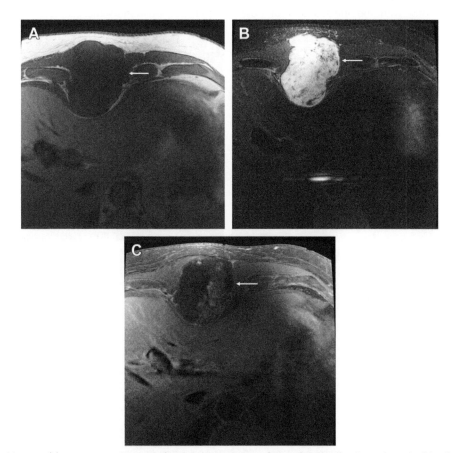

Fig. 1. A 41-year-old man presenting with focal right anterior-inferior chest wall pain and a palpable abnormality on physical examination. (*A*) Axial fast spin-echo T1-weighted MR imaging demonstrates a large mass (*arrow*) in the anterior chest wall slightly to the right of midline that is isointense to the adjacent muscle. (*B*) This mass is markedly hyperintense on axial fast spin-echo fat-suppressed T2-weighted MR imaging with a few scattered regions of internal low signal intensity representing mineralization. (*C*) On axial postcontrast fast spin-echo fat-suppressed T1-weighted MR imaging, regions of heterogeneous enhancement are present. Biopsy revealed chondrosarcoma.

adolescents.[19] When osteosarcomas arise in a primary fashion from the chest wall, the most frequently affected structures include the ribs, clavicle, and scapula.[11] A painful chest wall mass is usually reported at the time of presentation. Two different age peaks have been described for osteosarcomas arising from the chest wall: an osseous form that affects young adults and a less common extraosseous form that is encountered in patients older than 50 years.[3]

On T1-weighted images, the nonmineralized regions of osteosarcomas demonstrate variable signal intensity[6] but are often hyperintense to muscle.[3] On T2-weighted images, the nonmineralized regions demonstrate high signal intensity.[3,6] Large cystic regions may be identified within tumors.[20] Tumor mineralization is usually hypointense on both T1- and T2-weighted imaging. Heterogeneous enhancement after the administration of IV contrast is typical (**Fig. 2**).

Ewing Sarcoma Family of Tumors

The ESFT is a group of neoplasms that includes Ewing sarcoma and primitive neuroectodermal tumor, postulated to arise from embryonal neural crest cells[11] and highly aggressive in nature.[21,22] These tumors represent the most common primary chest wall lesions in children and young adults and the third most common overall malignant chest wall tumor.[12] Tumors typically arise from the ribs, scapula, clavicle, and sternum and most commonly affect individuals between the ages of 20 and 30 years.[11] All tumors included in this group contain the identical balanced reciprocal translocation between chromosomes 11 and 22, t(11; 22) (q24;q12).[23,24]

On MR imaging, these tumors typically result in heterogeneous signal intensity on T1-weighted images (usually iso- or hyperintense to muscle), with regions of hemorrhage demonstrating high signal

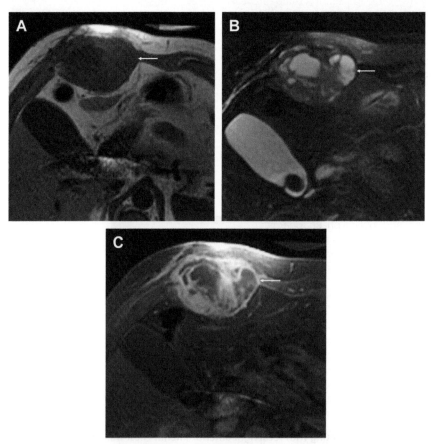

Fig. 2. A 38-year-old man presenting with focal right anterior-inferior chest wall pain. (*A*) Axial fast spin-echo T1-weighted MR imaging demonstrates a large mass (*arrow*) in the right anterior chest wall that is heterogeneous with internal regions that are both isointense and hyperintense to the adjacent muscle. (*B*) This mass demonstrates irregular foci of high signal intensity on axial fast spin-echo fat-suppressed T2-weighted MR imaging. (*C*) On axial postcontrast fast spin-echo fat-suppressed T1-weighted MR imaging, regions of heterogeneous enhancement are present peripherally and internally. Biopsy revealed osteosarcoma.

intensity. Tumors are heterogeneously hyperintense to muscle on T2-weighted images. Most lesions demonstrate intense enhancement after the administration of IV contrast (**Fig. 3**). In general, small tumors tend to be homogeneous, whereas large lesions are more likely to demonstrate regions of heterogeneity due to hemorrhage or necrosis.[11]

Multiple Myeloma and Plasmacytoma

Tumors comprised of malignant plasmacytes are characteristic of several malignancies, including MM, solitary plasmacytoma of bone (SPB), and extramedullary plasmacytoma (EMP).[3] Commonly affected structures and clinical symptoms are somewhat different between these lesions. MM is most common in patients 50 to 70 years of age, whereas SPB and EMP typically affect patients 40 to 80 years of age.[11] MM and SPB affect bones with active hematopoiesis, including the skull, thoracic skeleton, spine, pelvis, proximal

humeri, and femora. Although EMP may involve any soft tissue structure, a majority are found in the upper aerodigestive tract.[25] Typical clinical symptoms reported at the time of presentation include bone pain, renal failure, and anemia for MM; focal pain at site of tumor for SPB; and epistaxis and rhinorrhea for EMP.[25]

MM and SPB (**Fig. 4**) are typically iso- or hypointense to muscle on T1-weighted images and hyperintense to muscle on T2-weighted images.[6] EMP manifests as a soft tissue mass that is low signal on T1-weighted images and high signal intensity on T2-weighted images.[26] Diffuse enhancement of all neoplasms is typical after the administration of IV contrast.

BENIGN OSSEOUS TUMORS

Benign osseous tumors of the chest wall are less frequently encountered than malignant neoplasms. Most of these lesions are osseous or

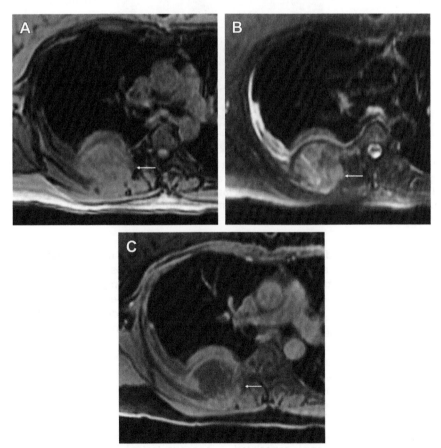

Fig. 3. A 29-year-old woman presenting with right posterior chest wall pain. (*A*) Axial spoiled gradient-recalled (SPGR) T1-weighted MR imaging demonstrates a large mass (*arrow*) involving the right posterior chest wall and pleura that is hyperintense to the adjacent muscle. (*B*) This mass is heterogeneously hyperintense to muscle on axial fat-suppressed T2-weighted imaging. (*C*) On axial postcontrast SPGR fat-suppressed T1-weighted MR imaging, there is predominantly peripheral enhancement due to the presence of central necrosis.

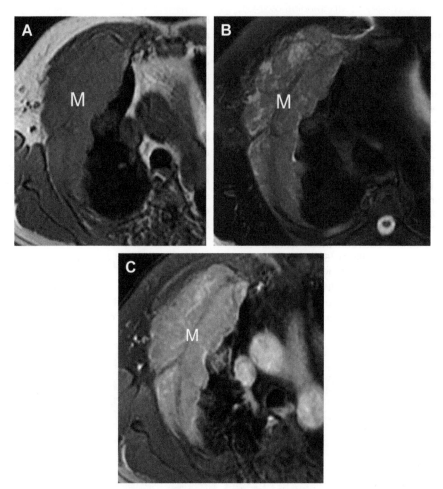

Fig. 4. A 52-year-old man presenting with diffuse right chest pain. (*A*) Axial T1-weighted MR imaging demonstrates a large mass (M) involving the right anterior and anterolateral chest wall that is isointense to the adjacent muscle. (*B*) This mass is diffusely hyperintense on axial fast spin-echo fat-suppressed T2-weighted MR imaging. (*C*) On axial postcontrast fat-suppressed T1-weighted MR imaging, diffuse enhancement of the mass is present. Biopsy revealed plasmacytoma.

cartilaginous in etiology and include fibrous dysplasia, osteochondroma, aneurysmal bone cysts (ABCs), and giant cell tumor (GCT).

Fibrous Dysplasia

Fibrous dysplasia is a benign lesion of bone that represents the failure of mesenchymal osteoblasts to undergo normal maturation and differentiation.[5] Lesions are monostotic in 70% to 80% of cases and polyostotic in 20% to 30% of cases. The most commonly affected osseous structures of the chest wall include the ribs,[27] usually the lateral or posterior aspects.[1] Involvement of the clavicle is less common. Monostotic disease is associated with an age range of 10 to 70 years, although it is most common in patients between 20 and 30 years of age. Most patients are asymptomatic; however, pathologic fractures may result in pain.[5] Malignant

transformation is rare, although development of tumors, such as osteosarcoma and fibrosarcoma, after radiation therapy has been described.[5]

MR imaging is beneficial in demonstrating the full extent of osseous disease. Tumors usually manifest as expansile lesions that are confined to the bone. Fibrous dysplasia is iso- to hypointense to muscle on T1-weighted images and variable in signal intensity on T2-weighted images, ranging from low signal intensity to high signal intensity.[5,6,28–30]

Osteochondroma

Osteochondromas are the most common benign osseous lesion[1] and represent hamartomatous, cartilage-capped osseous protuberances that arise from affected bone.[6] When osteochondromas occur in the chest wall, lesions are typically also encountered elsewhere within the body.[6]

The most frequently affected structures include the ribs and scapula,[5] and osteochondromas account for 8% of all rib lesions.[31] When occurring in the rib, there is a predilection for the costochondral junctions.[5] Patients may present with focal rib pain[32] or ventral scapular pain due to bursa formation.[33] Osteochondromas may be complicated by fractures and other osseous deformities, vascular injury, neural compression, and malignant transformation. Specific features that should raise concern for malignant transformation include pain at the tumor site, osseous erosion, regions of irregular mineralization, and thickening of the cartilage cap.[5]

Osteochondromas are isointense to the medullary cavity of the affected osseous structure on T1-weighted images. Similar to cartilaginous components of other tumors, the cartilaginous cap of osteochondroma is isointense to muscle on T1-weighted images and hyperintense to muscle on T2-weighted images. Malignant transformation should be considered if the thickness of the cartilage cap measures greater than 2 cm in adults or 3 cm in children.[34]

Aneurysmal Bone Cyst

ABCs, which can originate as primary tumors or as secondary changes in other neoplasms,[6] represent networks of multiple blood-filled cysts lined by fibroblasts, multinucleated giant cells, or osteoclasts.[5] These lesions are most common in patients under 30 years of age. The most common sites of chest wall involvement include the posterior elements of the spine, such as the lamina, articular processes, and spinous processes.[5]

Most ABCs appear as lobulated or septated masses with a well-defined low signal intensity rim on MR imaging.[35,36] Heterogeneous signal intensity on both T1- and T2-weighted images is due to the presence of hemorrhagic components (**Fig. 5**).[6] Fluid-fluid levels may be present; however, other tumors, such as GCTs, simple bone cysts, and chondroblastomas, may also demonstrate fluid-fluid levels.[37] ABCs may demonstrate rapid growth, osseous destruction, and extension into adjacent soft tissues; in the setting of such features, these tumors may be indistinguishable from sarcomas and other malignancies.

Giant Cell Tumor

GCTs are benign lesions composed of vascular sinuses lined or filled with abundant spindle and giant cells.[6] These tumors are usually diagnosed between the ages of 21 and 40 years and are more common in women than in men.[5] When GCTs occur in the chest wall, the most common location is the subchondral region of flat and tubular bones, including the sternum, clavicle, and ribs.[5]

GCTs usually demonstrate low to intermediate signal intensity on both T1- and T2-weighted images (**Fig. 6**). The low signal intensity may represent deposition of dense collagen and hemosiderin within the lesion.[38,39] Changes similar to ABCs also may be found concurrently in GCTs.[6] Fluid-fluid levels are less common, however, in GCTs than ABCs.[40–42]

SOFT TISSUE TUMORS

Malignant and benign soft tissue neoplasms of the chest wall represent a heterogeneous group of lesions that may be divided into the following groups based on the tissue of origin: adipocytic, vascular, peripheral nerve sheath, fibroblastic-myofibroblastic, fibrohistiocytic, and cutaneous.[6]

Adipocytic: Liposarcoma

Liposarcomas are the second most common chest wall malignancy of soft tissue origin.[43] These tumors account for approximately 15% of all sarcomas, although only 10% of involve the chest wall.[11] Liposarcomas are most common in men between the ages of 40 and 60 years but also may affect children.[12] Histopathologically, these tumors are composed of lipoblasts that range from poorly differentiated round cells to mature adipose tissue. Five pathologic subtypes of liposarcomas are recognized by the WHO: well-differentiated, dedifferentiated, myxoid, pleomorphic, and mixed.[44] The most common subtype is well-differentiated liposarcoma, which represents 50% of all lesions.[7]

Well-differentiated liposarcomas are typically composed of 50% to 75% adipose tissue, which results in high signal intensity on T1-weighted and low signal intensity on T2-weighted images (**Fig. 7**). Depending on the volume of fat, it may be difficult to distinguish well-differentiated liposarcoma from lipoma. Several features have been identified, however, that are suggestive of well-differentiated liposarcoma; these include lesion size greater than 10 cm, thick internal septations, nodular regions of nonadipose tissue, and adipose tissue comprising less than 75% of the tumor.[45] Nonadipose tissue components may demonstrate enhancement after the administration of IV contrast, although this is variable.[45] One study showed that thick, irregular septations demonstrated intense enhancement, whereas thin septations showed faint enhancement.[46] The other histologic subtypes of liposarcoma typically demonstrate less fat. For instance, pleomorphic sarcomas may contain no visible fat on MR imaging.[44,47] Myxoid liposarcomas demonstrate

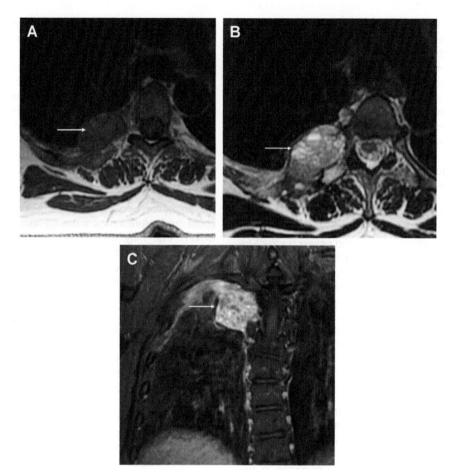

Fig. 5. A 27-year-old woman presenting with ill-defined right posterior chest wall pain. (*A*) Axial fast spin-echo T1-weighted MR imaging demonstrates a lobulated mass (*arrow*) arising from a right posterior rib that is predominantly hyperintense to the adjacent muscle. (*B*) This mass is very heterogeneous on axial fast spin-echo T2-weighted MR imaging with regions of high signal intensity and air-fluid levels. (*C*) On coronal postcontrast T1-weighted MR imaging, the majority of the mass demonstrates enhancement. Biopsy revealed ABC.

moderately high signal intensity on T1-weighted images and high signal intensity on T2-weighted images. Dedifferentiated liposarcoma should be suspected if a previously well-differentiated liposarcoma develops areas of low signal intensity on T1-weighted images and high signal intensity on T2-weighted images and if those areas enhance after IV administration of contrast material.

Adipocytic: Lipoma

Lipomas are the most common overall soft tissue tumor and represent well-circumscribed encapsulated masses composed of adipocytes that are similar to normal fatty tissue found within the chest wall. These lesions are most common in individuals 50 to 70 years of age and in obese patients.[5] Lipomas may vary in size and appearance based on their location in the chest wall. Most lipomas are deep lipomas and are usually larger in size

and not as well circumscribed as superficial lipomas. All lipomas are predominantly composed of adipose tissue; however, other components, such as connective tissue septa and calcifications, are present in one-third of cases.[45,48]

Lipomas are typically homogeneous lesions that demonstrate high signal intensity on T1-weighted images and low signal intensity on T2-weighted images. Uniform loss of signal intensity is typical on fat-suppression sequences.[2] Internal septations may be present and are usually low in signal intensity on T1-weighted images.[6] After the administration of IV contrast, lipomas do not enhance, although internal septations may enhance when present.[45,48]

Vascular: Angiosarcoma

Angiosarcomas are malignant neoplasms of endothelial origin that demonstrate vasoformative

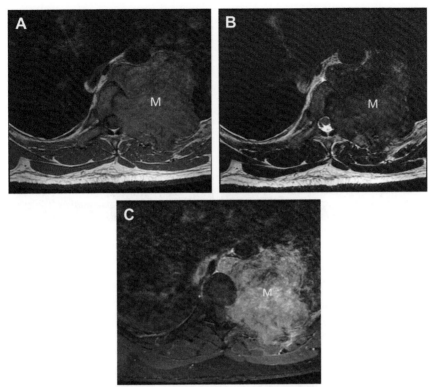

Fig. 6. A 37-year-old woman presenting with left posterior chest wall pain. (*A*) Axial fast spin-echo T1-weighted MR imaging demonstrates a large mass (M) arising from the left posterior chest wall and involving the adjacent vertebral body that is hyperintense to the adjacent muscle. (*B*) This mass is heterogeneous on axial fast spin-echo T2-weighted MR imaging but in general is hyperintense to muscle. (*C*) On axial postcontrast fast spin-echo fat-suppressed T1-weighted MR imaging, the mass demonstrates diffuse enhancement. Biopsy revealed GCT.

architecture.[11] These tumors are the most aggressive soft tissue malignancy of vascular origin and manifest as large, painful, and rapidly enlarging chest wall lesions lesions.[6] Affected patients may present with clinical signs and symptoms, such as hemorrhage, anemia, or coagulopathy.[49] Angiosarcoma is most strongly associated with chronic lymphedema,[50] although this association is present in only 10% of cases.[6] Of those cases associated with lymphedema, most are found after mastectomy.[51] When angiosarcomas occur in the chest wall, the most common location is the breast in a patient with breast cancer.[11]

The most common appearance on MR imaging is a soft tissue mass with heterogeneous signal intensity on T1- and T2-weighted images.[6] Intense enhancement after the administration of IV contrast is typical. Discrete vessels may be identified within the lesion and are usually encountered in the peripheral aspect of the tumor. Additional features, such as fibrous thickening, soft-tissue nodules, and fluid collections adjacent to chest wall muscles, are typically present in angiosarcoma as well as other neoplasms that are associated with lymphedema.[11]

Vascular: Hemangioma

Hemangiomas are composed of dilated, tortuous, and thin-walled vessels that may occur within the chest wall or extend into the chest wall after arising from intrathoracic structures, such as the mediastinum. Hemangiomas may be divided histopathologically into groups based on the predominant type of vascular channel present in the lesion: capillary, cavernous, arteriovenous, or venous.[51] Many lesions demonstrate various combinations of vascular components, however, as well as several nonvascular tissues, such as fat, smooth muscle, fibrous tissue, hemosiderin, and thrombus.[6] A majority of cavernous lesions are cutaneous in location; noncutaneous lesions account for only 0.8% of all benign vascular lesions.[52] Of all types, dystrophic vascular calcifications or phleboliths are present most frequently in cavernous hemangiomas.[53]

Hemangiomas typically demonstrate regions of high signal intensity on T1- and T2-weighted images due to the presence of vascular tissue intermixed with regions of fat.[44] Intramuscular hemangiomas may appear as poorly marginated

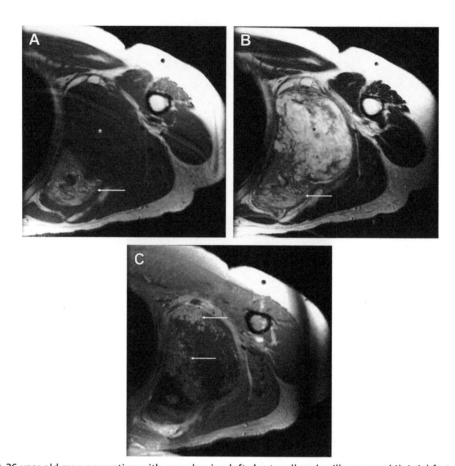

Fig. 7. A 36-year-old man presenting with an enlarging left chest wall and axillary mass. (*A*) Axial fast spin-echo T1-weighted MR imaging demonstrates a large mass in the left chest wall that is heterogeneous with a large anterior component (*asterisk*) that is isointense to muscle and a small posterior component (*arrow*) that is hyperintense to muscle and indicative of fat. (*B*) On axial fast spin-echo T2-weighted MR imaging, the posterior component (*arrow*) remains somewhat hyperintense but the anterior component (*asterisk*) becomes markedly hyperintense to muscle. (*C*) On axial postcontrast fast spin-echo fat-suppressed T1-weighted MR imaging, patchy regions of internal enhancement (*arrows*) are identified. Biopsy revealed well-differentiated liposarcoma.

lesions with intensity similar to skeletal muscle on T1-weighted images. Linear regions of high signal intensity are common and likely represent stagnant blood in cavernous or cystic spaces. These tumors are well marginated and are hyperintense to subcutaneous fat on T2-weighted images (**Fig. 8**). Rapidly flowing blood may result in signal voids.[54,55]

Peripheral Nerve Sheath: Malignant Peripheral Nerve Sheath Tumor

Malignant peripheral nerve sheath tumors (MPNSTs) are spindle cell sarcomas of nerve sheath origin that tend to affect major and medium-sized nerves. These lesions represent 5% to 10% of all soft tissue sarcomas and are most common in patients 20 to 50 years of age.[6] MPNSTs are associated with neurofibromatosis type 1 in most cases.[56] Pain reported in the setting

of a neurofibroma is suggestive of malignant transformation.[11]

MPNSTs typically manifest as invasive masses located adjacent to a peripheral nerve that are iso- or hyperintense to muscle on T1-weighted images and hyperintense to muscle on T2-weighted images.[11] Lesions may be heterogeneous based on the necrosis, hemorrhage, and cellularity present.[57] After the administration of IV contrast, enhancement is typically heterogeneous.[58] In the setting of malignant transformation of a neurofibroma, the characteristic target-like appearance on T2-weighted images may be lost.[11]

Nerve Tumors: Schwannoma

Schwannomas are benign tumors of nerve sheath origin that are most common in patients 20 to 50 years of age.[6] When these lesions occur in the chest wall, spinal nerve roots and intercostal

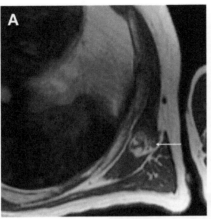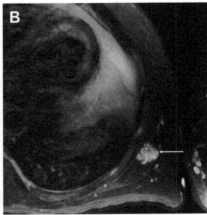

Fig. 8. A 32-year-old man presenting with a palpable abnormality in the left posterolateral chest wall. (*A*) Axial fast spin-echo T1-weighted MR imaging demonstrates an intramuscular mass (*arrow*) in the left chest wall that is heterogeneous but contains foci of high signal intensity indicative of fat. (*B*) This lesion is better defined on axial fast spin-echo fat-suppressed T2-weighted MR imaging and demonstrates high signal intensity. These MR imaging findings are consistent with an intramuscular hemangioma.

nerves are usually the source. These lesions are typically slow growing and result in painless masses measuring less than 5 cm.[6] Histopathologically, distinct areas designated as Antoni A and Antoni B regions have been described. Antoni A regions are organized hypercellular regions containing spindle cells and Antoni B regions are hypocellular regions containing myxoid components.

Schwannomas are typically iso- to hypointense to muscle on T1-weighted images and demonstrate heterogeneous signal intensity on T2-weighted images. After the administration of IV contrast, small tumors usually demonstrate intense and homogeneous enhancement (**Fig. 9**). As schwannomas increase in size, denegeneration, cyst formation, hemorrhage, fibrosis, and calcification are commonly seen. Because these findings are less common in neurofibromas, such features can be used to differentiate between these lesions.[45] The target sign, consisting of central low signal and peripheral high signal on T2-weighted images and central enhancement on postgadolinium images, is less common than in neurofibromas and has been reported in 0% to 54% of cases.[59–61] The fascicular sign, consisting of heterogeneous low signal intensity with a ringlike pattern on T2-weighted images, was reported in one series as more common in schwannoma than in neurofibroma (63% vs 25%).[61]

Nerve Tumors: Neurofibroma

Neurofibromas are benign tumors of nerve sheath origin that are most common in patients 20 to 30 years of age. Three distinct patterns of disease have been described: localized, diffuse, and plexiform. The localized form represents 90% of lesions, most of which are solitary. Plexiform

neurofibromas characterize neurofibromatosis type 1. Unlike schwannomas, neurofibromas do not contain Antoni A or Antoni B regions and secondary changes are uncommon.[25] In contrast to schwannomas, neurofibromas are inseparable from the affected nerves; therefore, resection of the nerve is necessary at the time of surgery.[62]

Neurofibromas are iso- to hypointense to muscle on T1-weighted images. The aforementioned target sign is more common in neurofibromas than in schwannomas and has been reported in 50% to 70% of lesions (**Fig. 10**).[59–61]

Fibroblastic-Myofibroblastic: Elastofibroma Dorsi

Elastofibroma dorsi is a soft tissue pseudotumor that typically occurs in the deep dorsal regions between the thoracic wall and the lower third of the scapula under the serratus anterior and latissimus dorsi muscles.[63] Bilaterality is present in 10% to 66% of cases.[45] Elastofibroma is more common in women than in men by a ratio of 4:1. Although a wide age range of 41 to 80 years has been reported, the average age at diagnosis is 60 years. Most patients are asymptomatic.

On MR imaging, elastofibromas typically appear as focal masses that are isointense to muscle on both T1- and T2-weighted images.[6] Regions of fat may be present in a fascicular pattern.[64]

Fibroblastic-Myofibroblastic: Fibromatosis

Fibromatosis, also known as desmoid tumor, is a soft tissue neoplasm composed of well-differentiated fibroblasts in an abundant collagenous matrix with peripheral cellularity.[65] Lesions

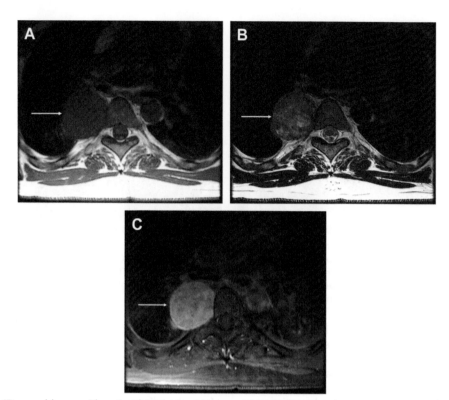

Fig. 9. A 47-year-old man with an incidental paraspinal mass detected on CT pulmonary angiogram. (*A*) Axial fast spin-echo T1-weighted MR imaging demonstrates a well-circumscribed, rounded mass (*arrow*) in the right paraspinal region that is hypointense to muscle. (*B*) This lesion becomes heterogeneous and hyperintense to muscle on axial fast spin-echo T2-weighted MR imaging. (*C*) On axial postcontrast fast spin-echo fat-suppressed T1-weighted MR imaging, diffuse enhancement is present. The location and MR imaging findings were suggestive of a schwannoma, which was confirmed with biopsy.

may arise from muscle, fascia, or aponeurosis and have been reported at the site of previous traumatic injury or surgical scar.[6] Fibromatosis has been reported to primarily arise from the chest wall in 10% to 28% of cases[11] and accounts for 54% of low-grade chest wall sarcomas.[8] Lesions are most common in adolescents and young adults,[8,66–69] although older individuals may also be affected.

Fibromatosis typically manifests as an ill-defined mass that grows in an infiltrative manner. On MR imaging, lesions demonstrate homogeneous low to intermediate signal intensity on T1-weighted images but are more heterogeneous on T2-weighted images, with varying signal intensity (very low, intermediate, and very high) depending on the amounts and proportion of collagen, spindle cells, and myxoid matrix (**Fig. 11**). Low signal intensity bands have been reported in fibromatosis, up to 86% in one report, and likely represent dense collagen bundles. Although fibromatosis may demonstrate moderate to marked heterogeneous enhancement, the collagen bundles do not enhance.

Fibrohistiocytic: Undifferentiated Pleomorphic Sarcoma

Undifferentiated pleomorphic sarcoma (UPS), also known as malignant fibrous histiocytoma, is classified as a fibrohistiocytic malignancy and represents the most common malignant soft tissue neoplasm of the chest wall in adults.[45] Women are affected slightly more frequently than men, and the mean age at the time of diagnosis is 55 years.[70] UPS originates in deep fascia or skeletal muscle but only rarely arises from the chest wall. Three histopathologic subtypes of UPS have been described by the WHO: (1) high-grade pleomorphic sarcoma, (2) pleomorphic sarcoma with giant cells, and (3) pleomorphic sarcoma with prominent inflammation.[6]

On MR imaging, UPS demonstrates intermediate to low signal intensity and is isointense to muscle on T1-weighted images. On T2-weighted images, UPS shows intermediate to high signal intensity and is iso- to hyperintense to fat (**Fig. 12**). Tumors demonstrate variable signal intensity due

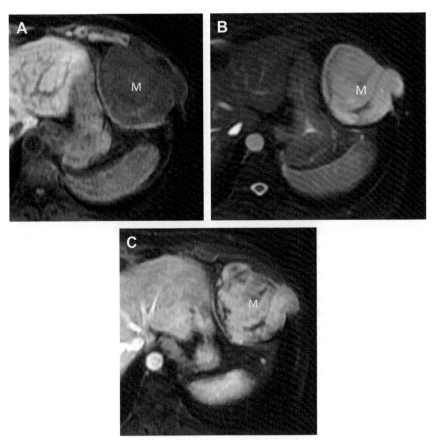

Fig. 10. A 39-year-old man presenting with focal left anterolateral chest wall pain and a palpable abnormality on physical examination. (*A*) Axial spoiled gradient-recalled (SPGR) fat-suppressed T1-weighted MR imaging demonstrates a large mass (M) in the left anterolateral chest wall that is hyperintense to the adjacent muscle. (*B*) This mass is markedly hyperintense on axial fat-suppressed T2-weighted MR imaging with a few bandlike regions of internal low signal intensity. (*C*) On axial postcontrast SPGR fat-suppressed T1-weighted MR imaging, the majority of the mass demonstrates enhancement although the internal bandlike regions do not enhance. Biopsy revealed neurofibroma.

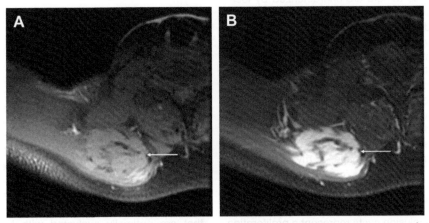

Fig. 11. (*A*) Axial fast spin-echo fat-suppressed T1-weighted MR imaging demonstrates a somewhat ill-defined mass (*arrow*) in the upper right posterior chest wall that is slightly hyperintense to the adjacent muscle. A few internal bandlike regions show low signal intensity. (*B*) On axial postcontrast fast spin-echo fat-suppressed T1-weighted MR imaging, there is intense enhancement of the majority of the mass, although the bandlike regions do not enhance. Biopsy revealed fibromatosis.

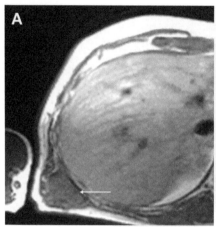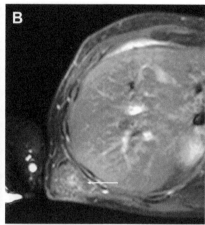

Fig. 12. (*A*) Axial fast spin-echo T1-weighted MR imaging demonstrates a focal mass (*arrow*) in the right postero-lateral chest wall that is isointense to the adjacent muscle. (*B*) On axial postcontrast fast spin-echo fat-suppressed T1-weighted MR imaging, heterogeneous enhancement is present. Biopsy revealed UPS.

to the presence of fibrous tissue components with high collagen content (resulting in low signal intensity with all pulse sequences), myxoid tissue components (resulting in low signal intensity on T1-weighted images and high signal intensity on T2-weighted images), and hemorrhagic components (resulting in variable signal intensity).[7]

Cutaneous: Dermatofibrosarcoma Protuberans

Dermatofibrosarcoma protuberans (DFSP) is a malignant lesion of the dermis composed of spindle cells that typically spreads to involve the subcutaneous tissues and muscles. DFSP is now classified as a primary tumor of the skin by the WHO but is considered by some investigators a soft tissue malignancy arising from the cutaneous layer.[6,7] These tumors are characterized by local invasion and recurrence after therapy. Most lesions are identified in adolescents. This neoplasm may be divided into 2 types: a fibrosarcomatous variant that is characterized by an aggressive course and a more indolent classic variant.

On MR imaging, these tumors range in size and appearance from a small nodule to a large mass. DFSP is hypointense to muscle on T1-weighted images and hyperintense to fat on T2-weighted images.[71] Lesions may demonstrate heterogenenity due to necrosis, hemorrhage, or myxoid changes (**Fig. 13**).[72]

Cutaneous: Epidermal Inclusion Cyst

Epidermal inclusion cysts represent a proliferation of epidermal cells contained within a dermal space that fills with keratin debris and is surrounded by stratified squamous epithelium.[6] The most common locations within the body include the scalp, face, neck, trunk, and back in approximately 90% of cases.[73]

On MR imaging, epidermal inclusion cysts typically manifest as well-defined masses with characteristic features: (1) variable low signal intensity with or without a high signal intensity cystlike background on T2-weighted images; (2) high signal intensity foci on T1-weighted images; and (3) thin peripheral rim enhancement.[6] The variable low signal intensity described on T2-weighted images is likely due to the heterogeneous nature and composition of the cysts. The high signal intensity foci on T1-weighted images are favored to represent calcium. These features can be used to differentiate epidermal inclusions cysts from other cystic lesions of the chest wall.[74]

METASTATIC DISEASE

Metastatic disease involving the osseous structures of the chest wall may be present early on in the setting of aggressive primary malignancies or in the terminal stages of extensive disease. Chest wall metastases may manifest in many different ways. Some lesions demonstrate imaging features more specific to certain primary tumors. For instance, lesions may be predominantly sclerotic in breast or prostate cancer, lytic and expansile in the setting of renal cell carcinoma, and lytic with MM.[3] Such features are often better visualized on MDCT than MR imaging. In some cases, metastases may demonstrate imaging characteristics similar to the primary tumor that are optimally evaluated with MR imaging. For instance, metastases due to lymphoma typically demonstrate low signal intensity on T1-weighted images and high signal intensity on T2-weighted images.[3]

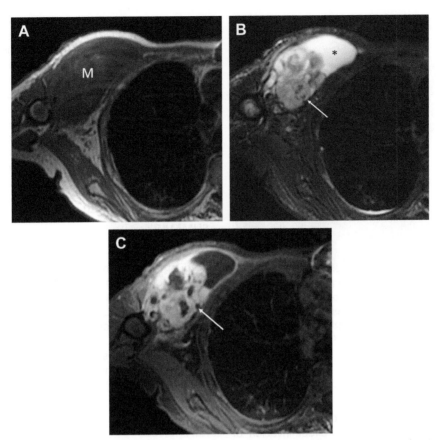

Fig. 13. A 47-year-old man presenting with focal right anterior chest wall pain and an enlarging palpable abnormality. (A) Axial T1-weighted MR imaging demonstrates a large, somewhat heterogeneous mass (M) in the right anterior chest wall that is predominantly isointense to the adjacent muscle, although some internal components are slightly hyperintense to muscle. (B) This mass demonstrates greater internal complexity on axial fat-suppressed T2-weighted MR imaging with a high signal intensity cystic component (*asterisk*) and a heterogeneous solid component (*arrow*). (C) On axial postcontrast spoiled gradient-recalled (SPGR) fat-suppressed T1-weighted MR imaging, regions of heterogeneous enhancement are present in the solid component and along the peripheral aspect of the mass. Biopsy revealed DFSP.

Metastases involving the soft tissues typically are seen only in the setting of extensive metastatic disease elsewhere in the body. Chest wall metastatic disease is considered a poor prognostic indicator and is associated with decreased survival rates.[75] Various patterns of metastatic spread have been described, including direct extension, hematogenous spread, and lymphatic spread. Breast cancer is one of the most common primary malignancies to involve the soft tissues, and the recurrence rate has been reported as 5% to 20%.[75,76]

CHEST WALL INVASION

The osseous chest wall may be directly invaded by aggressive intrathoracic malignancies, the most common of which to do so are lung cancers. MDCT and MR imaging have demonstrated variable ability to detect spread of lung cancer into the chest wall. MR imaging is, however, considered superior to MDCT in the ability to discern chest wall invasion, especially in the setting of superior sulcus or Pancoast tumors. MR imaging findings suggestive of chest wall invasion include infiltration or disruption of the normal extrapleural fat plane on T1-weighted images or high signal intensity of the parietal pleura on T2-weighted sequences (**Fig. 14**).[77,78] Short tau inversion recovery sequences may demonstrate high signal intensity within chest wall structures whose signal is otherwise suppressed by this sequence.[78] The administration of IV contrast material may assist in confirming chest wall invasion.[78] Techniques, such as cine MR during breathing, may be used to identify chest wall invasion, because fixation of the tumor to the chest wall suggests involvement, but free movement of the tumor along the parietal pleura suggests absence of invasion.[79]

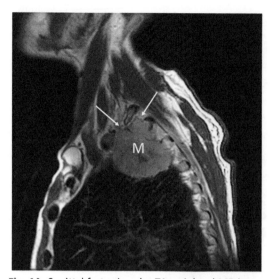

Fig. 14. Sagittal fast spin-echo T1-weighted MR imaging of a 66-year-old man with non–small cell lung carcinoma (M) of the right upper lobe demonstrates disruption of the normal extrapleural fat planes and invasion of the chest wall (*arrows*). MR imaging is considered superior to MDCT in identifying chest wall invasion.

LYMPHOMA

Lymphomatous involvement of the chest wall is rare but usually results from direct invasion of Hodgkin lymphoma (HL) or large B-cell lymphoma originating in the mediastinum, axilla, or bone. Direct invasion occurs in 6.4% of patients with HL. Primary malignant lymphoma comprises only 2.4% of primary chest wall tumors.[80] Overall, chest wall involvement occurs in 9.6% of patients during the course of their disease.[81] One study of patients with HL demonstrated that patients with chest wall involvement had significantly poorer outcomes than patients without chest wall invasion.[82]

On cross-sectional imaging, HL usually presents as an infiltrative mass in the parasternal soft tissues as a result of direct extension of disease from anterior mediastinal lymph nodes.[83] MR imaging is useful in evaluating chest wall masses due to its superior soft tissue contrast resolution and is more sensitive than CT for detecting chest wall involvement by lymphoma. Lymphoma is usually isointense to mildly increased in signal intensity on T1-weighted imaging and hyperintense on T2-weighted imaging.[84]

BIOPSY AND HISTOPATHOLOGIC SAMPLING

Because the MR imaging features of chest wall masses are frequently nonspecific, histopathologic sampling via fine-needle aspiration, incisional

biopsy, or excisional biopsy may be necessary to establish a definitive diagnosis.[1] The selection of a specific technique is usually dependent on several factors, including the size of the chest wall lesion, the extent of resection necessary at surgery, and whether reconstruction is desired.[12] Therefore, discussion regarding the anticipated treatment plan should be performed prior to histopathologic sampling. Chest wall masses measuring less than 5 cm usually undergo excisional biopsy, whereas lesions measuring greater than 5 cm may be sampled via fine-needle aspiration or incisional biopsy.[12]

SUMMARY

Chest wall tumors are uncommon lesions that account for approximately 5% of thoracic malignancies. Given the relative rarity of these neoplasms, radiologists may be uncertain as to appropriate management. Although some osseous and soft tissue tumors of the chest wall may demonstrate key features on MR imaging, a multidisciplinary approach using a combination of clinical presentation, imaging findings, and histopathologic features is key to correcting diagnosing these lesions.

REFERENCES

1. Incarbone M, Pastorino U. Surgical treatment of chest wall tumors. World J Surg 2001;25:218–30.
2. O'Sullivan P, O'Dwyer H, Flint J, et al. Soft tissue tumours and mass-like lesions of the chest wall: a pictorial review of CT and MR findings. Br J Radiol 2007;80(955):574–80.
3. O'Sullivan P, O'Dwyer H, Flint J, et al. Malignant chest wall neoplasms of bone and cartilage: a pictorial review of CT and MR findings. Br J Radiol 2007; 80(956):678–84.
4. Shah AA, D'Amico TA. Primary chest wall tumors. J Am Coll Surg 2010;210:360–6.
5. Tateishi U, Gladish GW, Kusumoto M, et al. Chest wall tumors: radiologic findings and pathologic correlation: part 1. Benign tumors. Radiographics 2003;23:1477–90.
6. Nam SJ, Kim S, Lim BJ, et al. Imaging of primary chest wall tumors with radiologic-pathologic correlation. Radiographics 2011;31(3):749–70.
7. Murphey MD. World Health Organization classification of bone and soft tissue tumors: modifications and implications for radiologists. Semin Musculoskelet Radiol 2007;11(3):201–14.
8. Athanassiadi K, Kalavrouziotis G, Rondogianni D, et al. Primary chest wall tumors: early and long-term results of surgical treatment. Eur J Cardiothorac Surg 2001;19:589–93.

9. Jeung MY, Gangi A, Gasser B, et al. Imaging of chest wall disorders. Radiographics 1999;19(3): 617–37.

10. Siegel MJ. Magnetic resonance imaging of musculoskeletal soft tissue masses. Radiol Clin North Am 2001;39:701–20.

11. Tateishi U, Gladish GW, Kusumoto M, et al. Chest wall tumors: radiologic findings and pathologic correlation: part 2. Malignant tumors. Radiographics 2003;23:1491–508.

12. Davis EA, Marshall MB. Review of chest wall tumors: a diagnostic, therapeutic, and reconstructive challenge. Semin Plast Surg 2011;25(1):16–24.

13. Stanic V, Vulovic T, Novakovic M, et al. Radical resection of giant chondrosarcoma of the anterior chest wall. Vojnosanit Pregl 2008;65:64–8.

14. Somers J, Faber LP. Chondroma and chondrosarcoma. Semin Thorac Cardiovasc Surg 1999;11: 270–7.

15. D'Aprile MR, Stasolla A, Guerrisi R, et al. Extraskeletal myxoid chondrosarcoma of the thoracic wall. J Exp Clin Cancer Res 2003;22:333–5.

16. Varma DG, Ayala AG, Carrasco CH, et al. Chondrosarcoma: MR imaging with pathologic correlation. Radiographics 1992;12:687–704.

17. Kransdorf MJ, Meis JM. Extraskeletal osseous and cartilaginous tumors of the extremities. Radiographics 1993;13:853–84.

18. de Lange EE, Pope TL Jr, Fechner RE. Dedifferentiated chondrosarcoma: radiographic features. Radiology 1986;161:489–92.

19. Wittg JC, Bickels J, Priebat D, et al. Osteosarcoma: a multidisciplinary approach to diagnosis and treatment. Am Fam Physician 2002;65:1123–32.

20. Sundaram M, McGuire MH, Herbold DR. Magnetic resonance imaging of osteosarcoma. Skeletal Radiol 1987;16:23–9.

21. Shamberger RC, Grier HE. Ewing's sarcoma/primitive neuroectodermal tumor of the chest. Semin Pediatr Surg 2001;10:153–60.

22. Goto T, Hozumi T, Kondo T. Ewing's sarcoma. Gan To Kagaku Ryoho 2004;31:346–50.

23. Dehner LP. Primitive neuroectodermal tumor and Ewing's sarcoma. Am J Surg Pathol 1993;17:1–13.

24. Ladanyi M, Heinemann FS, Huvos AG, et al. Neural differentiation in small round cell tumors of bone and soft tissue with the translocation t(11;22)(q24;q12): an immunohistochemical study of 11 cases. Hum Pathol 1990;21:1245–51.

25. Dores GM, Landgren O, McGlynn KA, et al. Plasmacytoma of bone, extramedullary plasmacytoma, and multiple myeloma: incidence and survival in the United States, 1992–2004. Br J Haematol 2009;144(1):86–94.

26. Hanrahan CJ, Christensen CR, Crim JR. Current concepts in the evaluation of multiple myeloma with MR imaging and FDG PET/CT. Radiographics 2010;30(1):127–42.

27. Hughes EK, James SL, Butt S, et al. Benign primary tumours of the ribs. Clin Radiol 2006;61(4):314–22.

28. Utz JA, Kransdorf MJ, Jelinek JS, et al. MR appearance of fibrous dysplasia. J Comput Assist Tomogr 1989;13:845–51.

29. Kransdorf MJ, Moser RP Jr, Gilkey FW. Fibrous dysplasia. Radiographics 1990;10:519–37.

30. Jee WH, Choi KH, Choe BY, et al. Fibrous dysplasia: MR imaging characteristics with radiopathologic correlation. AJR Am J Roentgenol 1996;167:1523–7.

31. Tang WM, Luk KD, Leong JC. Costal osteochondroma: a rare cause of spinal cord compression. Spine (Phila Pa 1976) 1998;23(17):1900–3.

32. Tomo H, Ito Y, Aono M, et al. Chest wall deformity associated with osteochondroma of the scapula: a case report and review of the literature. J Shoulder Elbow Surg 2005;14:103–6.

33. Okada K, Terada K, Sashi R, et al. Large bursa formation associated with osteochondroma of the scapula: a case report and review of the literature. Jpn J Clin Oncol 1999;29(7):356–60.

34. Woertler K, Lindner N, Gosheger G, et al. Osteochondroma: MR imaging of tumor-related complications. Eur Radiol 2000;10(5):832–40.

35. Beltran J, Simon DC, Levy M, et al. Aneurysmal bone cysts: MR imaging at 1.5 T. Radiology 1986;158: 689–90.

36. Zimmer WD, Berquist TH, Sim FH, et al. Magnetic resonance imaging of aneurysmal bone cyst. Mayo Clin Proc 1984;59:633–6.

37. Hudson TM, Hamlin DJ, Fitzsimmons JR. Magnetic resonance imaging of fluid levels in an aneurysmal bone cyst and in anticoagulated human blood. Skeletal Radiol 1985;13:267–70.

38. Murphey MD, Nomikos GC, Flemming DJ, et al. Imaging of giant cell tumor and giant cell reparative granuloma of bone: radiologic-pathologic correlation. Radiographics 2001;21(5):1283–309.

39. Kwon JW, Chung HW, Cho EY, et al. MRI findings of giant cell tumors of the spine. AJR Am J Roentgenol 2007;189(1):246–50.

40. Cooper KL, Beabout JW, Dahlin DC. Giant cell tumor: ossification in soft-tissue implants. Radiology 1984;153:597–602.

41. Dahlin DC. Caldwell lecture. Giant cell tumor of bone: highlights of 407 cases. AJR Am J Roentgenol 1985;144:955–60.

42. Lee MJ, Sallomi DF, Munk PL, et al. Pictorial review: giant cell tumours of bone. Clin Radiol 1998;53:481–9.

43. Kransdorf MJ. Malignant soft-tissue tumors in a large referral population: distribution of diagnoses by age, sex, and location. AJR Am J Roentgenol 1995;164(1):129–34.

44. Lee TJ, Collins J. MR imaging evaluation of disorders of the chest wall. Magn Reson Imaging Clin N Am 2008;16:355–79.

45. Kransdorf MJ, Bancroft LW, Peterson JJ, et al. Imaging of fatty tumors: distinction of lipoma and well-differentiated liposarcoma. Radiology 2002;224(1): 99–104.

46. Hosono M, Kobayashi H, Fujimoto R, et al. Septum-like structures in lipoma and liposarcoma: MR imaging and pathologic correlation. Skeletal Radiol 1997; 26(3):150–4.

47. Peterson JJ, Kransdorf MJ, Bancroft LW, et al. Malignant fatty tumors: classification, clinical course, imaging appearance and treatment. Skeletal Radiol 2003;32(9):493–503.

48. Bancroft LW, Kransdorf MJ, Peterson JJ, et al. Benign fatty tumors: classification, clinical course, imaging appearance, and treatment. Skeletal Radiol 2006;35(10):719–33.

49. Meis-Kindblom JM, Kindblom LG. Angiosarcoma of soft tissue: a study of 80 cases. Am J Surg Pathol 1998;22:683–97.

50. Coldwell DM, Baron RL, Charnsangavej C. Angiosarcoma: diagnosis and clinical course. Acta Radiol 1989;30:627–31.

51. Kransdorf MJ, Murphey MD. Vascular and lymphatic tumors. In: Kransdorf MJ, Murphey MD, editors. Imaging of soft tissue tumors. 2nd edition. Philadelphia (PA): Lippincott Williams & Wilkins; 2006. p. 150–88.

52. Enzinger FM, Weiss SW. Benign tumors and tumor-like lesions of blood vessels. In: Enzinger FM, Weiss SW, editors. Soft tissue tumors. 3rd edition. St Louis (MO): Mosby; 1995. p. 579–626.

53. Mulliken JB, Glowacki J. Hemangiomas and vascular malformations in infants and children: a classification based on endothelial characteristics. Plast Reconstr Surg 1982;69(3):412–22.

54. Kaplan PA, Williams SM. Mucocutaneous and peripheral soft-tissue hemangiomas: MR imaging. Radiology 1987;163:163–6.

55. Cohen EK, Kressel HY, Perosio T, et al. MR imaging of soft-tissue hemangiomas: correlation with pathologic findings. AJR Am J Roentgenol 1988;150: 1079–81.

56. Sordillo PP, Helson L, Hajdu SI, et al. Malignant schwannoma: clinical characteristics, survival, and response to therapy. Cancer 1981;47:2503–9.

57. Moon WK, Im JG, Han MC. Malignant schwannomas of the thorax: CT findings. J Comput Assist Tomogr 1993;17:274–6.

58. Levine E, Huntrakoon M, Wetzel LH. Malignant nerve-sheath neoplasms in neurofibromatosis: distinction from benign tumors by using imaging techniques. AJR Am J Roentgenol 1987;149:1059–64.

59. Suh JS, Abenoza P, Galloway HR, et al. Peripheral (extracranial) nerve tumors: correlation of MR imaging and histologic findings. Radiology 1992;183(2):341–6.

60. Jee WH, Oh SN, McCauley T, et al. Extraaxial neurofibromas versus neurilemmomas: discrimination with MRI. AJR Am J Roentgenol 2004;183(3):629–33.

61. Varma DG, Moulopoulos A, Sara AS, et al. MR imaging of extracranial nerve sheath tumors. J Comput Assist Tomogr 1992;16(3):448–53.

62. Kehoe NJ, Reid RP, Semple JC. Solitary benign peripheral-nerve tumours: review of 32 years' experience. J Bone Joint Surg Br 1995;77(3):497–500.

63. Nagamine N, Nohara Y, Ito E. Elastofibroma in Okinawa: a clinicopathologic study of 170 cases. Cancer 1982;50(9):1794–805.

64. Battaglia M, Vanel D, Pollastri P, et al. Imaging patterns in elastofibroma dorsi. Eur J Radiol 2009;72(1):16–21.

65. Bridge JA, Sreekantaiah C, Mouron B, et al. Clonal chromosomal abnormalities in desmoid tumors: implications for histopathogenesis. Cancer 1992; 69(2):430–6.

66. Feld R, Burk DL Jr, McCue P, et al. MRI of aggressive fibromatosis: frequent appearance of high signal intensity on T2-weighted images. Magn Reson Imaging 1990;8:583–8.

67. Ackman JB, Whitman GJ, Chew FS. Aggressive fibromatosis. AJR Am J Roentgenol 1994;163:544.

68. Casillas J, Sais GJ, Greve JL, et al. Imaging of intra- and extraabdominal desmoid tumors. Radiographics 1991;11:959–68.

69. O'Keefe F, Kim EE, Wallace S. Magnetic resonance imaging in aggressive fibromatosis. Clin Radiol 1990;42:170–3.

70. Tateishi U, Kusumoto M, Hasegawa T, et al. Primary malignant fibrous histiocytoma of the chest wall: CT and MR appearance. J Comput Assist Tomogr 2002; 26(4):558–63.

71. Torreggiani WC, Al-Ismail K, Munk PL, et al. Dermatofibrosarcoma protuberans: MR imaging features. AJR Am J Roentgenol 2002;178(4):989–93.

72. Kransdorf MJ, Meis-Kindblom JM. Dermatofibrosarcoma protuberans: radiologic appearance. AJR Am J Roentgenol 1994;163(2):391–4.

73. Vincent LM, Parker LA, Mittelstaedt CA. Sonographic appearance of an epidermal inclusion cyst. J Ultrasound Med 1985;4(11):609–11.

74. Hong SH, Chung HW, Choi JY, et al. MRI findings of subcutaneous epidermal cysts: emphasis on the presence of rupture. AJR Am J Roentgenol 2006; 186(4):961–6.

75. Haffty BG, Hauser A, Choi DH, et al. Molecular markers for prognosis after isolated postmastectomy chest wall recurrence. Cancer 2004;100:252–63.

76. Cuenca RE, Allison RR, Sibata C, et al. Breast cancer with chest wall progression: treatment with photodynamic therapy. Ann Surg Oncol 2004;11: 322–7.

77. Padovani B, Mouroux J, Seksik L, et al. Chest wall invasion by bronchogenic carcinoma: evaluation with MR imaging. Radiology 1993;187:33–8.

78. Freundlich IM, Chasen MH, Varma DG. Magnetic resonance imaging of pulmonary apical tumors. J Thorac Imaging 1996;11:210–22.

79. Sakai S, Murayama S, Murakami J, et al. Bronchogenic carcinoma invasion of the chest wall: evaluation with dynamic cine MRI during breathing. J Comput Assist Tomogr 1997;21:595–600.

80. King RM, Pairolero PC, Trastek VF, et al. Primary chest wall tumors: factors affecting survival. Ann Thorac Surg 1986;41:597–601.

81. Press GA, Glazer HS, Wasserman TH, et al. Thoracic wall involvement by Hodgkin disease and non-Hodgkin lymphoma: CT evaluation. Radiology 1985;157:195–8.

82. Hodgson DC, Tsang RW, Pintilie M, et al. Impact of chest wall and lung invasion on outcome of stage 1–2 Hodgkin's lymphoma after combined modality therapy. Int J Radiat Oncol Biol Phys 2003;57: 1374–81.

83. Guermazi A, Brice P, de Kerviler EE, et al. Extranodal Hodgkin disease: spectrum of disease. Radiographics 2001;21(1):161–79.

84. Knisely BL, Broderick LS, Kuhlman JE. MR imaging of the pleura and chest wall. Magn Reson Imaging Clin N Am 2000;8:125–41.

Hyperpolarized Gas MR Imaging
Technique and Applications

Justus E. Roos, MD[a],*, Holman P. McAdams, MD[a],
S. Sivaram Kaushik, PhD[b,c], Bastiaan Driehuys, PhD[c]

KEYWORDS

- MR imaging • Lung imaging • Hyperpolarized gas • Pulmonary ventilation
- Pulmonary gas exchange • Xenon (^{129}Xe)

KEY POINTS

- Hyperpolarized (HP) helium (^{3}He) and xenon (^{129}Xe) MR imaging of the lungs provides sensitive contrast mechanisms to probe changes in pulmonary ventilation, microstructure, and gas exchange.
- Recent scarcity in the supply of ^{3}He shifted the field of HP gas imaging to the use of less expensive and naturally available ^{129}Xe.
- ^{129}Xe has been shown to be well-tolerated in healthy volunteers and patients with various pulmonary diseases.
- Current technology allows ^{129}Xe to be imaged 3-dimensionally in all 3 compartments of the lung (airspace, barrier, red blood cells) and provides a new view of pulmonary gas exchange.

INTRODUCTION

Lung diseases affect the conducting airways, the gas exchange parenchyma, or both. As a result, they have a high impact on patients' morbidity, and quality of life. Chronic obstructive pulmonary disease (COPD), for example, is an umbrella term for progressive and irreversible obstructive diseases that affect the airways as well as the parenchyma. After cardiovascular diseases and cancer, COPD is predicted to be the third leading cause of death in the United States.[1] Similarly, airway diseases such as asthma have a high prevalence and a large economic impact with $56 billion in associated health care costs.[2] Furthermore, interstitial lung diseases, although less prevalent than COPD

or asthma, also have a high morbidity. This morbidity is partially attributable to a lack of viable therapeutic options to treat the underlying diseases.[3] However, equally problematic is the lack of sensitive biomarkers that can be used to diagnose these diseases earlier, better monitor progression, and show early therapeutic response.

The current gold standard for diagnosis and monitoring treatment of pulmonary diseases is spirometric pulmonary function testing (PFTs). However, by assessing the lung only on a global basis, PFT metrics generally lack the ability to detect functional changes associated with the small airways and gas exchange regions. This insensitivity of PFTs to the functioning of the distal lung parenchyma (**Fig. 1**) has led these regions to be referred to as the 'silent

Dr B. Driehuys is a founder and shareholder of Polarean, Inc. Dr J.E. Roos, Dr H.P. McAdams, and Dr S.S. Kaushik have nothing to disclose. This work was funded by NIH/NHLBI R01 HL105643 with additional support from the Duke Center for In Vivo Microscopy, an NIH/NIBIB national Biomedical Technology Resource Center (P41 EB015897).

[a] Department of Radiology, Duke University Medical Center, Box 3808, Durham, NC 27710, USA; [b] Department of Biomedical Engineering, Duke University, Durham, NC, USA; [c] Department of Radiology, Center for In Vivo Microscopy, Duke University Medical Center, Durham, NC, USA
* Corresponding author.
E-mail address: Justus.roos@duke.edu

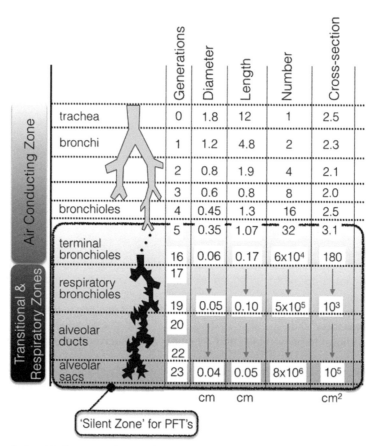

	Generations	Diameter	Length	Number	Cross-section
trachea	0	1.8	12	1	2.5
bronchi	1	1.2	4.8	2	2.3
	2	0.8	1.9	4	2.1
	3	0.6	0.8	8	2.0
bronchioles	4	0.45	1.3	16	2.5
	5	0.35	1.07	32	3.1
terminal bronchioles	16	0.06	0.17	6×10^4	180
	17				
respiratory bronchioles	19	0.05	0.10	5×10^5	10^3
	20				
alveolar ducts	22				
alveolar sacs	23	0.04	0.05	8×10^6	10^5
		cm	cm		cm^2

Air Conducting Zone

Transitional & Respiratory Zones

'Silent Zone' for PFT's

Fig. 1. Anatomic relationship between the purely air conducting zone and the transitional/respiratory zones. Pulmonary function test (PFTs) lack the ability to detect early changes at the level of the small airways, the so-called silent zone for PFTs. (*Adapted from* Weibel ER. Morphometry of the human lung. Heidelberg (Germany): Springer; 1963.)

zone.'[4] Additionally, these metrics largely rely on subject effort, causing significant measurement uncertainty and variability. Hence, current therapy is guided largely by patients' symptoms and survival.[5–7] Given the large burden on our health care system and the growing prevalence of pulmonary disease, there exists a need for improved diagnostic tools and quantitative metrics to better diagnose and quantify pulmonary disease progression and help to accurately measure response to therapy.

To overcome the lungs' many compensatory mechanisms and improve sensitivity to early disease, it is necessary to exploit regional information obtained by imaging. To this end, hyperpolarized (HP) gas MR imaging provides a noninvasive, ionizing radiation–free method to image pulmonary structure and function.[8–13] Although the early days of HP gas MR imaging saw extensive development and progress using the noble gas ^{3}He, its recent scarcity and concomitant increase in price ($\sim$\$2000/L)[14] has caused a transition to the less expensive and naturally available ^{129}Xe ($\sim$\$30/L,

natural abundance). An added advantage of ^{129}Xe is obtained by virtue of its solubility in pulmonary tissues, which leads to 2 signal sources, distinct from the xenon in the airspaces. ^{129}Xe can be detected separately in the pulmonary barrier tissues and the red blood cells (RBCs) in the capillary network, compartments in which it exhibits distinct resonant signal frequencies. These 3 ^{129}Xe resonances can provide quantitative regional information on the fundamental function of the lung, gas exchange.[15]

This article briefly touches on the history of HP gas MR imaging, describes the key technical properties, and discusses current and future applications and opportunities for pulmonary imaging.

HISTORY AND SAFETY

In 1994, the first HP gas MR imaging studies were carried out ex vivo using the noble gas isotope ^{129}xenon (^{129}Xe).[16] In 1997, Mugler and colleagues[17] used ^{129}Xe to conduct the first ground breaking studies in humans. Although this represented a rapid advancement from mouse to clinical translation, these studies were limited by relatively low ^{129}Xe polarization (1%–2%), which resulted in low signal intensities. This limitation caused research interest to transition quickly to the other stable inert gas isotope. ^{3}He, which has a larger gyromagnetic ratio than ^{129}Xe (32.4 MHz/T vs 11.77 MHz/T), offered a simpler and more mature polarization technology ($\sim$30%), and corresponding larger signal intensities. Additionally, unlike ^{129}Xe that, in large enough alveolar concentrations (>70%),[18] is known to exhibit anesthetic properties, ^{3}He does not have any physiologic side effects, and was considered to be a better starting point for clinical imaging. Indeed, the known anesthetic properties of xenon led to it being regulated as a drug, and further increased the barriers to its use in research. Interestingly, it would later be recognized that the tissue solubility of ^{129}Xe that contribute to its anesthetic properties actually provided new and exciting opportunities for imaging of the lung beyond what is possible with ^{3}He.

^{3}He MR imaging entered clinical research in 1996[19,20] and soon expanded to multicenter clinical studies.[21] The results of the ventilation studies showed significant correlation to conventional PFTs in patients with COPD, asthma, and cystic fibrosis. Diffusion-weighted imaging yielded the apparent diffusion coefficient (ADC), which is a sensitive marker of alveolar enlargement, and this marker was significantly increased in subjects with emphysema.[8,9,22–24]

The problem with ^{3}He HP MR imaging is 2-fold. First, the only source of ^{3}He comes from the decay of tritium, which is exclusively derived from the past production of nuclear warheads in the United States. The supply from the current stockpile is becoming progressively depleted and access increasingly limited. Second, a large portion of the current stockpile has been allocated for homeland security applications to detect emitted neutrons from smuggled plutonium. These reasons have driven up costs significantly to approximately $800 to $2000 per liter depending on academic versus commercial use.[14] With these greater costs and lesser availability, ^{3}He HP MR imaging, although having contributed greatly to the creation of this field, is not sustainable economically.

Recent progress in ^{129}Xe polarization technology led Patz and colleagues[25] to reintroduce ^{129}Xe MR imaging in humans. Xenon has a long history of safe use as a contrast agent in CT lung imaging studies,[26] which was confirmed by Driehuys and colleagues,[27] who rigorously tested the safety and tolerability of inhaling multiple, undiluted 1-L

volumes of HP ^{129}Xe. No major adverse effects were reported in total of 44 study subjects including healthy volunteers and COPD patients. Among the reported symptoms were mild dizziness, paresthesia/hypoesthesia, and euphoria, which were transient for approximately 1 to 2 minutes. No subject showed changes in laboratory tests or electrocardiogram. With the advent of more efficient polarizers, resulting in improved ^{129}Xe polarization,[28] one can expect better image quality with a lesser volume of xenon, and the described symptoms are likely to be diminished further. In fact, a second safety study by Shukla and co-workers[29] showed that inhalation of only 0.5 L volumes caused subjects to experience few or no symptoms.

TECHNIQUE

Traditional MR imaging of the lungs is fraught with a number of difficulties. Conventional MR scanners are primarily tuned to excite hydrogen protons (^{1}H) that are present in abundance in water molecules. However, the lungs have only very low ^{1}H density ($\sim$20%) compared with other anatomic structures. Combined with a long relaxation time, the signal available for imaging is minimal. Further complicating the image acquisition is the inhomogeneous magnetic environment of the lung, which introduces significant susceptibility artifacts that further challenge conventional MR acquisitions. However, these problems of MR-based lung imaging are not faced by the external gaseous contrast media (^{3}He or ^{129}Xe), which instead image the airways and airspaces within the lungs rather than the surrounding tissues (**Fig. 2**). This greatly reduces the problems of unfavorable longitudinal and transverse relaxation times faced by ^{1}H MR imaging in the lung. On the other hand, MR imaging of a gas is challenging because its density is typically about 4 orders of magnitude less than that of protons (^{1}H density of water $\sim$100 mol/L vs ^{129}Xe gas density $\sim$0.01 mol/L). This lower density reduces commensurately the available signal intensity and would seem to make gas MR imaging impossible. To circumvent this limitation, a physical process called hyperpolarization is used to increase the magnetization of these particular gases by about 5 orders of magnitude. Hyperpolarization more than overcomes their low density and makes MR-based imaging of these inhaled gases feasible within a single breath-hold.

Gas Polarization

Physics

The physics around polarizing gases dates back to the atomic physics publications in the 1960s.[30,31]

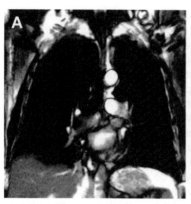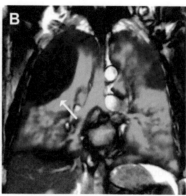

Fig. 2. Coronal mid lung proton MR imaging without (*A*) and with (*B*) hyperpolarized ^{129}Xe gas contrast (*green overlay*). It is obvious that proton MR imaging and the lungs are not really close friends: Conventional MR imaging excites and detects hydrogen nuclei (protons) in water. The lungs have a very low proton density and those that are present are difficult to image given their unfavorable relaxation characteristics. However, beyond the challenge of imaging parenchymal structure by MR imaging, there is an enormous need to image its function. This led to the development of contrast techniques using noble gases, such as ^{3}He or ^{129}Xe, which nicely demonstrate the lack of ventilation in a large right upper lobe bullae (*arrow*) in this patient.

This technology remained of purely intellectual interest until the introduction of high-power lasers afforded the ability to polarize large volumes of gases on reasonable time scales. This paved the way for the use of HP gases in medical imaging. The schematic shown in **Fig. 3** describes the sequence of events involved in increasing the nuclear spin polarization of either ^{3}He or ^{129}Xe. This involves 2 processes: (1) optical pumping and (2) spin exchange.[30,31]

As shown in **Fig. 3**A depicting 6 nuclear spins, under normal conditions, roughly one-half of the nuclear spins within the gas volume are aligned parallel to the direction of the main magnetic field and one-half against it. This situation leads to zero signal because the MR signal is determined by the difference in the number of spins aligned in either direction, that is, polarization. Hence, the most ideal scenario that would give us the most signal would have all the nuclear spins pointed along 1 direction, or 100% polarized. If we were to put this ensemble of spins into a large magnetic field like that of a 1.5-T or 3.0-T scanner, it would cause slightly more spins to align with rather than against the field. This difference, although sufficient for imaging with ubiquitous sources like water, is not nearly sufficient for imaging dilute gases like ^{3}He or ^{129}Xe. An alternative way of viewing our hypothetical system is to note that we need only to add 3 quanta of angular momentum to turn every downward pointed nuclear spin to one that is up and thereby align every nuclear spin in the same direction. Thus, hyperpolarization involves simply adding angular momentum to the system.

To achieve this, circularly polarized laser light is used as a carrier of angular momentum. However, nuclei cannot directly absorb laser light, so we use an intermediary to absorb the light and its angular momentum. Specifically, laser light is tuned to the principal resonance of an alkali metal atom such as rubidium (Rb), which causes its single outer shell valence electron to become aligned. This process is known as optical pumping (see **Fig. 3**B).[32,33] Only alkali metal atoms with electron spins that are down can absorb the light, so simply illuminating the alkali vapor with circularly polarized resonant light converts the entire sample to the spin up direction. Once a valence electron spin has been flipped up, it remains in this state until collisions cause it to depolarize. Then, it simply absorbs another photon and returns to the aligned state.

Subsequently, through collisions between polarized electron spins of the alkali metal Rb and the ^{129}Xe or ^{3}He nuclei, the alignment from Rb valence electron is transferred to the noble gas nucleus. This process is referred as spin exchange (see **Fig. 3**C).[30–33] After the spin exchange collision, the Rb electrons become aligned again by absorbing additional laser light and continue to build polarization within the available noble gas nuclei. Currently available optical pumping and spin exchange techniques deliver polarizations of approximately 40% to 80% for ^{3}He and approximately 10% to 40% for ^{129}Xe. Recently, very high peak ^{129}Xe polarization levels have been demonstrated in diluted mixtures.[34]

Gas polarization technique
A simplified schematic for xenon polarization is shown in **Fig. 4**. *Optical pumping* is carried out using Rb, which is contained within a glass optical cell. This optical cell is housed in an oven, surrounded by 2 Helmholtz coils that generate a small, but homogeneous 20 G magnetic field.

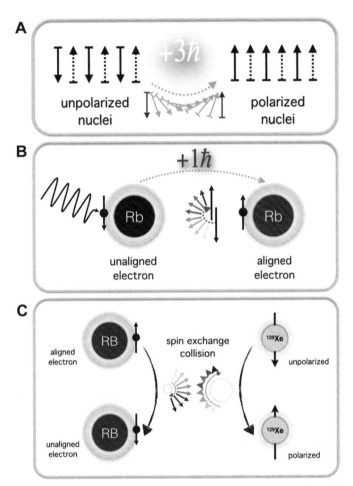

Fig. 3. Schematics explain sequence involved in gas polarization. Under normal conditions, one-half of the nuclear spins within the gas volume are pointed up, along the magnetic field direction, and half are pointed down. This leads to zero polarization. If we put this sample in a large magnetic field (1.5–3.0 T), it is slightly more favorable for spins to be up, but this leads to polarization of only a few parts per million. In hyperpolarization, we seek to have nearly all nuclei spins polarized in one direction. (*A*) From a physics perspective, all that is needed to transform this unpolarized sample of 3 down and 3 up spins, is to add 3 quanta of angular momentum (*A*) to flip the down spins to up, and polarize the sample. (*B*) We cannot directly flip nuclear, but we can flip electron spins in an alkali metal atom rubidium, which by absorbing angular momentum from laser photons, allows its outer shell valence electron to become spin polarized. This process is known as optical pumping (see **Fig. 3B**). (*C*) Mother Nature takes care of the rest when ^{129}Xe or ^{3}He nuclei collide with Rb and transfer polarization from its valence electron to the nuclear spin of the noble gas atom. This process is known as spin exchange.

The Rb in the optical cell is heated to approximately 150°C to produce a Rb vapor pressure equal to about 1 ppm of the total gas density in the cell. During this time, 10 to 100 W of circularly polarized laser light tuned to the D1 transition of Rb illuminates the optical cell. The Rb vapor absorbs a significant fraction (>50%) this incident laser light, which polarizes the valence electron spins on the Rb atoms in the vapor.

Spin exchange is initiated when a mixture of 1% ^{129}Xe, 89% ^{4}He, and 10% N_2 is directed to flow through the optical cell and interact with the optically pumped Rb atoms. The buffer gases (helium and nitrogen) serve to pressure broaden the Rb absorption cross-section to enable a large fraction of laser light to be productively absorbed. Rb–^{129}Xe spin exchange transfers electron spin polarization to the ^{129}Xe nuclei through a combination of binary collisions and the formation of transient Van der Waals complexes. The gas flow rate through the system is regulated such that ^{129}Xe emerges from the cell highly polarized. To now separate the ^{129}Xe from the ^{4}He and N_2 buffer gases, it is accumulated cryogenically in a cold finger immersed in liquid nitrogen. Because xenon has a higher freezing point than both these gases

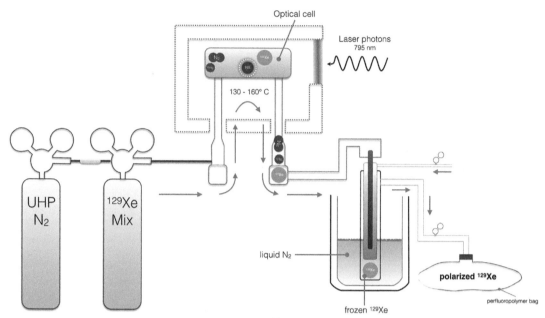

Fig. 4. Schematic of the device used to hyperpolarize ^{129}Xe. The optical pumping and spin exchange process occurs in the optical cell in a flowing mixture of 1% hyperpolarized (HP) ^{129}Xe, 89% ^{4}He, and 10% N_2. Once the mixture flows out of the optical cell, ^{129}Xe can be separated from the ^{4}He N_2 buffer gases by exploiting the fact that xenon freezes readily at the 77°K temperature of liquid nitrogen, while the other gases remain gaseous. Once a sufficient quantity of HP ^{129}Xe has been frozen and accumulated, it is thawed and evacuated into a perfluoropolymer bag for delivery to the patient and subsequent imaging. In these bags, the HP state has about a 1 hour half-life, allowing ample time for delivery.

(161 K), it is selectively frozen out and separated from the helium and nitrogen, which are vented out of the system. Once sufficient xenon has been accumulated, the frozen xenon is thawed, and the gaseous, polarized xenon is dispensed into a perfluoropolymer bag. The xenon polarization is then measured using a low-field nuclear MR-based system and the delivered to the patient. Commercially available systems can produce liter quantities xenon polarized to 10% to 15% in 1 hour. New discoveries in polarization physics are certain to enhance both the production rate and ^{129}Xe polarization in the near future.

This dose of xenon is then administered to the subject in the MR imaging scanner. Before inhalation, the subject is coached to inhale to total lung capacity and exhale to functional residual capacity, twice. The contents of the bag are then inhaled through a 6-mm ID Tygon tube that is connected to a mouth piece. Typical scans use between 200 and 1000 mL of ^{129}Xe and may be mixed with a buffer gas like helium or nitrogen to create a full inhalation volume.

Magnetic Resonance Scanner Configuration

A conventional MR scanner is typically configured to work primarily on the proton frequency. However,

through minor commercially available additions to the MR hardware and software, any scanner can be used to image HP gases. As xenon has a gyromagnetic ratio of 11.77 MHz/T, which is almost a factor of ~4 lower than that of protons (42.5 MHz/T), at typical field strengths of 1.5 T, it has a much lower resonance frequency of 17.66 MHz. Because most scanners typically use a narrow-banded radiofrequency (RF) amplifier optimized only for exciting at the proton frequency, nonproton nuclei such as xenon require a separate broad-banded RF amplifier to be installed. Similarly, the receive side of the scanner is typically also tuned to operate just at the proton frequency and thus must also be broad banded. Fortunately, such upgrades are available from all major scanner vendors and known as a "multinuclear package." As with most MR applications, a dedicated transmit–receive coil is also necessary, and must of course be designed to operate at the xenon frequency. It is preferred that such coils are "proton blocked" to enable an anatomic image to be acquired using the scanners body coil without moving the patient. These RF coils are available commercially (Clinical MR Solutions, Brookfield, WI; Rapid Biomedical, Rimpar, Germany) and at our institution we use a quadrature vest coil that delivers optimal signal-to-noise ratio (Clinical MR Solutions).

Proton MR imaging has the advantage of a renewable thermal signal, which affords it the utility of a multitude of MR pulse sequences. However, the nonthermal signal of HP gases enforces a number of constraints in the choice of pulse sequences.[35] First, once inhaled, the HP signal has a finite lifetime in the lung (T_1), which is typically around 20 seconds. Note that the T_1 for HP gases refers to timescale with which the polarized state decays down to negligibly small thermal equilibrium values, rather than the conventional beneficial recovery of longitudinal magnetization. The T_1 of xenon in lung is primarily affected by dipolar interactions with paramagnetic, molecular oxygen. Fortunately, T_1 effects are rendered somewhat negligible by acquiring images as rapidly as the scanner will allow. A second significant consideration is that the RF pulses used to excite the xenon signal also deplete its magnetization by the cosine of the flip angle applied. Hence, a traditional spin echo pulse sequence using 90° and 180° RF pulses cannot generally be used for HP gas imaging. Second, being a gaseous contrast agent, xenon also has high diffusivity that can depend on the local gas composition (0.14 cm^2/s at infinite dilution).[23,36] This means that the gradients applied just to acquire the image can actually induce diffusion-based attenuation of the signal if not properly considered. Last, clinical imaging using HP gases require that the acquisition be completed in a short breath-hold ($\sim$ 15 s). These factors confine HP gas imaging to fast pulse sequences with low flip angles that can adequately sample all of k-space while minimizing image blurring. This means that most HP gas imaging is done using fast gradient echo–based sequences.

CLINICAL APPLICATIONS
Ventilation Imaging

The technical robustness and performance of HP ^{3}He gas MR imaging of the lungs was confirmed in multiple clinical studies since its introduction in 1997.[19,20] HP ^{3}He MR imaging was predominately applied to produce spin density images of the gas distribution to quantify regions that lack any ventilation, namely, ventilation defects. These defects

A

B

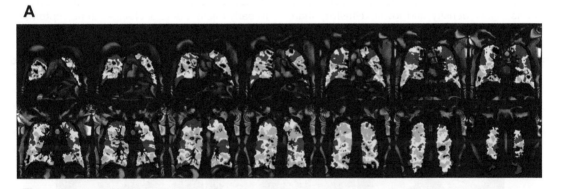

Fig. 5. Quantified ventilation defects using a 4-color ventilation mask with red representing the most impaired ventilation in a asthma patient before (A) and after (B) bronchodilator therapy. From these images, the ventilation defect percentage (VDP) can be calculated. In this patient, with an forced expiratory volume in 1 second (FEV$_1$) of 31%, the prebronchodilator VDP is 30%; after the bronchodilator, the FEV$_1$ remained at 31%, and VDP reduced significantly to 19%. Based on American Thoracic Society criteria, this patient would represent a nonresponder to bronchodilatation by PFT criteria, although quantified HP gas ventilation confirms a significant and positive effect to bronchodilator therapy.

may be caused by obstruction of airways as seen in diseases like asthma, or it may be owing to alveolar tissue destruction as seen in emphysema. Given the wide dynamic range of signal intensities in the ventilation images, these intensities can be grouped into 4 clusters to analyze the signal distribution. Clusters of low or absent MR signal within the lungs corresponded well with ventilation defects and allowed to detect and quantify functional ventilation impairment like in asthma, COPD, or cystic fibrosis patients (**Fig. 5**). Because data acquisition is completed during a single breath-hold, this renders static ventilation information from early in the wash-in period. Other dynamic ventilation properties, such as gas flow characteristics including delayed gas filling, are not as readily attainable, although significant progress has been made recently in this arena.[37]

Traditionally, because of the significantly larger polarization available using HP ^{3}He compared with ^{129}Xe, the ^{3}He image quality was superior. More recently, significant advances in the polarization technology and careful tuning of the MR acquisition have yielded ^{129}Xe ventilation images that rival those obtained with ^{3}He. As for ventilation defects, despite its lower signal-to-noise ratio, ^{129}Xe with its higher density and lower diffusivity than ^{3}He seems to be more sensitive to ventilation defects.[38] Currently, using a somewhat larger volume of ^{129}Xe (up to 1 L per scan) counterbalances the

decreased signal-to-noise ratio of ^{129}Xe compared with ^{3}He (normally 0.1–0.3 L per scan; **Fig. 6**).

Diffusion-Weighted Imaging

Diffusion-weighted MR imaging has been extensively validated, and widely used with HP gases to calculate the ADC of the gas.[8,9,22–24] The ADC image is obtained by acquiring gas images with and without applying diffusion-sensitizing gradients. The value of this contrast derives from the fact that the diffusion of the gases is highly constrained by the architecture of the normal lung. However, in diseases such as emphysema, where airspaces become significantly enlarged, the gases are free to diffuse (**Fig. 7**). Thus, diffusion weighting can differentiate normal from enlarged airspaces by the degree of signal attenuation observed. The signal intensities in the weighted and nonweighted ventilation images are then used to calculate the ADC on a voxel-by-voxel basis. Thus, ADC maps exhibit low values in healthy lung, whereas in emphysematous lungs elevated ADC values are often observed. In fact, in addition to revealing emphysematous changes, ^{3}He or ^{129}Xe ADC values have been shown to be sensitive to early microstructural changes in asymptomatic smokers[8] and in second-hand smokers.[39] Even within healthy individuals, ADC MR imaging has been shown to be sensitive to age-related

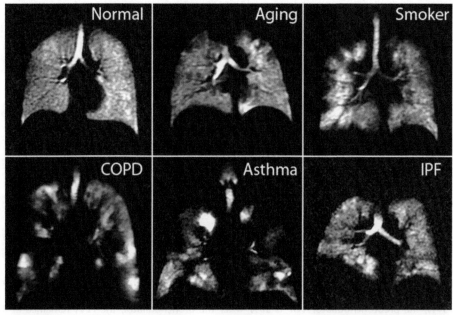

Fig. 6. Hyperpolarized ^{3}He ^{129}Xe images of healthy volunteer, an old but otherwise healthy individual, a smoker without chronic obstructive pulmonary disease (COPD), COPD, asthma and idiopathic pulmonary fibrosis (IPF) patients. HP ^{129}Xe images depict accurately different ventilation patterns related to underlying pulmonary disease.

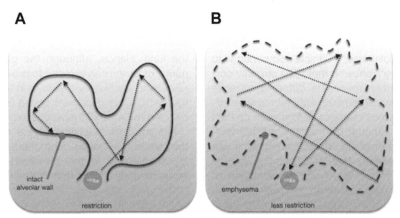

Fig. 7. Diffusion-weighted imaging of hyperpolarized ^{129}Xe can reveal airspace enlargement. The schematics compare diffusion of gas atoms in normal lung airspaces (*A*) versus enlarged airspaces (*B*). In normal airspaces the diffusion of ^{129}Xe is constrained by the normal alveolar architecture. However, when alveolar spaces become enlarged such as occurs in emphysema, ^{129}Xe diffusion is no longer constrained, and measured apparent diffusion coefficients (ADC) become higher.

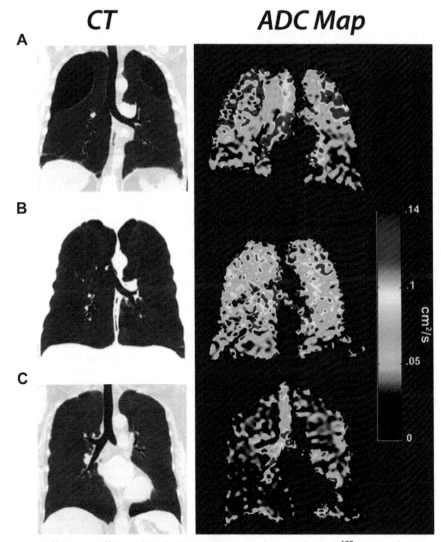

Fig. 8. Apparent diffusion coefficient (ADC) MR imaging using hyperpolarized ^{129}Xe gas. The color scale shows escalating enlargement of airspaces from normal lung tissue (*blue*) to severe bullous emphysematous parenchymal destruction (*red*). Note the parenchymal destruction depicted by CT (*A*, bullous emphysema; *B*, centrilobular and panlobular emphysema; *C*, normal lung) paralleling the change of ADC values.

changes in alveolar size.[40] Clinical comparisons to CT densitometry[41] showed that ADC strongly correlates with carbon monoxide diffusing capacity and that ADC measurements may reveal subclinical emphysematous changes before seen on high resolution CT.[8] Although the majority of ADC imaging to date has involved ^{3}He MR imaging, it has been shown recently that ADC imaging is also feasible with ^{129}Xe. **Fig. 8** shows examples of ^{129}Xe ADC images acquired in patients with COPD. It illustrates the highly elevated ADC value seen in emphysematous bullae, but also a more subtle distribution in patients where disease is less severe.[23]

FUTURE APPLICATIONS
^{129}Xe Dissolving Imaging

Compared with helium, xenon has a lower gyromagnetic ratio, and images have moderately lower signal-to-noise ratio. However, the useful and unique property of ^{129}Xe that sets it apart from ^{3}He comes by virtue of its moderate solubility in pulmonary tissues (**Fig. 9**).[18,42] As a result, xenon diffuses into the alveolar capillary membrane, and when it does, it experiences a distinct frequency shift from the gas phase of about 3.5 kHz (on a 1.5-T scanner) or 198 ppm in relative terms. Xenon diffuses further into the capillary blood stream, where it transiently binds with the hemoglobin in the RBCs, and when it does, it experiences a larger chemical shift of 217 ppm. These 2 resonances of xenon are known as the 'dissolved phase,' and because xenon follows the same gas transfer pathway as oxygen, these resonances to the first order give us information about gas exchange in

the lung. Hence, although the gas-phase resonance of xenon can be used to provide information relating to ventilatory distribution and microstructure (ADC), the dissolved phase resonances can be used to probe diffusive gas exchange.

Imaging this dissolved phase comes with its own set of challenges. First, the magnetization or signal intensity in the dissolved-phase is only approximately 2% of that in the alveolar spaces, or the gas phase. Second, in addition to the lower signal intensity, the T_2^* of the dissolved phase is extremely rapid, at approximately 2 ms.[43] Last, because the dissolved phase resonances are approximately 200 ppm from the gas phase, which on a 1.5-T scanner is about 3.8 kHz, the RF excitation pulses must be made sufficiently frequency selective so as to not excite the larger gas phase magnetization pool.

Because of these limitations, the early efforts in imaging the dissolved-phase employed indirect methods such as xenon polarization transfer contrast.[44] Because the xenon resonances are in dynamic exchange with one another, RF pulses applied to the dissolved phase caused slight attenuation of the gas phase signal. This concept was used to indirectly map out the dissolved phase distribution. However, with the onset of increased polarization and rapid pulse sequences, this method soon gave way to approaches that imaged the dissolved ^{129}Xe directly. By using frequency selective RF pulses and a 3-dimensional radial pulse sequence, the first dissolved phase images in humans were acquired in 2010.[45] These images were of a lower resolution owing to the small signal intensity of dissolved phase ^{129}Xe, but already showed intriguing aspects of lung

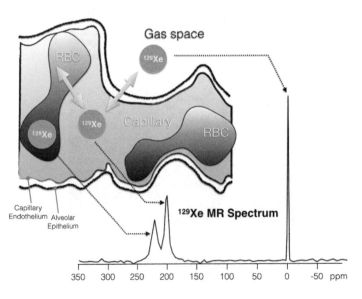

Fig. 9. Hyperpolarized ^{129}Xe can be separately detected in airspaces, interstitial tissues, and red blood cells (RBCs). A small fraction of the inhaled ^{129}Xe dissolves in pulmonary tissues and blood plasma (referred to as the barrier tissues), and changes its MR frequency dramatically compared with ^{129}Xe left in the airspaces. When ^{129}Xe diffuses further into the RBCs, it changes its detection frequency again. Because ^{129}Xe follows essentially the same pathway as oxygen, these spectroscopic properties of ^{129}Xe present an enormously powerful means to assess directly pulmonary gas exchange.

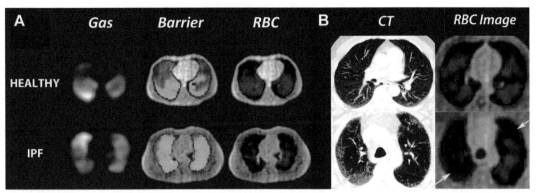

Fig. 10. Dissolved hyperpolarized ^{129}Xe MR imaging in a healthy individual and a patient with idiopathic pulmonary fibrosis (IPF). (*A*) Recent improvements in 3-dimensional imaging acquired radially, breath-hold images of inhaled ^{129}Xe now enable simultaneous depiction of ^{129}Xe in airspaces as well as ^{129}Xe transferred to the barrier and RBC compartments. (*B*) Note that in the patient with IPF, numerous focal defects are visible in the Xe–RBC transfer images. These defects correspond nicely with fibrotic changes seen on CT (*yellow arrows*).

function. Soon after the introduction of this direct dissolved phase imaging approach, Mugler and colleagues,[46] showed the merit of acquiring the 'source' gas phase distribution in the same breath. This ability allowed for the quantification of the dissolved phase distribution. This strategy was soon extended to using a radial acquisition strategy, which afforded the ability to quantify the impact of posture on the gas transfer distribution.[15]

However, because the pathway xenon follows to reach the RBCs is identical to that of oxygen, it is the ability to detect separately ^{129}Xe transfer to RBCs that is of fundamental importance. The value of doing so, even on a whole lung basis, was demonstrated recently. Spectra of ^{129}Xe in the dissolved phase were acquired in subjects with idiopathic pulmonary fibrosis and exhibited greatly reduced ^{129}Xe transfer to the RBCs compared with that observed in healthy volunteers.[15] This work thus showed that separating the dissolved ^{129}Xe resonances was critical to enable probing diffusion limitation caused by interstitial thickening in the lung. ^{129}Xe measurements correlated strongly with carbon monoxide diffusing capacity, but also showed that the frequency of the ^{129}Xe RBC resonance may be a sensitive probe of blood oxygenation at the level of the capillary bed. Although this work provided a global marker for gas exchange impairment, it also highlighted the need to detect separately xenon uptake in the barrier tissues and RBCs by imaging.

Separate imaging of ^{129}Xe in barrier and RBCs is a problem that shares similarities to separating fat and water in ^{1}H MR imaging. Because the 2 resonances are similarly spaced, one can borrow from the vast library of fat–water separation algorithms. One such approach was employed by Qing and colleagues,[47] who used the hierarchical IDEAL algorithm to image all 3 resonances of xenon in a single breath. Alternatively, the 1-point Dixon strategy has also shown promise, and may be more robust against the short T_2^* of the dissolved phase ^{129}Xe signal. This technique was also recently shown to allow imaging all 3 resonances of xenon in a single breath.[48] One such example of images of xenon in all 3 compartments is shown in **Fig. 10**. Note that in the patient with idiopathic pulmonary fibrosis, numerous focal defects are visible in the Xe–RBC transfer images. These defects correspond well to fibrotic changes seen on CT.

SUMMARY

Although the field of pulmonary medicine has relied on PFTs for more than 100 years, increasing evidence is mounting that these data are not sufficient. Instead, functional imaging now offers a rich world of information that is more sensitive to changes in lung structure and function than PFTs. Although MR imaging may not have been historically the first choice with which to image the lungs, HP ^{3}He and ^{129}Xe have begun to change this view. These gases have provided new, sensitive contrast mechanisms to probe changes in pulmonary ventilation, microstructure, and gas exchange. Given the recent scarcity in the supply of helium and the associated increase in price, the field has adopted the less expensive and naturally available xenon. Xenon has been shown to be well-tolerated in healthy volunteers and subjects with disease, and recent technical advances have ensured that the xenon image quality in on par with that of helium. The added advantage of xenon is that it exhibits 2 distinct new resonances that permit tracking its diffusion into the barrier tissues and the RBCs. Careful investigation of the amplitude, width, and the frequency of these resonances carries additional important information about alveolar oxygenation that is only now beginning to be understood. Perhaps, most important, the past several years have now demonstrated that the day has arrived where ^{129}Xe can be imaged 3-dimensionally in all 3 compartments of the lung (airspace, barrier, RBC) to provide a fundamental view of pulmonary gas exchange without requiring ionizing radiation. With a plethora of contrast mechanisms, HP gases and ^{129}Xe in particular stand to be an excellent probe of pulmonary structure and function, and provide sensitive and noninvasive biomarkers for a wide variety of pulmonary diseases. Interestingly, combined with recent advancements in structural imaging of the lung using ^{1}H MR imaging,[49] and 3-dimensional perfusion measurements, the day may finally be dawning that MR becomes the modality of choice for evaluating cardiopulmonary function comprehensively and noninvasively.

REFERENCES

1. Hoyert DL, Xu J. Deaths: preliminary data for 2011. Natl Vital Stat Rep 2012;61(6):1–51.
2. Barnett SB, Nurmagambetov TA. Costs of asthma in the United States: 2002–2007. J Allergy Clin Immunol 2011;127(1):145–52.
3. Nalysnyk L, Cid-Ruzafa J, Rotella P, et al. Incidence and prevalence of idiopathic pulmonary fibrosis: review of the literature. Eur Respir Rev 2012; 21(126):355–61.
4. Hogg JC, Chu F, Utokaparch S, et al. The nature of small-airway obstruction in chronic obstructive pulmonary disease. N Engl J Med 2004;350(26): 2645–53.
5. Ashutosh K, Haldipur C, Boucher ML. Clinical and personality profiles and survival in patients with COPD. Chest 1997;111(1):95–8.
6. Mahler DA, Mackowiak JI. Evaluation of the short-form 36-item questionnaire to measure health-related quality of life in patients with COPD. Chest 1995;107(6):1585–9.
7. Nishimura K, Izumi T, Tsukino M, et al. Dyspnea is a better predictor of 5-year survival than airway obstruction in patients with COPD. Chest 2002; 121(5):1434–40.
8. Fain SB, Panth SR, Evans MD, et al. Early emphysematous changes in asymptomatic smokers: detection with 3HE MR imaging 1. Radiology 2006; 239(3):875–83.
9. Kirby M, Mathew L, Wheatley A, et al. Chronic obstructive pulmonary disease: longitudinal hyperpolarized 3He MR imaging 1. Radiology 2010; 256(1):280–9.
10. McAdams HP, Palmer SM, Donnelly LF, et al. Hyperpolarized 3He-enhanced MR imaging of lung transplant recipients: preliminary results. AJR Am J Roentgenol 1999;173(4):955–9.
11. McMahon CJ, Dodd JD, Hill C, et al. Hyperpolarized 3helium magnetic resonance ventilation imaging of the lung in cystic fibrosis: comparison with high resolution CT and spirometry. Eur Radiol 2006;16(11):2483–90.
12. Mentore K, Froh DK, de Lange EE, et al. Hyperpolarized HHe 3 MRI of the lung in cystic fibrosis. Acad Radiol 2005;12(11):1423–9.
13. Salerno M, de Lange EE, Altes TA, et al. Emphysema: hyperpolarized helium 3 diffusion MR imaging of the lungs compared with spirometric indexes—initial experience1. Radiology 2002;222(1):252–60.
14. Kramer D. For some, helium-3 supply picture is brightening. Physics Today 2011.
15. Kaushik SS, Freeman MS, Yoon SW, et al. Measuring diffusion limitation with a perfusion-limited gas—hyperpolarized 129Xe gas-transfer spectroscopy in patients with idiopathic pulmonary fibrosis. J Appl Physiol (1985) 2014;117(6):577–85.
16. Albert MS, Cates GD, Driehuys B, et al. Biological magnetic resonance imaging using laser-polarized 129Xe. Nature 1994;370(6486):199–201.
17. Mugler JP, Driehuys B, Brookeman JR. MR imaging and spectroscopy using hyperpolarized 129Xe gas: preliminary human results. Magn Reson Med 1997; 37:809–15.
18. Kennedy RR, Stokes JW, Downing P. Anaesthesia and the 'inert' gases with special reference to xenon. Anaesth Intensive Care 1992;20(1):66–70.
19. Ebert M, Grossmann T, Heil W, et al. Nuclear magnetic resonance imaging with hyperpolarised helium-3. Lancet 1996;347(9011):1297–9.
20. MacFall JR, Charles HC, Black RD, et al. Human lung air spaces: potential for MR imaging with hyperpolarized He-3. Radiology 1996;200(2):553–8.
21. van Beek EJ, Dahmen AM, Stavngaard T, et al. Hyperpolarised 3He MRI versus HRCT in COPD and normal volunteers: PHIL trial. Eur Respir J 2009; 34(6):1311–21.
22. Chen XJ, Möller HE, Chawla MS, et al. Spatially resolved measurements of hyperpolarized gas properties in the lung in vivo. Part I: diffusion coefficient. Magn Reson Med 1999;42(4):721–8.
23. Kaushik SS, Cleveland ZI, Cofer GP, et al. Diffusion-weighted hyperpolarized 129Xe MRI in healthy volunteers and subjects with chronic obstructive pulmonary disease. Magn Reson Med 2011;65(4):1154–65.
24. Swift AJ, Wild JM, Fichele S, et al. Emphysematous changes and normal variation in smokers and COPD patients using diffusion 3He MRI. Eur J Radiol 2005; 54(3):352–8.
25. Patz S, Hersman FW, Muradian I, et al. Hyperpolarized (129)Xe MRI: a viable functional lung imaging modality? Eur J Radiol 2007;64(3):335–44.

26. Latchaw RE, Yonas H, Pentheny SL, et al. Adverse reactions to xenon-enhanced CT cerebral blood flow determination. Radiology 1987;163(1):251–4.

27. Driehuys B, Martinez-Jimenez S, Cleveland ZI, et al. Chronic obstructive pulmonary disease: safety and tolerability of hyperpolarized 129Xe MR imaging in healthy volunteers and patients. Radiology 2012; 262(1):279–89.

28. Ruset IC, Ketel S, Hersman FW. Optical pumping system design for large production of hyperpolarized Xe 129. Phys Rev Lett 2006;96(5):53002.

29. Shukla Y, Wheatley A, Kirby M, et al. Hyperpolarized 129Xe magnetic resonance imaging: tolerability in healthy volunteers and subjects with pulmonary disease. Acad Radiol 2012;19(8):941–51.

30. Bouchiat MA, Carver TR, Varnum CM. Nuclear polarization in He 3 gas induced by optical pumping and dipolar exchange. Phys Rev Lett 1960.

31. Kastler A. The optical production and the optical detection of an inequality of population of the levels of spatial quantification of atoms. Application to the experiments. J Phys Radium 1950.

32. Goodson BM. Nuclear magnetic resonance of laser-polarized noble gases in molecules, materials, and organisms. J Magn Reson 2002;155(2):157–216.

33. Walker TG, Happer W. Spin-exchange optical pumping of noble-gas nuclei. Rev Mod Phys 1997; 69(2):629–42.

34. Nikolaou P, Coffey AM, Walkup LL, et al. Near-unity nuclear polarization with an open-source 129Xe hyperpolarizer for NMR and MRI. Proc Natl Acad Sci U S A 2013;110:14150–5.

35. Zhao L, Albert MS. Biomedical imaging using hyperpolarized noble gas MRI: pulse sequence considerations. Nucl Instrum Methods Phys Res A 1998;402:454–60.

36. Driehuys B, Walker J, Pollaro J, et al. ³He MRI in mouse models of asthma. Magn Reson Med 2007; 58(5):893–900.

37. Marshall H, Deppe MH, Parra-Robles J, et al. Direct visualisation of collateral ventilation in COPD with hyperpolarised gas MRI. Thorax 2012;67(7):613–7.

38. Svenningsen S, Kirby M, Starr D, et al. Hyperpolarized (3) He and (129) Xe MRI: differences in asthma before bronchodilation. J Magn Reson Imaging 2013;38(6):1521–30.

39. Wang C, Mugler JP, de Lange EE, et al. Lung injury induced by secondhand smoke exposure detected with hyperpolarized helium-3 diffusion MR. J Magn Reson Imaging 2014;39(1):77–84.

40. Fain SB, Altes TA, Panth SR, et al. Detection of age-dependent changes in healthy adult lungs with diffusion-weighted 3He MRI. Acad Radiol 2005; 12(11):1385–93.

41. Diaz S, Casselbrant I, Piitulainen E, et al. Validity of apparent diffusion coefficient hyperpolarized 3He-MRI using MSCT and pulmonary function tests as references. Eur J Radiol 2009;71(2):257–63.

42. Weathersby PK, Homer LD. Solubility of inert gases in biological fluids and tissues: a review. Undersea Biomed Res 1980;7(4):277–96.

43. Mugler JP, Altes TA, Ruset IC, et al. Image-based measurement of T2* for dissolved-phase Xe129 in the human lung. Berkeley (CA): International Society for Magnetic Resonance in Medicine; 2012.

44. Ruppert K, Brookeman JR, Hagspiel KD, et al. Probing lung physiology with xenon polarization transfer contrast (XTC). Magn Reson Med 2000;44(3):349–57.

45. Cleveland ZI, Cofer GP, Metz G, et al. Hyperpolarized 129Xe MR imaging of alveolar gas uptake in humans. PLoS One 2010;5(8):e12192.

46. Mugler JP, Altes TA, Ruset IC, et al. Simultaneous magnetic resonance imaging of ventilation distribution and gas uptake in the human lung using hyperpolarized xenon-129. Proc Natl Acad Sci U S A 2010;107:21707–12.

47. Qing K, Ruppert K, Jiang Y, et al. Regional mapping of gas uptake by blood and tissue in the human lung using hyperpolarized xenon-129 MRI. J Magn Reson Imaging 2014;39(2):346–59.

48. Kaushik SS, Robertson SH, Freeman MS, et al. Imaging hyperpolarized 129Xe uptake in pulmonary barrier and red blood cells using a 3D Radial 1-point Dixon approach: results in healthy volunteers and subjects with pulmonary fibrosis. Berkeley (CA): International Society for Magnetic Resonance in Medicine; 2014.

49. Johnson KM, Fain SB, Schiebler ML, et al. Optimized 3D ultrashort echo time pulmonary MRI. Magn Reson Med 2013;70(5):1241–50.

Lung Cancer Assessment Using MR Imaging
An Update

Yoshiharu Ohno, MD, PhD[a,b,*], Hisanobu Koyama, MD, PhD[c],
Takeshi Yoshikawa, MD, PhD[a,b], Sumiaki Matsumoto, MD, PhD[a,b],
Kazuro Sugimura, MD[c]

KEYWORDS

• Lung cancer • MR imaging • Nodules • Staging • Therapeutic effect

KEY POINTS

• Non–contrast enhanced (CE) MR imaging techniques can improve differentiation of malignant from benign nodules compared with routine clinical protocols.

• Dynamic MR imaging with three-dimensional GRE sequence and ultrashort TE has the potential to play a complementary role in the characterization of pulmonary nodules and as a viable alternative to dynamic CE CT, FDG-PET, and/or PET/CT.

• Because multidetector row CT is widely used clinically, potential use of MR imaging in T-factor assessment may be limited; when MR imaging is used in this setting, STIR turbo SE imaging and three-dimensional CE GRE sequence may be helpful.

• For N-factor assessment, STIR turbo SE imaging can improve diagnostic performance compared with DWI and FDG-PET and/or PET/CT, although DWI is considered at least as valuable as PET or PET/CT.

• For M-factor assessment, whole-body MR imaging with and without DWI is as effective as FDG-PET or PET/CT in routine clinical practice.

OUTLINE

Since the 1980s many physicists and radiologists have been trying to evaluate the efficacy of MR imaging for various lung diseases, and for mediastinal and pleural diseases. Until 2000, however, thoracic MR imaging had shown limited clinical relevance, and could not be substituted for computed tomography (CT) and other modalities. It was therefore generally used for select clinical indications. During the first decade of this century, numerous basic and clinical researchers in radiology reported technical advances in sequencing, scanners and coils, adoption of parallel imaging techniques, use of contrast media, and development of postprocessing tools. In addition, several promising new techniques, including short inversion time inversion recovery (STIR) turbo spin echo (SE) imaging, diffusion-weighted imaging (DWI), and pulmonary functional MR imaging,

Drs Ohno, Yoshikawa, Matsumoto and Sugimura have research grants from Toshiba Medical Systems Corporation, Philips Electronics Japan, Bayer Pharma, Daiichi-Sankyo, Co. Ltd, and/ or Eizai, Co., Ltd.
[a] Division of Functional and Diagnostic Imaging Research, Department of Radiology, Kobe University Graduate School of Medicine, 7-5-2 Kusunoki-cho, Chuo-ku, Kobe, Hyogo 650-0017, Japan; [b] Advanced Biomedical Imaging Research Center, Kobe University Graduate School of Medicine, 7-5-2 Kusunoki-cho, Chuo-ku, Kobe, Hyogo 650-0017, Japan; [c] Division of Diagnostic Radiology, Department of Radiology, Kobe University Graduate School of Medicine, 7-5-2 Kusunoki-cho, Chuo-ku, Kobe, Hyogo 650-0017, Japan.
* Corresponding author. Division of Functional and Diagnostic Imaging Research, Department of Radiology, Kobe University Graduate School of Medicine, 7-5-2 Kusunoki-cho, Chuo-ku, Kobe, Hyogo 650-0017, Japan.
E-mail addresses: yosirad@kobe-u.ac.jp; yosirad@med.kobe.ac.jp; yoshiharuohno@aol.com

have been extensively researched and developed, leading to a re-examination of MR imaging as a new research and diagnostic tool for various pulmonary diseases, especially lung cancer. As a result, state-of-the-art thoracic MR imaging now has the potential to be used as a substitute for traditional imaging techniques and/or to play a complementary role in patient management.

This article focuses on these recent advances in MR imaging for lung cancer imaging, especially for pulmonary nodule assessment, lung cancer staging, prediction of postoperative lung function, prediction of therapeutic response, and recurrence. The potential and limitations for routine clinical application of these advances are also discussed and compared with those of other modalities, such as CT, PET, and PET/CT.

INTRODUCTION

Lung cancer is one of the most common cancers worldwide with the highest mortality for men and women,[1] and frequently manifests as a lung nodule or mass. Radiologically identified lung lesions that are less than 30 mm in diameter are known as pulmonary nodules, whereas those larger than 30 mm are called masses. Diagnosis and further characterization of pulmonary nodules is one of the most important areas of pulmonary medicine for appropriate management. Early diagnosis is important because non–small cell lung cancer (NSCLC), which currently accounts for 80% of all lung cancers, can be cured surgically if detected at an early stage.[2] However, most patients with NSCLC present late in the course of their illness, often at an inoperable, advanced stage.[3–5]

Apart from characterization, another potential application of MR imaging is tumor staging. NSCLC is usually staged with the tumor, lymph node, and metastasis (TNM) staging system, which has been recommended by the Union Internationale Contre le Cancer, the American Joint Committee on Cancer, and the International Association for the Study of Lung Cancer. However, small cell lung carcinoma, which constitutes approximately 13% to 20% of all lung cancers,[6] is staged with a two-stage system developed by the Veteran's Administration Lung Cancer study group. Irrespective of the type of staging system, radiologic examinations including CT, MR imaging, PET with 2-[fluorine-18] fluoro-2-deoxy-D-glucose (FDG-PET), and FDG-PET combined with CT (FDG-PET/CT) are important for pretherapeutic assessment in conjunction with pathologic information from transbronchial/CT-guided/mediastinoscopic biopsies.

Recent technical advances in MR systems, application of parallel imaging, introduction of new MR techniques, and use of contrast media have markedly improved the diagnostic accuracy of MR imaging in this setting. Also, FDG-PET combined or fused with MR imaging (FDG-PET/MR imaging) is now being evaluated in several studies as an emerging technique. This article focuses on these recent advances in MR imaging, and its potential clinical applications and limitations particularly in pulmonary nodule assessment and lung cancer staging.

PULMONARY NODULE AND MASS ASSESSMENT

Most solitary pulmonary nodules are incidental findings on chest radiographs obtained for unrelated diagnostic work-ups. In addition, a growing number are being detected on chest CTs as a direct result of increased use of CT examinations in routine clinical practice. Results of national lung cancer screening trials and previous CT-based lung cancer screening studies have led to a growing need for management of pulmonary nodules.[7] Although CT facilitates detection of an unsuspected lung cancer, the major drawback is exposure to ionizing radiation and a concomitant increase in the detection of benign and indeterminate nodules. This upsurge in the frequency of nodule detection is associated with an increase in the number of follow-up studies, further radiologic examinations, and/or of interventional procedures and associated costs. MR imaging is associated with no radiation, and is being evaluated as a possible alternative or complementary technique for management of such nodules in addition to traditionally used techniques.

Since the clinical application of MR imaging in the chest, SE or turbo SE sequences have aided in the detection of numerous pulmonary nodules including lung cancers, pulmonary metastases, and low-grade malignancies, such as carcinoids and lymphomas. Such lesions usually show low or intermediate signal intensity on T1-weighted imaging (T1WI) and slightly high intensity on T2-weighted imaging (T2WI). Previous reports[8–18] have suggested that T2WI and pre– and post–contrast-enhanced (CE) T1WI are useful for diagnosis of specific types of nodule or masses, such as bronchoceles, tuberculomas, mucin-containing tumors, hamartomas, and aspergillomas based on their specific MR findings, although significant overlap occurs between benign and malignant nodules or masses.

To overcome this limitation, STIR turbo SE imaging and DWI were introduced in 2008 as promising sequences for nodule assessment.[19,20] Koyama and colleagues[19] demonstrated that

STIR turbo SE imaging was significantly better than non-CE T1WI or T2WI for differentiating malignant from benign solitary pulmonary nodules, with sensitivity, specificity, and accuracy of 83.3%, 60.6%, and 74.5%, respectively. DWI involves estimation of apparent diffusion coefficient (ADC), which evaluates the diffusivity of water molecules within tissue for b values ranging from 0 s/mm^2 to a maximum value of 500 s/mm^2 to 1000 s/mm^2 in routine clinical practice. With ADC evaluation, the range of sensitivity and specificity of DWI in this setting has been reported to be 70.0% to 88.9% and 61.1% to 97.0%, respectively.[20–22] One study evaluated signal intensity of lesion to spinal cord ratio at high b value DWI and suggested that this parameter is more useful than ADC. The authors found lesion to spinal cord ratio to have a sensitivity, specificity, and accuracy of 83.3%, 90.0%, and 85.7%, respectively, and noted that the accuracy of this new parameter was significantly higher than that of ADC (85.7% vs 50.0%).[22] It would therefore be advantageous to use the previously mentioned non-CE MR imaging techniques (STIR turbo SE imaging and DWI) in routine clinical protocols along with other sequences to improve differentiation between malignant and benign nodules. This approach can be considered at least as efficacious as FDG-PET or PET/CT (**Figs. 1** and **2**).[22]

In addition to the previously mentioned non-CE MR imaging techniques, dynamic CE MR imaging can lead to further improvement of diagnostic performance. Since dynamic CE MR imaging was first reported,[17,18] various MR imaging techniques have been used for this purpose, and have evolved with improvements in MR imaging systems, sequences, and the use of injectors and development of new software. There are currently three major methods for dynamic MR imaging of the lung. These broad categories include two-dimensional SE or turbo SE sequences and various types of two-dimensional and three-dimensional gradient-echo (GRE) sequences. It is recommended that the enhancement patterns within nodules and/or parameters determined from signal intensity-time course curves be assessed visually.[23–31] The diagnostic performance of dynamic MR imaging techniques in distinguishing malignant from benign nodules has been reported to have a sensitivity ranging from 94% to 100%, specificity of 70% to 96%, and accuracy of more than 94%.[23–31] In addition, a meta-analysis found that there were no significant differences in diagnostic performance of dynamic CE CT, dynamic CE MR imaging, FDG-PET, and single-photon emission tomography (SPECT),[23] although dynamic MR imaging with the three-dimensional GRE sequence and ultrashort echo time (TE) proved to be superior in a direct and prospective comparison study of dynamic CE CT and coregistered FDG-PET/CT (see **Figs. 1** and **2**).[30] The use of dynamic MR imaging with the three-dimensional GRE sequence and ultrashort TE is therefore more likely to be effective than other methods and may lead to improved diagnostic performance of dynamic CE MR imaging. This method has the potential to play a complementary role in the characterization of pulmonary nodules and as a viable alternative to dynamic CE CT, FDG-PET, and/or PET/CT.

LUNG CANCER STAGING

TNM classification is essential for lung cancer management, and it is hoped that this classification be as accurate as possible to direct appropriate management. Currently, thin-section CE CT is deemed effective for assessment of tumor extent because of its multiplanar capability and higher spatial resolution, whereas FDG-PET and PET/CT are used for accurate diagnosis of metastatic lymph nodes and distant metastatic sites except brain metastasis.[32–35] In contrast to the previously mentioned modalities, MR imaging has been used in limited scenarios since 1991.[36] With recent advances in MR imaging techniques, it is now possible to improve TNM staging accuracy in patients with lung cancer.[37,38] In this section, historical, traditional, and newly applied MR imaging techniques for TNM staging are introduced and discussed in the hope that they will help improve imaging protocols for patients with lung cancer in daily clinical practice.

T-Factor Assessment on MR Imaging

In relation to T-factor assessment, the Radiologic Diagnostic Oncology Group published a comparative study of CT and non-CE MR imaging for TNM staging of 170 patients with NSCLC in 1991.[36] This study found that operability assessment based on differentiating T3-T4 from T1-T2 tumors on non-CE MR imaging (sensitivity, 56.0%; specificity, 80.0%) was not significantly different from that of CT (sensitivity, 63.0%; specificity, 84.0%).[36]

New MR imaging techniques have been added to improve MR imaging–based T-factor assessment since 1997. Sakai and colleagues[39] used dynamic cine MR imaging during breathing rather than static MR imaging, resulting in improved diagnosis of chest wall invasion. This study assessed the movement of the tumor along the parietal pleura during the respiratory cycle displayed as a cine loop in a manner similar to that used for dynamic expiratory multisection CT.[40] In another study,[39] the sensitivity, specificity, and accuracy of dynamic cine MR imaging for the

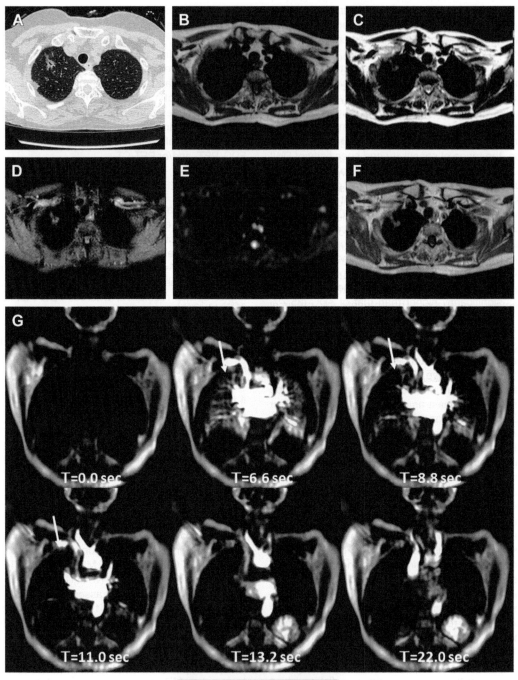

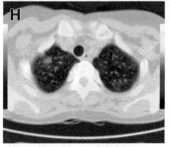

detection of chest wall invasion were 100%, 70%, and 76%, respectively, whereas those of conventional CT and static MR imaging were 80%, 65%, and 68%.[39] Dynamic cine MR imaging in conjunction with static MR imaging can therefore be considered a useful method for chest wall invasion assessment.

Another promising technique, first reported in 2001, is CE MR angiography for assessment of cardiovascular or mediastinal invasion.[41,42] In comparison with CE CT and cardiac-gated T1WI, it has a higher sensitivity, specificity, and accuracy for detection of mediastinal and hilar invasion ranging from 78% to 90%, 73% to 87%, and 75% to 88%, respectively.[42] CE MR angiography based on three-dimensional CE GRE sequence can thus help improve the diagnostic capability of MR imaging for T-factor assessment in routine clinical practice.

N-Factor Assessment on MR Imaging

The performance of MR imaging for N-factor assessment was previously not considered to be significantly different from CT because diagnostic criteria for differentiation of metastatic from nonmetastatic lymph nodes primarily depended on lymph node size. Therefore, in previous publications, the multiplanar capability of MR imaging was regarded as the only advantage in the detection of lymph nodes in such areas as the aortopulmonary window and subcarinal regions, which were difficult to assess on the commonly used axial images in CT.[36,43]

To improve the diagnostic performance of N-factor assessment on MR imaging, cardiac- and/or respiratory-triggered conventional or black-blood STIR turbo SE imaging has been tested since 2002, and has demonstrated its superiority over CE CT, FDG-PET, or PET/CT and other MR imaging sequences.[38,39,44–49] STIR turbo SE imaging consists of a simple sequence that is easily incorporated into clinical protocols to yield T1 and T2 relaxation times. On STIR turbo SE images, metastatic lymph nodes show high signal intensity and nonmetastatic lymph nodes demonstrate low signal intensity (**Fig. 3**).

According to previously published results,[44–49] sensitivity of quantitatively and qualitatively assessed STIR turbo SE imaging ranged, on a per-patient basis, from 83.7% to 100.0%, specificity from 75.0% to 93.1%, and accuracy from 86.0% to 92.2%, and these values were equal to or higher than those for CE CT, FDG-PET, or PET/CT. Yet another study showed that the quantitative and qualitative sensitivity, specificity, and accuracy of STIR turbo SE imaging were not significantly different from FDG-PET/CT. However, the combination of FDG-PET/CT with STIR turbo SE imaging was found to be significantly more effective in detecting nodal involvement on a per-patient basis (96.9% specificity, 90.3% accuracy) than FDG-PET/CT alone (65.6% specificity, 81.7% accuracy).[48]

In 2008, DWI was introduced as another promising MR imaging technique for this purpose.[49–52] Sensitivity, specificity, and accuracy of DWI reportedly range, on a per-patient basis, from 77.4% to 80.0%, 84.4% to 97.0%, and 89.0% to 95.0%, respectively, and these results seem to be similar to or better than those for FDG-PET or PET/CT (see **Fig. 3**).[49–52] Ohno and colleagues[49] prospectively and directly compared these modalities to determine the clinical relevance of MR imaging–based N-factor assessment compared with FDG-PET/CT. In this study, sensitivity and/or accuracy of STIR turbo SE imaging (quantitative sensitivity, 82.8%; qualitative sensitivity, 77.4%; quantitative accuracy, 86.8%) proved to be significantly higher than those of DWI (74.2%, 71.0%, and 84.4%, respectively) and FDG-PET/CT (quantitative sensitivity, 74.2%). This means that quantitative and qualitative assessment of the N stage of patients with NSCLC obtained with STIR turbo SE MR imaging is more sensitive and more accurate than those obtained with DWI and FDG-PET/CT.[49] According to these results and considering the limitations of DWI and FDG-PET/CT for detection of small metastatic foci or lymph nodes, STIR turbo SE imaging may be the better MR imaging

Fig. 1. A 67-year-old woman with organizing pneumonia proved pathologically and on follow-up examinations. (*A*) On thin-section CT, a 15-mm part solid right upper lobe nodule was suspected of being a lung adenocarcinoma. The nodule has low signal intensity on T1-weighted imaging (*B*), intermediate intensity on T2-weighted imaging (*C*), and high signal intensity on STIR turbo spin echo imaging (*D*). High signal intensity on STIR imaging favors a malignant nodule. (*E*) DWI shows the nodule to have low to intermediate signal intensity, favoring a benign nodule. (*F*) Contrast-enhanced T1-weighted imaging shows contrast enhancement of the nodule, favoring a malignant cause. (*G*) Dynamic MR imaging with ultrashort TE shows the nodule as a perfusion defect in the lung parenchyma (*arrow*) in early phases (T = 6.6, 8.8, and 11.0 seconds) and minimal enhancement in the later phases (T = 13.2 and 22.0 seconds). (*H*) FDG-PET/CT shows faint uptake within the nodule. Hence, STIR and T1-weighted contrast-enhanced sequence were false-positive in this case, whereas DWI and dynamic MR imaging with ultrashort TE were true-negative.

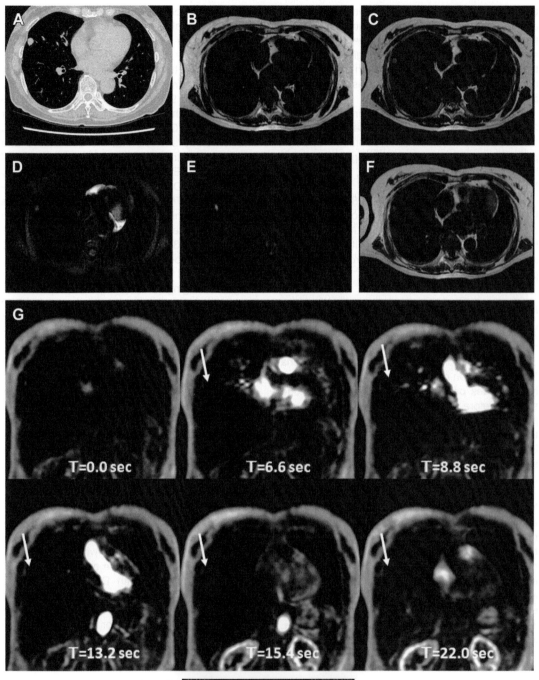

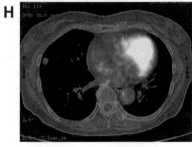

technique to use before surgical treatment or lymph node sampling for accurate pathologic TNM staging and after treatment.[49] Further technical improvements in DWI are needed to overcome its current limitations and enable it to function in a complementary role to STIR turbo SE imaging in routine clinical practice.

M-Factor Assessment on MR Imaging

M-factor assessment for detection of metastasis in patients with lung cancer has major implications for management and prognosis, and an accurate diagnosis in this respect may help clinicians provide the most appropriate treatment and/or management for patients with lung cancer. For M-factor assessment, intrathoracic and extrathoracic metastases have to be evaluated. For this purpose, chest radiography, CT, MR imaging, bone scintigraphy, and PET or PET/CT are used in routine clinical practice. When MR imaging is used in this setting, a clear understanding of the diagnostic performance of state-of-the-art MR imaging for intrathoracic and extrathoracic metastases assessment is necessary.[37,38]

Intrathoracic metastasis assessment

Chest radiography and CT are often regarded as the first choice for assessment of intrathoracic metastasis; other commonly used modalities include PET/CT. Since 1992, several investigators have tried to determine the capability of MR imaging in evaluating metastatic lung nodules in the context of primary lung cancer or other primary malignancies by using various sequences with 1.5- and 3.0-T scanners.[19,53–61] In addition, combination of the previously mentioned MR imaging techniques to differentiate malignant nodules (metastatic and primary malignancies) from benign nodules has been evaluated. The detection rate or sensitivity of MR imaging using various sequences on 1.5- and 3.0-T systems has ranged from 36.0% to 96.0%.[19,53–61] The study with the largest population to date compared CT with 1.5-T MR imaging and demonstrated that although the overall detection rate of thin-section CT (97%) was superior to

that of respiratory-triggered STIR turbo SE imaging (82.5%), there was no significant difference between the two in the detection rate for all types of malignant nodules.[19] Therefore, the currently available MR imaging technique can have a complementary role in intrathoracic metastasis detection. More importantly, these findings emphasize the need to carefully check for nodules on thoracic MR images of oncology patients.

Extrathoracic metastasis assessment

For evaluation of extrathoracic metastases, CE CT, bone scintigraphy, brain CE MR imaging, and PET or PET/CT have been used in routine clinical practice in accordance with published guidelines or recommendations.[32–35] Whole-body MR imaging has become clinically feasible after the introduction of fast imaging and moving table equipment. Since 2007, it has been regarded as a single, cost-effective imaging test using 1.5- and 3-T systems for patients with not only lung cancer, but also other malignancies.[37,38,47,62–65] Furthermore, whole-body DWI has been recommended as a promising new tool for whole-body MR imaging examination of oncologic patients.[63–65] Comparison of the diagnostic performance of whole-body MR imaging for M-factor assessment with FDG-PET or PET/CT has shown that the diagnostic capability of whole-body MR imaging with or without DWI (sensitivity, 52.0%–80.0%; specificity, 74.3%–94.0%; accuracy, 80.0%–87.7%) was equal to or significantly higher than that of FDG-PET or PET/CT (sensitivity, 48.0%–80.0%; specificity, 74.3%–96%; accuracy, 73.3%–88.2%).[47,62–65] However, one drawback associated with the use of whole-body DWI in this setting needs to be carefully considered. The specificity (87.7%) and accuracy (84.3%) of whole-body DWI alone on a per-patient basis was found to be significantly lower than FDG-PET/CT (specificity, 94.5%; accuracy, 90.4%).[63] Another study found that the diagnostic accuracy of whole-body MR imaging combined with DWI (87.8%) was not significantly different from that of FDG-PET/CT (**Fig. 4**), although that of whole-

Fig. 2. A 73-year-old woman with biopsy-proved adenocarcinoma. (*A*) On thin-section CT, a part solid nodule with a diameter of 12 mm is located in the right middle lobe, and was suspected of being a lung adenocarcinoma. T1-weighted imaging shows low signal intensity (*B*) and T2-weighted imaging shows high intensity (*C*) in the right middle lobe nodule. (*D*) STIR turbo spin echo imaging shows the nodule to have high signal intensity, suspicious for malignancy (true-positive). (*E*) Diffusion-weighted imaging shows high intensity, favoring malignant nodule (true-positive). (*F*) This was also supported by contrast-enhanced T1-weighted imaging, which demonstrates contrast enhancement (true-positive). (*G*) The nodule on dynamic MR imaging with ultrashort TE demonstrates considerable enhancement in the early and late phases (*arrow*) (T = 6.6, 8.8, 11.0, 13.2, and 22.0 seconds). This nodule was diagnosed as malignant on dynamic MR imaging (true-positive). (*H*) FDG-PET/CT shows faint uptake within the nodule (false-negative).

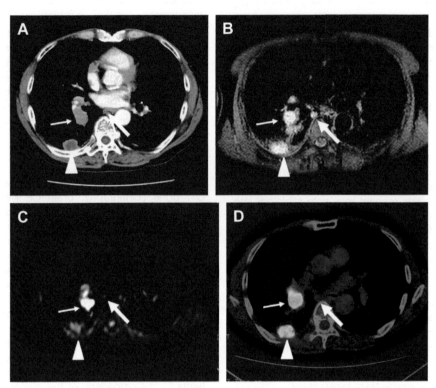

Fig. 3. A 69-year old man with lung cancer proved to have N2 disease. (*A*) Contrast-enhanced CT shows primary lung cancer (*arrowhead*) in the right lower lobe. Right hilar lymph node enlargement (*small arrow*) with a short axis diameter of 13 mm was suspected to be a metastatic lymph node. A subcarinal lymph node (*large arrow*) with a short axis diameter of 5 mm was considered to be a nonmetastatic lymph node. This case was therefore assessed as N1 disease, although the N-stage could not be accurately evaluated. (*B*) STIR turbo spin echo image shows primary lung cancer (*arrowhead*) as a high signal intensity area in the right lower lobe. Right hilar lymph node (*small arrow*) and the subcarinal lymph node (*large arrow*) both appear as high signal intensity areas and were favored to represent metastatic lymph nodes. This case was appropriately assessed as N2 disease on STIR turbo spin echo imaging. (*C*) Diffusion-weighted image shows primary lung cancer (*arrowhead*) as a high signal intensity area in the right lower lobe. Right hilar lymphadenopathy (*small arrow*) appears as a high signal intensity area and was diagnosed as a metastatic lymph node, whereas the subcarinal lymph node (*large arrow*) was not detected because of artifacts. This case was incorrectly downstaged as N1 disease based on diffusion-weighted imaging. (*D*) FDG-PET/CT shows primary lung cancer (*arrowhead*) and right hilar lymphadenopathy (*small arrow*) as high FDG uptake areas, whereas the subcarinal lymph node (*large arrow*) is shown as a low FDG uptake area. This case was incorrectly staged as N1 disease on FDG-PET/CT. The involvement of subcarinal node was confirmed based on pathologic examination.

body MR imaging without DWI (85.8%) was lower than that of FDG-PET/CT.[63] Therefore, it is advisable to use whole-body DWI as part of whole-body MR imaging examination to improve the diagnostic accuracy of M-factor assessment of patients with NSCLC.[37,38,63]

More recently, whole-body PET/MR imaging obtained with a hybrid PET/MR imaging system or presented as PET fused with MR imaging has become clinically feasible (see **Fig. 4**). A few investigators have conducted preliminary tests of its use in patients with lung cancer and reportedly found no significant difference in diagnostic capability between PET/MR imaging and PET/CT for M-factor assessment and for T- and N-factor assessments.[66–68] However, all these studies only assessed FDG uptake and anatomic information from PET/MR imaging data and PET/CT, but not signal intensities on a variety of MR images. It has been shown that with newly developed sequences, whole-body MR imaging on a 3-T MR imaging system can identify recurrence after treatment in patients with lung cancer,[69] similar to PET/CT. However, this study only used whole-body MR imaging and not hybrid PET/MR imaging or PET combined with MR imaging. Therefore, it remains to be seen if evaluation of signal intensity changes at all suspected sites on PET/MR imaging may result in better diagnostic performance than PET/CT in the near future.

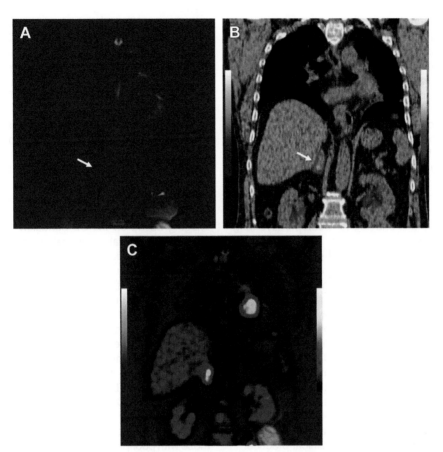

Fig. 4. A 75-year-old man with right adrenal gland metastasis from lung cancer. (*A*) Whole-body STIR turbo spin echo image shows the right adrenal gland to have high signal intensity (*arrow*). FDG-PET/CT (*B*) and whole-body PET/MR imaging (*C*) also show a high FDG uptake area within the right adrenal gland (*arrow*). All modalities are suspicious for right adrenal gland metastasis. However, conspicuity of adrenal gland metastasis is better on PET/MR imaging than whole-body MR imaging and PET/CT.

POSTOPERATIVE LUNG FUNCTION PREDICTION USING MR IMAGING

Primary lung cancer is frequently associated with chronic obstructive pulmonary disease and other cardiopulmonary diseases. Because surgical resection of lung cancer in such cases is associated with high rates of morbidity and mortality, a frequent clinical dilemma is whether lung resection is appropriate for patients with primary lung cancer in specific clinical situations, even if patients are eligible for lung resection. To reach a decision in routine clinical practice, standard lung function tests are currently used with CT and/or nuclear medicine examinations for anatomic or perfusion-based prediction.[35,70–74]

To this end, pulmonary functional MR imaging has been undergoing tests since 2004 and its use has been compared with that of quantitative or qualitative assessment using CT and semiquantitative assessment of perfusion scan, perfusion SPECT, and/or SPECT fused with CT (SPECT/CT). Currently, it has been suggested that two approaches for using MR imaging for the prediction of postoperative lung function can be considered useful: three-dimensional CE perfusion MR imaging,[75–78] and oxygen (O_2)-enhanced MR imaging.[79]

When compared with thin-section CT, perfusion scan, SPECT, and SPECT/CT, the predictive capability of quantitatively assessed three-dimensional CE perfusion MR imaging is better than that of qualitatively assessed thin-section CT, perfusion scan, and perfusion SPECT, and almost the same as that of quantitatively assessed thin-section CT and perfusion SPECT/CT.[76–78] In addition, the discrepancy between actual and predicted postoperative lung function when using three-dimensional CE perfusion MR imaging is reportedly less than 10%, which is small enough for clinical purposes.[76–78] In addition, this technique can use the same dataset used for dynamic CE MR imaging with an ultrashort TE, which is also used for pulmonary nodule assessment and does not require additional examination time. Therefore, when appropriate software and techniques are available, three-dimensional CE perfusion MR imaging should be performed and has the potential to replace perfusion scan, SPECT, and SPECT/CT for perfusion-based prediction of postoperative lung function in the future.

In contrast to the several comparative studies of three-dimensional CE perfusion MR imaging, only one study has reported the predictive capability of O_2-enhanced MR imaging for postoperative lung function in comparison with quantitative and qualitative thin-section CT and perfusion scan.[79] This study found that O_2-enhanced MR imaging showed significant and excellent correlation with actual postoperative lung function ($r \geq 0.90$; $P<.0001$) similar to quantitatively assessed thin-section CT. Also, the correlation coefficients for both techniques were better than those for qualitatively assessed thin-section CT and perfusion scan ($r \leq 0.88$; $P<.0001$). The prediction error for O_2-enhanced MR imaging was almost equal to that for quantitatively assessed thin-section CT, smaller than that for qualitatively assessed thin-section CT and perfusion scan, and small enough for potential implementation in clinical practice.[79] Although further investigation using large prospective cohorts is warranted to determine the real significance of O_2-enhanced MR imaging techniques for this purpose, pulmonary functional MR imaging can be regarded as a promising tool and as a future potential substitute for CT and nuclear medicine examinations for candidates undergoing lung resection.

THERAPEUTIC EFFECT PREDICTION AND ASSESSMENT USING MR IMAGING

The standard evaluation of treatment response in the oncologic field is based on the response evaluation criteria in solid tumors (RECIST), which depends on size changes of tumors on CT.[80] However, several studies have suggested that CE T1WI, dynamic CE MR imaging including perfusion MR imaging technique, and DWI are effective in predicting and evaluating treatment response in thoracic oncology patients.[17,26,81–89]

Based on the results of a previously published hyperthermia study[90] and a paper discussing the use of traditional CE T1WI in patients with lung cancer,[17] traditional CE T1WI, which was used to evaluate changes in tumor size by taking enlargement of the necrosis area into account, was first tested in 2000 for therapeutic response assessment after conservative therapy and was suggested to be useful for this purpose.[81] At that time, however, the use of MR imaging for lung cancer was limited, and the results of this study were not followed up. However, dynamic CE MR imaging was introduced as an effective technique for assessment of tumor angiogenesis,[26] which prompted investigators to evaluate or predict therapeutic effect, prognosis, and recurrence by using semiquantitative or quantitative parameters obtained from CE MR imaging.[81–86,89]

In addition to contrast enhancement evaluation using traditional CE T1WI and dynamic CE MR imaging based on the CE perfusion MR imaging technique, several investigators have reported that ADC is effective in early tumor response evaluation and tumor response prediction.[87–89] Early changes in the ADC were found to correlate significantly with ultimate tumor size reduction.[87] Moreover, patient groups with an increase in ADC showed longer median progression-free and overall survival than the groups with a stable or reduced ADC.[87] Finally, the ADC on DWI reportedly has better potential than maximum standardized uptake value on FDG-PET/CT in distinguishing patients with NSCLC with partial response from those with no change or with disease progression, and in differentiating those with better prognosis from those with poor prognosis.[88] These results suggest that the ADC may be able to function as an imaging-based biomarker for patients with lung cancer.

The promising results of dynamic CE MR imaging and DWI for prediction and treatment response evaluation in lung cancer suggest that parameters provided by these techniques can provide additional information based on biologic behavior of tumors. Changes in tumor vascularity, tissue density, and microstructure result from a variety of therapeutic effects of radiotherapy, chemotherapy, or both. Therefore, standardization of MR imaging sequences, image processing, and semiquantitative or quantitative analyses are warranted to show the real significance of these techniques in this setting, and possibly to use for establishing more accurate response criteria in the not too distant future.

SUMMARY

It has now become possible to routinely use advanced MR imaging systems, fast imaging and/or parallel imaging techniques, superior contrast resolution with and without contrast media, and quantitative and qualitative analyses of MR imaging to answer a variety of clinical questions in patients with lung cancer. It seems, however, that further development of protocols, more clinical trials, and the more widespread use of advanced analysis tools are needed to determine the true significance of MR imaging in patients with lung cancer. In addition, previously and more recently published results indicate that MR imaging may well be able to perform a complementary role or function as a substitute for CT, FDG-PET, PET/CT, and other nuclear medicine examinations. It is hoped that future study results will validate this use of MR imaging.

REFERENCES

1. Siegel R, Naishadham D, Jemal A. Cancer statistics, 2012. CA Cancer J Clin 2012;62:10–29.

2. Melamed MR, Flehinger BJ, Zaman MB. Impact of early detection on the clinical course of lung cancer. Surg Clin North Am 1987;67:909–24.

3. Nahmias C, Hanna WT, Wahl LM, et al. Time course of early response to chemotherapy in non–small cell lung cancer patients with 18F-FDG PET/CT. J Nucl Med 2007;48:744–51.

4. Geddes DM. The natural history of lung cancer: a review based on rates of tumour growth. Br J Dis Chest 1979;73:1–17.

5. Spiro SG, Silvestri GA. One hundred years of lung cancer. Am J Respir Crit Care Med 2005;172:523–9.

6. Allen MS, Darling GE, Pechet TT, et al, ACOSOG Z0030 Study Group. Morbidity and mortality of major pulmonary resections in patients with early-stage lung cancer: initial results of the randomized, prospective ACOSOG Z0030 trial. Ann Thorac Surg 2006;81:1013–9.

7. National Lung Screening Trial Research Team, Aberle DR, Adams AM, et al. Reduced lung-cancer mortality with low-dose computed tomographic screening. N Engl J Med 2011;365:395–409.

8. Sakai F, Sone S, Maruyama A, et al. Thin-rim enhancement in Gd-DTPA-enhanced magnetic resonance images of tuberculoma: a new finding of potential differential diagnostic importance. J Thorac Imaging 1992;7:64–9.

9. Sakai F, Sone S, Kiyono K, et al. MR of pulmonary hamartoma: pathologic correlation. J Thorac Imaging 1994;9(1):51–5.

10. Fujimoto K, Meno S, Nishimura H, et al. Aspergilloma within cavitary lung cancer: MR imaging findings. AJR Am J Roentgenol 1994;163(3):565–7.

11. Blum U, Windfuhr M, Buitrago-Tellez C, et al. Invasive pulmonary aspergillosis. MRI, CT, and plain radiographic findings and their contribution for early diagnosis. Chest 1994;106(4):1156–61.

12. Chung MH, Lee HG, Kwon SS, et al. MR imaging of solitary pulmonary lesion: emphasis on tuberculomas and comparison with tumors. J Magn Reson Imaging 2000;11(6):629–37.

13. Gaeta M, Minutoli F, Ascenti G, et al. MR white lung sign: incidence and significance in pulmonary consolidations. J Comput Assist Tomogr 2001;25(6):890–6.

14. Gaeta M, Vinci S, Minutoli F, et al. CT and MRI findings of mucin-containing tumors and pseudotumors of the thorax: pictorial review. Eur Radiol 2002;12(1):181–9.

15. Ohno Y, Sugimura K, Hatabu H. MR imaging of lung cancer. Eur J Radiol 2002;44(3):172–81.

16. Sieren JC, Ohno Y, Koyama H, et al. Recent technological and application developments in computed tomography and magnetic resonance imaging for improved pulmonary nodule detection and lung cancer staging. J Magn Reson Imaging 2010;32(6):1353–69.

17. Kono M, Adachi S, Kusumoto M, et al. Clinical utility of Gd-DTPA-enhanced magnetic resonance imaging in lung cancer. J Thorac Imaging 1993;8(1):18–26.

18. Kusumoto M, Kono M, Adachi S, et al. Gadopentate-dimeglumine-enhanced magnetic resonance imaging for lung nodules. Differentiation of lung cancer and tuberculoma. Invest Radiol 1994;29(Suppl 2):S255–6.

19. Koyama H, Ohno Y, Kono A, et al. Quantitative and qualitative assessment of non-contrast-enhanced pulmonary MR imaging for management of pulmonary nodules in 161 subjects. Eur Radiol 2008; 18(10):2120–31.

20. Mori T, Nomori H, Ikeda K, et al. Diffusion-weighted magnetic resonance imaging for diagnosing malignant pulmonary nodules/masses: comparison with positron emission tomography. J Thorac Oncol 2008;3(4):358–64.

21. Satoh S, Kitazume Y, Ohdama S, et al. Can malignant and benign pulmonary nodules be differentiated with diffusion-weighted MRI? AJR Am J Roentgenol 2008;191(2):464–70.

22. Uto T, Takehara Y, Nakamura Y, et al. Higher sensitivity and specificity for diffusion-weighted imaging of malignant lung lesions without apparent diffusion coefficient quantification. Radiology 2009;252(1):247–54.

23. Cronin P, Dwamena BA, Kelly AM, et al. Solitary pulmonary nodules: meta-analytic comparison of cross-sectional imaging modalities for diagnosis of malignancy. Radiology 2008;246(3):772–82.

24. Guckel C, Schnabel K, Deimling M, et al. Solitary pulmonary nodules: MR evaluation of enhancement patterns with contrast-enhanced dynamic snapshot gradient-echo imaging. Radiology 1996;200(3):681–6.

25. Ohno Y, Hatabu H, Takenaka D, et al. Solitary pulmonary nodules: potential role of dynamic MR imaging in management initial experience. Radiology 2002; 224(2):503–11.

26. Fujimoto K, Abe T, Muller NL, et al. Small peripheral pulmonary carcinomas evaluated with dynamic MR

imaging: correlation with tumor vascularity and prognosis. Radiology 2003;227(3):786–93.

27. Ohno Y, Hatabu H, Takenaka D, et al. Dynamic MR imaging: value of differentiating subtypes of peripheral small adenocarcinoma of the lung. Eur J Radiol 2004;52(2):144–50.

28. Schaefer JF, Vollmar J, Schick F, et al. Solitary pulmonary nodules: dynamic contrast-enhanced MR imaging–perfusion differences in malignant and benign lesions. Radiology 2004;232(2):544–53.

29. Kono R, Fujimoto K, Terasaki H, et al. Dynamic MRI of solitary pulmonary nodules: comparison of enhancement patterns of malignant and benign small peripheral lung lesions. AJR Am J Roentgenol 2007;188(1):26–36.

30. Ohno Y, Koyama H, Takenaka D, et al. Dynamic MRI, dynamic multidetector-row computed tomography (MDCT), and coregistered 2-[fluorine-18]-fluoro-2-deoxy-D-glucose-positron emission tomography (FDG-PET)/CT: comparative study of capability for management of pulmonary nodules. J Magn Reson Imaging 2008;27(6):1284–95.

31. Ohno Y, Nishio M, Koyama H, et al. Dynamic contrast-enhanced CT and MRI for pulmonary nodule assessment. AJR Am J Roentgenol 2014;202:515–29.

32. Gámez C, Rosell R, Fernández A, et al. PET/CT fusion scan in lung cancer: current recommendations and innovations. J Thorac Oncol 2006;1:74–7.

33. Silvestri GA, Gould MK, Margolis ML, et al, American College of Chest Physicians. Noninvasive staging of non-small cell lung cancer: ACCP evidenced-based clinical practice guidelines (2nd edition). Chest 2007;132:178S–201S.

34. Samson DJ, Seidenfeld J, Simon GR, et al, American College of Chest Physicians. Evidence for management of small cell lung cancer: ACCP evidence-based clinical practice guidelines (2nd edition). Chest 2007;132:314S–23S.

35. Silvestri GA, Gonzalez AV, Jantz MA, et al. Methods for staging non-small cell lung cancer: diagnosis and management of lung cancer, 3rd ed: American College of Chest Physicians evidence-based clinical practice guidelines. Chest 2013;143:e211S–50S.

36. Webb WR, Gatsonis C, Zerhouni EA, et al. CT and MR imaging in staging non-small cell bronchogenic carcinoma: report of the radiologic diagnostic oncology group. Radiology 1991;178(3):705–13.

37. Koyama H, Ohno Y, Seki S, et al. Magnetic resonance imaging for lung cancer. J Thorac Imaging 2013;28:138–50.

38. Ohno Y. New applications of magnetic resonance imaging for thoracic oncology. Semin Respir Crit Care Med 2014;35:27–40.

39. Sakai S, Murayama S, Murakami J, et al. Bronchogenic carcinoma invasion of the chest wall: evaluation with dynamic cine MRI during breathing. J Comput Assist Tomogr 1997;21(4):595–600.

40. Murata K, Takahashi M, Mori M, et al. Chest wall and mediastinal invasion by lung cancer: evaluation with multisection expiratory dynamic CT. Radiology 1994; 191(1):251–5.

41. Takahashi K, Furuse M, Hanaoka H, et al. Pulmonary vein and left atrial invasion by lung cancer: assessment by breath-hold gadolinium-enhanced three-dimensional MR angiography. J Comput Assist Tomogr 2000;24:557–61.

42. Ohno Y, Adachi S, Motoyama A, et al. Multiphase ECG-triggered 3D contrast-enhanced MR angiography: utility for evaluation of hilar and mediastinal invasion of bronchogenic carcinoma. J Magn Reson Imaging 2001;13:215–24.

43. Boiselle PM, Patz EF Jr, Vining DJ, et al. Imaging of mediastinal lymph nodes: CT, MR, and FDG PET. Radiographics 1998;18:1061–9.

44. Takenaka D, Ohno Y, Hatabu H, et al. Differentiation of metastatic versus non-metastatic mediastinal lymph nodes in patients with non-small cell lung cancer using respiratory-triggered short inversion time inversion recovery (STIR) turbo spin-echo MR imaging. Eur J Radiol 2002;44(3):216–24.

45. Ohno Y, Hatabu H, Takenaka D, et al. Metastases in mediastinal and hilar lymph nodes in patients with non-small cell lung cancer: quantitative and qualitative assessment with STIR turbo spin-echo MR imaging. Radiology 2004;231(3):872–9.

46. Ohno Y, Koyama H, Nogami M, et al. STIR turbo SE MR imaging vs. coregistered FDG-PET/CT: quantitative and qualitative assessment of N-stage in non-small-cell lung cancer patients. J Magn Reson Imaging 2007;26(4):1071–80.

47. Yi CA, Shin KM, Lee KS, et al. Non-small cell lung cancer staging: efficacy comparison of integrated PET/CT versus 3.0-T whole-body MR imaging. Radiology 2008;248(2):632–42.

48. Morikawa M, Demura Y, Ishizaki T, et al. The effectiveness of 18F-FDG PET/CT combined with STIR MRI for diagnosing nodal involvement in the thorax. J Nucl Med 2009;50(1):81–7.

49. Ohno Y, Koyama H, Yoshikawa T, et al. N stage disease in patients with non-small cell lung cancer: efficacy of quantitative and qualitative assessment with STIR turbo spin-echo imaging, diffusion-weighted MR imaging, and fluorodeoxyglucose PET/CT. Radiology 2011;261(2):605–15.

50. Nomori H, Mori T, Ikeda K, et al. Diffusion-weighted magnetic resonance imaging can be used in place of positron emission tomography for N staging of non-small cell lung cancer with fewer false-positive results. J Thorac Cardiovasc Surg 2008;135(4):816–22.

51. Hasegawa I, Boiselle PM, Kuwabara K, et al. Mediastinal lymph nodes in patients with non-small cell lung cancer: preliminary experience with diffusion-weighted MR imaging. J Thorac Imaging 2008; 23(3):157–61.

52. Pauls S, Schmidt SA, Juchems MS, et al. Diffusion-weighted MR imaging in comparison to integrated [18F]-FDG PET/CT for N-staging in patients with lung cancer. Eur J Radiol 2012;81(1):178–82.

53. Feuerstein IM, Jicha DL, Pass HI, et al. Pulmonary metastases: MR imaging with surgical correlation. A prospective study. Radiology 1992;182:123–9.

54. Kersjes W, Mayer E, Buchenroth M, et al. Diagnosis of pulmonary metastases with turbo-SE MR imaging. Eur Radiol 1997;7:1190–4.

55. Schroeder T, Ruehm SG, Debatin JF, et al. Detection of pulmonary nodules using a 2D HASTE MR sequence: comparison with MDCT. AJR Am J Roentgenol 2005; 185:979–84.

56. Both M, Schultze J, Reuter M, et al. Fast T1- and T2-weighted pulmonary MR-imaging in patients with bronchial carcinoma. Eur J Radiol 2005;53:478–88.

57. Regier M, Kandel S, Kaul MG, et al. Detection of small pulmonary nodules in high-field MR at 3 T: evaluation of different pulse sequences using porcine lung explants. Eur Radiol 2007;17:1341–51.

58. Bruegel M, Gaa J, Woertler K, et al. MRI of the lung: value of different turbo spin-echo, single-shot turbo spin-echo, and 3D gradient-echo pulse sequences for the detection of pulmonary metastases. J Magn Reson Imaging 2007;25:73–81.

59. Yi CA, Jeon TY, Lee KS, et al. 3-T MRI: usefulness for evaluating primary lung cancer and small nodules in lobes not containing primary tumors. AJR Am J Roentgenol 2007;189:386–92.

60. Frericks BB, Meyer BC, Martus P, et al. MRI of the thorax during whole-body MRI: evaluation of different MR sequences and comparison to thoracic multidetector computed tomography (MDCT). J Magn Reson Imaging 2008;27:538–45.

61. Sommer G, Tremper J, Koenigkam-Santos M, et al. Lung nodule detection in a high-risk population: comparison of magnetic resonance imaging and low-dose computed tomography. Eur J Radiol 2014;83:600–5.

62. Ohno Y, Koyama H, Nogami M, et al. Whole-body MR imaging vs. FDG-PET: comparison of accuracy of M-stage diagnosis for lung cancer patients. J Magn Reson Imaging 2007;26(3):498–509.

63. Ohno Y, Koyama H, Onishi Y, et al. Non-small cell lung cancer: whole-body MR examination for M-stage assessment–utility for whole-body diffusion-weighted imaging compared with integrated FDG PET/CT. Radiology 2008;248(2):643–54.

64. Takenaka D, Ohno Y, Matsumoto K, et al. Detection of bone metastases in non-small cell lung cancer patients: comparison of whole-body diffusion-weighted imaging (DWI), whole-body MR imaging without and with DWI, whole-body FDG-PET/CT, and bone scintigraphy. J Magn Reson Imaging 2009;30(2):298–308.

65. Sommer G, Wiese M, Winter L, et al. Preoperative staging of non-small-cell lung cancer: comparison of whole-body diffusion-weighted magnetic resonance imaging and 18F-fluorodeoxyglucose-positron emission tomography/computed tomography. Eur Radiol 2012;22(12):2859–67.

66. Schwenzer NF, Schraml C, Müller M, et al. Pulmonary lesion assessment: comparison of whole-body hybrid MR/PET and PET/CT imaging–pilot study. Radiology 2012;264:551–8.

67. Kohan AA, Kolthammer JA, Vercher-Conejero JL, et al. N staging of lung cancer patients with PET/MRI using a three-segment model attenuation correction algorithm: initial experience. Eur Radiol 2013;23:3161–9.

68. Heusch P, Buchbender C, Köhler J, et al. Thoracic staging in lung cancer: prospective comparison of 18F-FDG PET/MR imaging and 18F-FDG PET/CT. J Nucl Med 2014;55:373–8.

69. Ohno Y, Nishio M, Koyama H, et al. Comparison of the utility of whole-body MRI with and without contrast-enhanced Quick 3D and double RF fat suppression techniques, conventional whole-body MRI, PET/CT and conventional examination for assessment of recurrence in NSCLC patients. Eur J Radiol 2013;82:2018–27.

70. Pierce RJ, Copland JM, Sharpe K, et al. Preoperative risk evaluation for lung cancer resection: predicted postoperative product as a predictor of surgical mortality. Am J Respir Crit Care Med 1994;150:947–55.

71. Bolliger CT, Jordan P, Solèr M, et al. Exercise capacity as a predictor of postoperative complications in lung resection candidates. Am J Respir Crit Care Med 1995;151:1472–80.

72. Wyser C, Stulz P, Soler M, et al. Prospective evaluation of an algorithm for the functional assessment of lung resection candidates. Am J Respir Crit Care Med 1999;159:1450–6.

73. Mazzone PJ, Arroliga AC. Lung cancer: preoperative pulmonary evaluation of the lung resection candidate. Am J Med 2005;118:578–83.

74. Colice GL, Shafazand S, Griffin JP, et al, American College of Chest Physicians. Physiologic evaluation of the patient with lung cancer being considered for resectional surgery: ACCP evidenced-based clinical practice guidelines (2nd edition). Chest 2007;132(3 Suppl):161S–77S.

75. Iwasawa T, Saito K, Ogawa N, et al. Prediction of postoperative pulmonary function using perfusion magnetic resonance imaging of the lung. J Magn Reson Imaging 2002;15:685–92.

76. Ohno Y, Hatabu H, Higashino T, et al. Dynamic perfusion MRI versus perfusion scintigraphy: prediction of postoperative lung function in patients with lung cancer. AJR Am J Roentgenol 2004;182:73–8.

77. Ohno Y, Koyama H, Nogami M, et al. Postoperative lung function in lung cancer patients: comparative analysis of predictive capability of MRI, CT, and SPECT. AJR Am J Roentgenol 2007;189:400–8.

78. Ohno Y, Koyama H, Nogami M, et al. State-of-the-art radiological techniques improve the assessment of postoperative lung function in patients with non-small cell lung cancer. Eur J Radiol 2011;77:97–104.

79. Ohno Y, Hatabu H, Higashino T, et al. Oxygen-enhanced MR imaging: correlation with postsurgical lung function in patients with lung cancer. Radiology 2005;236:704–11.

80. Eisenhauer EA, Therasse P, Bogaerts J, et al. New response evaluation criteria in solid tumours: revised RECIST guideline (version 1.1). Eur J Cancer 2009; 45:228–47.

81. Ohno Y, Adachi S, Kono M, et al. Predicting the prognosis of non-small cell lung cancer patient treated with conservative therapy using contrast-enhanced MR imaging. Eur Radiol 2000;10:1770–81.

82. Ohno Y, Nogami M, Higashino T, et al. Prognostic value of dynamic MR imaging for non-small-cell lung cancer patients after chemoradiotherapy. J Magn Reson Imaging 2005;21:775–83.

83. de Langen AJ, van den Boogaart V, Lubberink M, et al. Monitoring response to antiangiogenic therapy in non-small cell lung cancer using imaging markers derived from PET and dynamic contrast-enhanced MRI. J Nucl Med 2011;52:48–55.

84. Giesel FL, Bischoff H, von Tengg-Kobligk H, et al. Dynamic contrast-enhanced MRI of malignant pleural mesothelioma: a feasibility study of noninvasive assessment, therapeutic follow-up, and possible predictor of improved outcome. Chest 2006;129:1570–6.

85. Giesel FL, Choyke PL, Mehndiratta A, et al. Pharmacokinetic analysis of malignant pleural mesothelioma-initial results of tumor microcirculation and its correlation to microvessel density (CD-34). Acad Radiol 2008;15:563–70.

86. Kelly RJ, Rajan A, Force J, et al. Evaluation of KRAS mutations, angiogenic biomarkers, and DCE-MRI in patients with advanced non-small-cell lung cancer receiving sorafenib. Clin Cancer Res 2011;17: 1190–9.

87. Yabuuchi H, Hatakenaka M, Takayama K, et al. Non-small cell lung cancer: detection of early response to chemotherapy by using contrast-enhanced dynamic and diffusion-weighted MR imaging. Radiology 2011;261:598–604.

88. Ohno Y, Koyama H, Yoshikawa T, et al. Diffusion-weighted MRI versus 18F-FDG PET/CT: performance as predictors of tumor treatment response and patient survival in patients with non-small cell lung cancer receiving chemoradiotherapy. AJR Am J Roentgenol 2012;198:75–82.

89. Nishino M, Hatabu H, Johnson BE, et al. State of the art: response assessment in lung cancer in the era of genomic medicine. Radiology 2014;271:6–27.

90. Hiraoka M, Akuta K, Nishimura Y, et al. Tumor response to thermoradiation therapy: use of CT in evaluation. Radiology 1987;164:259–62.

PET/MR Imaging for Chest Diseases

Review of Initial Studies on Pulmonary Nodules and Lung Cancers

Soon Ho Yoon, MD[a], Jin Mo Goo, MD, PhD[a,b,*], Sang Min Lee, MD[a], Chang Min Park, MD, PhD[a,b], Gi Jeong Cheon, MD, PhD[b,c]

KEYWORDS

- Hybrid imaging • PET • MR imaging • Lung cancer • Lung lesion detection • Lung cancer staging

KEY POINTS

- Integrated PET/MR imaging systems for the evaluation of lung cancer may be feasible owing to the development of new hardware systems with MR attenuation correction.
- PET/MR imaging showed highly correlated standardized uptake values of lesions and equivalent performance in terms of lesion detection and staging when compared with PET/CT according to several initial studies on this new hybrid modality.
- The synergistic benefits of integrated PET/MR imaging beyond simply adding the capabilities of the 2 modalities need to be validated with dedicated, time-efficient PET/MR imaging protocols.

INTRODUCTION

Multimodality imaging can be a powerful tool for the simultaneous evaluation of both anatomic and functional information and may potentially improve patient management, leading to better patient outcomes. The strengths of multimodality imaging have already been proven by the introduction of PET/computed tomography (CT) systems in oncologic imaging, which have enormously contributed to better diagnosis, treatment, and prediction of prognosis in cancer.[1,2] Indeed, the PET/CT system has become a vital imaging modality in the evaluation of lung cancers often preferred over previous conventional staging methods.[3–5] Recently, a new multimodality imaging combining PET and MR Imaging has been proposed as an alternative to PET/CT because it offers various kinds of contrast resolutions, which can reflect cellular density, perfusion, hypoxia, as well as metabolic features in addition to its inherent advantages of not requiring radiation exposure.[6,7] However, it is unclear as of yet whether the PET/MR imaging system can truly offer better diagnostic performance compared with the PET/CT system for chest diseases, particularly lung cancer, because there are considerable obstacles in pulmonary MR imaging owing to the low proton density of air, large magnetic inhomogeneity in the lung parenchyma, and cardiac and respiratory motion.[8] Although the underlying difficulties in pulmonary MR imaging have not yet been fully resolved, various designs of PET/MR imaging systems have already been implemented

This work was supported in part by a grant from Guerbet Korea.
[a] Department of Radiology, Institute of Radiation Medicine, Seoul National University Medical Research Center, Seoul National University College of Medicine, Seoul, Korea; [b] Cancer Research Institute, Seoul National University College of Medicine, Seoul, Korea; [c] Department of Nuclear Medicine, Seoul National University College of Medicine, Seoul, Korea
* Corresponding author. 101 Daehangno, Jongno-gu, Seoul 110-744, Korea.
E-mail address: jmgoo@plaza.snu.ac.kr

mri.theclinics.com

with several preliminary studies having been published on chest diseases. In this review, the PET/MR imaging system is briefly introduced and a series of recently published initial studies is reviewed to allow readers to better comprehend and specify the expected role of the PET/MR imaging system for chest diseases.

TECHNICAL ASPECTS OF PET/MR IMAGING
Hardware Design

Early generations of PET/MR imaging systems included the usage of software developed for the spatial registration of PET and MR images were acquired in 2 completely separate systems.[6] Although varying degrees of success have been achieved using many different computation algorithms,[9,10] this system suffered from innate limitations (ie, the bulk position of the patient's body tended to differ between PET and MR scanning as the patient was required to move and lie in different beds for PET and MR scanning, and there was an unavoidable temporal mismatch in the acquired images). Thus, to develop an integrated PET/MR imaging system that can overcome these limitations, modifications of the PET subsystem was necessary to make it insensitive to the strong magnetic fields of the MR imaging subsystem.[11]

Sequential System

To mitigate different body positioning required between the separate PET and MR imaging scanning, the sharing of a patient bed with sequential allocation of PET and MR imaging systems nearby was adopted for a new generation of PET/MR imaging systems, either in the same space (Ingenuity TF; Philips Healthcare, Best, Netherlands) or in 2 separate spaces (Discovery PET/CT and MR imaging system; GE Healthcare, Milwaukee, WI, USA). This secondary strategy also allowed a decrease in the temporal differences between PET and MR scanning because scanning was performed sequentially with a minimum delay for the movement of the patient bed. The Discovery PET/CT and MR imaging system adopted a trimodality system combining both PET/CT and MR imaging systems, and the Ingenuity TF system omitted the CT component of the PET/CT system and combined only the PET component with the MR imaging machine. The latter system was able to reduce the radiation dose compared with the trimodality system at the expense of CT-based attenuation correction and by using MR-based attenuation correction instead. With this evolution of PET/MR imaging systems, temporal and spatial mismatches were decreased compared with previous coregistered PET/MR images; however, sequential PET/MR imaging systems still were not free of temporal and spatial misalignments.[7]

Simultaneous System

Thus, there were 3 major challenges for the integration of the PET/MR imaging scanner into a single gantry. First, a magnetic field–insensitive photodetector was warranted because the photomultiplier tube used in pre-existing PET detectors was vulnerable to static, gradient magnetic fields, and abrupt changes in radiofrequency signals. Second, PET detectors mounted within MR scanners should not interfere with any MR signal or magnetic field gradient. Third, simultaneous acquisition of PET and MR images should be possible without mutual interference. Among these major technical difficulties, designing a PET system using avalanche photodiodes (APDs), which is a photodetector insensitive to magnetic fields, was the most crucial hurdle that needed to be cleared to enable the integration of the PET/MR imaging system. Recently, Biograph mMR (Siemens Healthcare, Erlangen, Germany), a fully integrated system using APDs in which PET and MR imaging scanning can be performed simultaneously, was developed. In addition, as time-of-flight (TOF) PET is not yet possible in PET systems using APDs, despite its magnetic insensitivity, a whole-body TOF PET/MR imaging system using a silicon photomultiplier detector has been also introduced recently (Signa PET/MR imaging; GE Healthcare). Theoretically, TOF should be able to improve the image quality of PET with higher structural detail and provide a better signal-to-noise ratio. Compared with the sequential type of arrangement, simultaneous PET/MR imaging systems have merits in minimizing potential anatomic and temporal mismatches and thus can offer more robust interpretation of PET/MR images.[7]

MR-based attenuation correction
Another important factor is the accurate attenuation correction of photons emitted from radiotracers throughout the body so as to quantify the activity concentration of radiotracers used in the PET system. As attenuation of the emitted photon occurs inhomogeneously according to the characteristics and heterogeneities of body tissue, an attenuation map needs to be created for quantification by assigning continuous attenuation coefficients. In the PET/CT system, linear attenuation coefficients of emitted photons at 511 keV can be assessed by converting the Hounsfield units of CT images. However, there is no direct relationship between the attenuation of emitted photons and the signal intensity on MR images.[12] The currently used strategy of MR attenuation

correction is image segmentation of body parts into 4 tissue classes using the Dixon-based MR sequence. MR images provided by the Dixon-based MR sequence enables the separation of the background, lung, fat, and soft tissue through the chemical shift phenomenon of fatty tissue relative to that of water.[13] Thereafter, an attenuation map of the body is created by assigning fixed values to the segmented tissue while ignoring the tissue heterogeneities in segmented areas.

Alignment

Robust anatomic registration between different imaging modalities is imperative to provide both anatomic and functional information of a disease. Voluntary as well as involuntary physiologic movements in the body are potential sources hampering correct alignment. The thorax is one of the most vulnerable body parts to misalignment because of cardiac motion and respiration. Although a conjunction of the CT and PET system enabled better anatomic registration and localization of abnormalities in addition to attenuation correction, sequential acquisitions followed by image registration of the PET/CT system was a fundamental limitation subject to errors in obtaining an exact alignment. As an example, curvilinear cold artifacts paralleling the dome of the diaphragm and misregistration of pulmonary lesions located in

the basal lung are well-known limitations that are difficult to avoid with the PET/CT system.[14] Because simultaneous image acquisition and registration would be the ideal strategy to fuse images acquired by different imaging modalities, the hybrid PET/MR imaging system is expected to have the potential to improve spatial registration (**Fig. 1**).

Three studies[15–17] have quantitatively analyzed the alignment of pulmonary malignancies or thoracic landmarks on hybrid PET/MR systems. Rakheja and colleagues[15] evaluated 6 pulmonary metastases and showed that not only radial volume-interpolated breath-hold examination (VIBE) but also short tau inversion recovery (STIR) sequences with axial free-breathing acquisition provided more accurate alignment than did PET/CT images (differences in distance of the isocenter; PET/VIBE image, 3.2 ± 1.5 mm; PET/STIR image, 2.3 ± 0.7 mm; PET/CT image, 5.5 ± 3.5 mm). In the study by Brendle and colleagues,[17] the alignment of either pulmonary malignancies or thoracic landmarks in 15 patients did not differ significantly between free-breathing PET/STIR and PET/CT images but differed significantly on co-registered PET/MR image (mean cumulative misalignments; PET/STIR image, 7.7 mm; PET/CT image, 7.0 mm; co-registered PET/MR image, 17.1 mm). Finally, Brendle and colleagues[17]

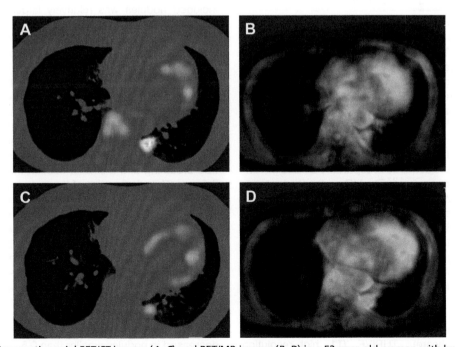

Fig. 1. Consecutive axial PET/CT images (*A, C*) and PET/MR images (*B, D*) in a 53-year-old woman with lung cancer in the left lower lobe. The location showing maximum metabolic uptake on PET image was the upper part of the nodule (*A*) rather than the center of nodule (*C*) as seen on CT image. Spatial registration was improved on PET/MR images (*B, D*) correctly matching the location showing maximum metabolic uptake with the center of the nodule.

reported that the anatomic registration of thoracic landmarks was more accurate with the free-breathing or expiratory breath-hold MR sequence than with the inspiratory MR sequence. In addition, the anatomic registration of the liver and spleen adjacent to the basal lung was similar between PET/STIR and PET/CT images but was significantly inferior in co-registered PET/MR images (mean cumulative misalignments of the liver and spleen; PET/STIR image, 6.3 and 7.2 mm; PET/CT image, 7.6 and 7.4 mm; co-registered PET/MR image, 13.1 and 11.7 mm).

INITIAL PET/MR IMAGING STUDIES OF CHEST DISEASE: A REVIEW

As there is only limited experience with the PET/MR imaging system for chest diseases, the authors reviewed PET/MR imaging studies to minimize the gap between theoretic expectations and preliminary observations. They performed a literature search of the MEDLINE and EMBASE databases to identify relevant publications on PET/MR imaging primarily focusing on chest disease using the keywords related with PET/MR, MR/PET, and lung, updated until July 2014. They supplemented their literature search by screening bibliographies of the retrieved publications as well as those of review articles.

Characteristics of the Included Studies

There were 12 studies evaluating chest diseases using co-registered or integrated PET/MR imaging systems (Table 1).[16,18–28] The primary focus of the studies was either detection of pulmonary nodules or the staging of lung cancers. The sample size for the integrated PET/MR imaging system was relatively small in all studies, ranging from 10 to 32.[16,19–24,26,28] On the contrary, the study population was larger in the studies dealing with co-registered PET/MR imaging systems, where the images were acquired in separate PET and MR imaging systems.[18,25,27] The MR protocol adopted in the PET/MR imaging studies for chest disease varied across the studies with the majority evaluating basic MR sequences for routine body imaging rather than dedicated MR sequences for pulmonary imaging, except for a series of studies in the same center.[21,22,26] The most frequently adopted MR sequence was a 3-dimensional (3D) T1-weighted spoiled gradient-recalled echo (GRE) sequence such as VIBE (Siemens Healthcare), liver acquisition with volume acceleration (LAVA; GE Healthcare), THRIVE (T1 high-resolution isotropic volume excitation; Philips Healthcare), or quick 3D (Toshiba Medical Systems, Tokyo, Japan). T1-weighted MR sequences in earlier studies were usually performed without contrast enhancement. Most studies performed PET/CT scanning first with subsequent PET/MR imaging scanning in the same patient, allowing a direct comparison of the PET/CT and PET/MR imaging systems except in one randomized 2-arm controlled study.[25] As the study populations in a series of PET/MR imaging studies were recruited in the same hospital, some of the included patients of earlier studies[21,22] may have overlapped with those in later studies.[26]

Detection, Size Measurement, and Interpretation of Pulmonary Nodules

Three studies evaluated the detectability of pulmonary nodules in sequential[24] and hybrid PET/MR imaging systems.[20,24] Although all of the studies adopted the 3D T1-weighted spoiled GRE sequence, interpretation of the results of those studies was not straightforward because details were inhomogeneous in terms of section thickness, use of contrast, and acquisition method, along with differences in the size distribution of the nodules.

Stolzmann and colleagues[24] evaluated the noncontrast-enhanced axial T1-weighted Dixon-base LAVA sequence with 6.8-mm section thickness and expiratory breath-hold on a sequential PET/MR imaging system. The median size of the included nodules was relatively larger than the other 2 studies (see Table 1). The detectability of this MR sequence was 87.9% (58/66) for all nodules, 97.2% (35/36) for fluorodeoxyglucose (FDG)-positive nodules, and 76.7 (23/30) for FDG-negative nodules. Chandarana and colleagues[20] used a unique state-of-the-art MR sequence on a hybrid PET/MR imaging system: noncontrast axial T1-weighted VIBE with radial K-space sampling, which is relatively robust against motion artifact. This sequence enabled MR image acquisition with free-breathing and a smaller section thickness of 2.5 mm. The median size of the included nodules was less than 1 cm in diameter, smallest among the 3 studies. The detectability of this MR sequence was 62.3% (43/69) for all nodules, 80.0% (36/45) for FDG-positive nodules, and 29.2% (7/24) for FDG-negative nodules. When evaluated with PET/MR fusion images, the detectability increased by up to 10% except in the case of FDG-negative nodules: 70.3% (97/138) for all nodules; 95.6% (86/90) for FDG-positive nodules; and 22.9% (11/48) for FDG-negative nodules. The detectability decreased in nodules smaller than 0.5 cm (38.0% [19/50]) compared with nodules 0.5 cm or larger in diameter (88.6% [78/88]). Rauscher and colleagues[28] performed a contrast-enhanced axial

Table 1
Baseline characteristics of PET/MR imaging studies on chest disease

Sources	Primary Focus	Machine	Patient No.[a]	Lesion No.	Lesion Distribution	MR Sequences
Morikawa et al,[18] 2009, University of Fukui	Lung cancer	Coregistered PET/1.5T MR	93	137	1.7 ± 0.5 cm	Axial STIR with electrocardiographically triggering
Schwenzer et al,[19] 2012, Eberhard-Karls University	Lung cancer	Biograph mMR	10	10	Stage I, 40%; II, 30%; III, 20%; IV, 10%	Non-CE coronal T1w GRE Dixon[b] Non-CE axial T1w VIBE, Coronal STIR
Stolzmann et al,[24] 2013, University Hospital Zurich	Pulmonary nodule	Discovery PET/CT + MR	34	66	Median, 1.8 cm (range, 0.2–6.9 cm)	Non-CE axial T1w LAVA Dixon
Schmidt et al,[16] 2013, Eberhard Karls University	Lung cancer	Biograph mMR	14	14	NS	Non-CE coronal T1w GRE Dixon[b] Coronal STIR, axial SS EPI DWI with FS
Heusch et al,[21] 2013, University Dusseldorf	Lung cancer	Biograph mMR	15	15	NS	Dedicated pulmonary MR sequences[c]
Yi et al,[25] 2013, Sungkyunkwan University School of Medicine	Lung cancer	Coregistered PET/1.5T MR	263	263	Stage I, 60%; II, 27%; IIIA, 13%	Axial T2w HASTE with FS and cardiac gating, SS EPI DWI with FS, CE T1w SE
Kohan et al,[23] 2013, Case Western Reserve University	Lung cancer	Ingenuity TF	11	11	NS	Non-CE coronal 3D T1w GRE[b]
Heusch et al,[22] 2013, University Dusseldorf	Lung cancer	Biograph mMR	18	18	NS	Dedicated pulmonary MR sequences[c]
Chandarana et al,[20] 2013, New York Medical College	Pulmonary nodule	Biograph mMR	32	69	Median, <1 cm (70%, <1 cm)	Non-CE axial radial T1w VIBE with FS
Heusch et al,[26] 2014, University Dusseldorf	Lung cancer	Biograph mMR	22	22	4.3 ± 2.7 cm	Dedicated pulmonary MR sequences[c]
Rauscher et al,[28] 2014, Technische Universität München	Pulmonary nodule	Biograph mMR	25	47	1.0 ± 1.1 cm (range, 0.2–6.0 cm)	Non-CE coronal T1w GRE Dixon[b] CE axial T1w VIBE with FS,
Ohno et al,[27] 2014, Kobe University Graduate School of Medicine	Lung cancer	Coregistered PET/3-T MR	70	70	Stage I, 41%; II, 31%; III, 16%; IV, 11%	Non-CE & CE coronal T1 Quick 3D with double FS, STIR

Abbreviations: CE, contrast-enhanced; FS, fat suppression; HASTE, half-Fourier acquisition with single-shot turbo spin echo; SE, spin echo; SS EPI, single-shot spin echo echo-planar imaging; T1w, T1-weighted; T2w, T2-weighted; TSE, turbo spin echo.
[a] Numbers of patients included for analysis.
[b] This MR sequence was performed for MR attenuation correction rather than anatomic evaluation.
[c] Dedicated pulmonary MR sequences included the non-CE coronal T1w GRE Dixon sequence, coronal T2w steady-state free precession sequence, axial T2w blade turbo SE sequence, axial SS EPI DWI, axial T1w fast low-angle shot GRE sequence, coronal T2w HASTE sequence, non-CE, CE coronal T1w VIBE sequence, axial T1w fast low-angle shot GRE with FS, and coronal STIR sequence.
Data from Refs.[16,18–28]

T1-weighted VIBE sequence with 5-mm section thickness and expiratory breath-hold on a hybrid PET/MR imaging system. The mean size of the included nodules was 1.0 cm. Their detectability was 61.7% (29/47) and was smaller for nodules less than 1 cm (45.4% [15/32]) compared with nodules 1 cm or larger (100% [14/14]).

With regard to the size of pulmonary nodules, one study compared nodules measured with the PET/CT system and sequential PET/MR system.[24] The measured axial diameters of pulmonary nodules was significantly smaller with a mean difference of 3 to 4 mm on water-only or in-phase images obtained using the Dixon-based LAVA sequence than on the CT images. There were 2 studies[19,22] reporting 3 cases with smaller measurements of the maximum diameter of lung cancer on hybrid PET/MR imaging compared with PET/CT, leading to inappropriate down-staging. When the detected nodules were interpreted on the hybrid PET/MR imaging system for the presence of malignancy, there was a tendency to over-call the nodules as indeterminate rather than a benign lesion, compared with CT.[28]

Comparison of Measured Standardized Uptake Values in Lung Lesions Between PET/ Computed Tomography and PET/MR imaging

Attenuation correction is an important process for the quantification of PET data essential in tumor evaluation and therapy monitoring. To validate this process, 7 studies[19–23,26,28] compared standardized uptake values (SUVs) obtained from PET/CT and PET/MR imaging in patients with oncologic diseases using a double scanning protocol of PET/CT followed by PET/MR imaging with one single injection of a standard dose of ^{18}F-FDG (Fig. 2, Table 2). PET/CT and PET/MR imaging scanning usually started approximately 60 minutes and 140 minutes after radiotracer injections, respectively. The median time for PET data acquisition was 2 to 3 minutes per bed position with the PET/CT system and 6 minutes per bed position with the PET/MR system, with the exception of a series of studies[21,22,26] that took 20 minutes for the thorax because they included many MR sequences for chest MR imaging. The mean SUV as well as maximum SUV tended to

be similar or higher on PET/MR imaging systems than on PET/CT systems. The measured maximum and mean SUVs were well correlated between the 2 systems when analyzed using correlation coefficients. The mean value of the relative measurement difference in measured SUVs between the systems ranged from 16% to 44% on a per-patient basis.

T Staging

Five studies[19,22,25–27] compared T staging of lung cancer based on PET/MR and PET/CT systems and found a high concordance between the 2 systems. Yi and colleagues[25] reported that a co-registered PET/1.5-T MR imaging system performed better in T staging, allowing correct up-staging in 5 of 37 patients, including 4 cases of up-staging owing to tumor size and one case of up-staging due to tumor invasion, albeit without statistical significance. T staging using a hybrid PET/MR system compared with the PET/CT system was completely identical in one study (16 of 16 patients) and similar in 2 studies[19,22] (8 of 10 patients; 12 of 15 patients). In the discrepant patients, there were cases in which PET/MR was more beneficial in determining the presence of pleural or mediastinal invasion, allowing correct up-staging or down-staging, although a few cases were inappropriately down-staged because of the smaller measurements on PET/MR imaging compared with PET/CT. A recent study evaluating a state-of-the-art co-registered PET/3-T MR imaging system[27] suggested that PET/MR imaging may be more helpful in T staging than PET/CT.

N Staging

Six studies[18,19,23,25–27] compared the PET/MR imaging system with the PET/CT system in terms of N staging for lung cancer. Among them, PET/MR images were acquired on hybrid PET/MR imaging systems in 2 studies,[19,26] on co-registered PET/MR imaging systems in 3 studies,[18,25,27] and on sequential PET/MR imaging system in one study.[23] Two studies[25,26] adopted not only STIR sequence but also the diffusion-weighted imaging (DWI) sequence for N staging, whereas the other 4 studies adopted only STIR sequence[18,19,27] or neither.[23]

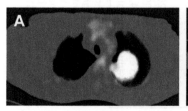 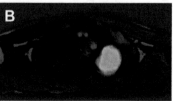

Fig. 2. Axial PET/CT image (A) and PET/MR image (B) in a 56-year-old man with lung cancer in the right upper lobe. The mass was 5.5 cm in diameter on both images with similar maximum SUV of 12.7 on PET/CT image and 13.0 on PET/MR image.

Table 2
Summary of studies correlating measured standardized uptake values of pulmonary lesions between PET/CT and PET/MR systems

Sources	Lesion No.	Region of Interest	Parameter	Measured SUV		Correlation Coefficient	Relative Measurement Difference
				PET/CT	PET/MR		
Schwenzer et al,[19] 2012, Eberhard-Karls University	10	Primary lung cancer (tumor-to-liver ratio)	Maximum	4.4 ± 2.0	8.0 ± 3.9	r = 0.93; P<.001[a]	44% ± 15%
Heusch et al,[21] 2013, University Dusseldorf	15	Primary lung cancer	Maximum (mean)	13.9 ± 6.4 (8.1 ± 3.6)	13.5 ± 7.6 (7.9 ± 4.3)	r = 0.89; P<.001[a] (r = 0.83; P<.001)	
Kohan et al,[23] 2013, Case Western Reserve University	27	Mediastinal lymph node	Maximum	NS	NS	r = 0.93; P<.001[a]	27%
Heusch et al,[22] 2013, University Dusseldorf	18	Primary lung cancer	Maximum (mean)	12.7 ± 4.6 (7.5 ± 2.7)	12.3 ± 4.8 (7.2 ± 2.8)	r = 0.93, P<.001[b] (r = 0.92, P<.001)	
Chandarana et al,[20] 2013, New York Medical College	21	Pulmonary nodule	Maximum	range, 1.7–14.0	range, 2.2–14.4	r = 0.96, P<.001[b]	16% ± 14%
Heusch et al,[26] 2014, University Dusseldorf	22	Primary lung cancer	Maximum (mean)	10.5 ± 5.3 (4.2 ± 2.3)	12.0 ± 5.7 (3.4 ± 1.5)	r = 0.86, P<.0001[b] (r =0.74; P<.0001)	
Rauscher et al,[28] 2014, Technische Universität München	22	Pulmonary nodule	Maximum (mean)	7.3 ± 5.8 (5.1 ± 4.0)	9.2 ± 8.3 (6.3 ± 5.5)	r = 0.91; P<.0001[a] (r = 0.90; P<.0001)	

Data are presented as mean ± standard deviation. Data in parentheses indicate data regarding the mean value of measured SUVs of pulmonary lesions.
Abbreviation: NS, not specified.
a Spearman's correlation coefficient.
b Pearson correlation coefficient.
Data from Refs.[19–23,26,28]

The 2 studies using the hybrid PET/MR imaging system reported that 1 of 10 cases[19] and 2 of 22 cases[26] were correctly N staged only with the PET/MR imaging system. The latter study also found higher diagnostic performance of the PET/MR imaging system on a per-node basis albeit without statistical significance. However, these gains in correct N staging with the PET/MR imaging system resulted from different tracer uptakes compared with the PET/CT system possibly associated with the delayed PET/MR scanning after tracer injection rather than an inherent advantage of the MR imaging sequence in detecting metastatic mediastinal lymph nodes.

There were 3 prospective studies using co-registered PET/MR images that reported somewhat conflicting results.[18,25,27] In the study by Morikawa and colleagues,[18] quantitative as well as qualitative assessment of nodal staging in co-registered PET/MR images provided higher specificity than with the PET/CT system on a per-node and per-patient basis (per-patient sensitivity and specificity of the PET/CT system, 90.2% and 65.6%; those of co-registered PET-STIR images, 86.9% and 96.9%). In a 2-arm prospective study,[25] the proportion of correctly up-staged patients in the co-registered PET-1.5-T MR imaging group was not significantly different from the PET/CT plus brain MR group in terms of N staging (32.4% [12/36] vs 30.8% [8/26]). In another single-arm study,[27] the co-registered PET-3-T MR imaging system appeared to allow a potential gain over the PET/CT system. However, it lacked detailed information because the study was presented only for a conference. Finally, Kohan and colleagues[23] investigated the diagnostic accuracies of PET/CT and sequential PET/MR systems regarding N staging of lung cancers. The study reported similar diagnostic performances in N staging on a per-patient basis between the 2 systems and a tendency toward higher N staging on a per-node basis with the PET/MR imaging system albeit without statistical significance. However, this result should be interpreted carefully because the MR sequence used for the evaluation of N staging was originally for the purpose of MR attenuation correction rather than anatomic evaluation.

M Staging

Because there is a paucity of studies[25] investigating the role of the PET/MR imaging system in detecting metastases focusing on lung cancer, 5 studies[29–33] that assessed the detectability of metastases in various malignancies on a hybrid PET/MR imaging system were additionally identified and reviewed by screening the bibliographies of review articles and retrieved publications. Among the 5 studies, most studies adopted at least T1-weighted VIBE or T2-weighted STIR sequence. Per-patient analysis was performed in 4 studies[29,30,32,33] and per-lesion analysis in one study.[31]

A 2-arm study[25] investigated the M staging of lung cancer and found that there were more frequent extrathoracic metastases found with the PET/CT system plus brain MR than with co-registered PET/MR images (57.7% [15/26 patients] versus 35.1% [13/37 patients]). In another study, Catalano and colleagues[29] compared the frequency of meaningful findings affecting clinical management between PET/CT and PET/MR imaging systems. The clinical management changed in 17.9% (24/134) of patients based on the findings detected using the PET/MR imaging system, whereas findings detected with the PET/CT system changed the clinical management in only 1.5% (2/134) of patients. The changed management with the PET/MR imaging system included the institution of chemotherapy to avoid futile surgery, avoidance of invasive diagnostic procedures, and institution of curative surgery. On a per-lesion analysis in the study by Tian and colleagues,[31] the PET/MR system performed equally as the PET/CT on the 278 malignant lesions. However, it missed 3 malignant lesions shown on PET/CT in the lungs and bone and detected 18 more malignant lesions in intra-abdominal organs and the digestive tract. Al-Nabhani and colleagues[32] also evaluated 50 patients with proven malignancies and possible metastases. Although the PET/CT and PET/MR imaging findings were concordant in 45 of 50 patients, there were 5 discrepant cases with regard to T staging, including correct T staging with the PET/MR imaging system in 4 patients and incorrect T staging in one patient with lung cancer. In a study by Schäfer and colleagues,[33] metastatic lesions were found only with the PET/MR system in the bone marrow, renal capsule, and liver in 4 of 19 patients, resulting in a potential change of their clinical management.

DISCUSSION

One of the most anticipated advantages of the PET/MR imaging system compared with the PET/CT system is the superior soft tissue contrast it provides, allowing a more accurate evaluation of invasion to adjacent tissue, such as the visceral pleura, chest wall, diaphragm, rib, and mediastinal structures.[34,35] Assessment of T staging in lung cancer depends on the tumor size and locoregional invasion. As expected, there were cases with correct down-staging or up-staging that benefited from the PET/MR imaging system in preliminary studies even though it included only a small number of patients. However, there is still some room for improvement of the MR sequences used for the PET/MR imaging system. Preliminary PET/MR imaging studies have never adopted dedicated pulmonary MR sequences, such as dynamic cine MR imaging,[36–38] thin-section single-shot turbo spin-echo with half-Fourier acquisition,[39] or contrast-enhanced MR angiography,[40] which have been previously reported to be potentially useful in determining local invasion.

In regard to size measurement, one study[41] addressed this issue comparing multidetector CT and 1.5-T MR imaging and reported results similar to those of a PET/MR imaging study.[24] The measured maximum diameter of pulmonary lesions was smaller with a mean difference of 2 mm, and incorrect T staging occurred when solely assessing the measured diameter on MR imaging regardless of the MR sequences used.

The understaging of lung cancer owing to the smaller measurement on the PET/MR imaging system, however, should not be a problem because the initial diagnosis in clinical practice is routinely made on a chest CT scan.[42] Considering these findings, PET/MR imaging systems, which provide more optimized MR sequences, may allow for more accurate T staging, especially in populations that might benefit the most, such as in patients with T2–T3 lung cancers suspected on CT (**Fig. 3**).

PET/CT is a mandatory noninvasive imaging modality for nodal staging of lung cancer owing to its high diagnostic performance.[42,43] However, inflammatory lymph nodes may be shown as FDG-positive lymph nodes on PET/CT, resulting in incorrect N staging especially in tuberculosis-endemic areas.[44] In the PET/MR imaging system, the key MR sequences for nodal staging of lung cancer are the STIR and DWI sequences.[45,46] Recent meta-analysis[47] comparing DWI with the PET/CT system for nodal staging of lung cancer showed that DWI has a higher pooled specificity

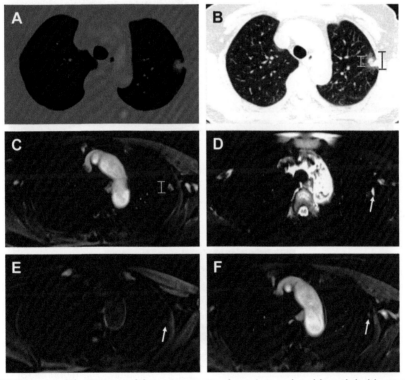

Fig. 3. Axial PET/CT image (*A*), CT image (*B*), postcontrast volume interpolated breath-hold examination (VIBE) images (*C, F*), half-Fourier acquisition single-shot turbo-spin-echo (HASTE) image (*D*), and precontrast VIBE image (*E*) in a 71-year-old woman with T2N0M0 lung cancer in the left upper lobe. The maximum diameter of part-solid nodule including peripheral ground glass opacity (*black bar*) and solid component (*white bar*) was 2.3 cm designating T1b stage on PET/CT system (*A, B*). The maximum diameter measured on postcontrast VIBE image (*C; white bar*) was 1.4 cm and smaller than that measured on CT image (*B*). A focal thickening of the adjacent visceral pleura showing subtle high signal intensity and enhancement (*arrow*) was identified on HASTE, precontrast and postcontrast VIBE images (*D–F*). T stage could be correctly up-staged as T2 on PET/MR system.

but a similar pooled sensitivity for N staging. In addition, the STIR sequence was reported to have a higher sensitivity or specificity than the PET/CT system.[45,46] Although a few preliminary studies examining the PET/MR imaging system showed similar diagnostic value as the PET/CT system, these key MR sequences in the evaluation of nodal metastasis were rarely applied. We think that a hybrid PET/MR imaging system adopting both STIR and DWI MR sequences may allow better identification of nodal metastasis, particularly in tuberculosis-endemic areas (**Figs. 4** and **5**).

From a clinical viewpoint, for mediastinal lymph nodes suspicious for metastasis on PET/CT, endobronchial or endoscopic ultrasound needle aspiration is recommended.[42] Both endobronchial and endoscopic ultrasound needle aspiration are minimally invasive procedures with a pooled sensitivity and specificity of the combined procedure of 0.86 (95% confidence interval [CI], 0.82–0.90) and 1.00 (95% CI, 0.99–1.00).[48] Moreover,

the diagnostic accuracy of the PET/CT system may have room for improvement.[49,50] Provided these results, there is uncertainty as to whether the PET/MR imaging system even with optimized MR sequences can offer additional diagnostic value over the current diagnostic strategy for N staging using PET/CT followed by endobronchial or endoscopic ultrasound needle aspiration.

Even though approximately 40% of patients with non-small-cell lung cancers have metastatic disease at distant organs at the time of initial diagnosis,[51] most of these patients have disseminated metastases and only 7% of patients have oligometastatic disease.[52] In the setting of lung cancer with overt disseminated metastasis, the PET/MR imaging system may detect additional distant metastases on a per-lesion basis compared with the PET/CT system. However, most metastases additionally detected in the PET/MR imaging tend to have less clinical importance in regard to M staging because most of the overt disseminated

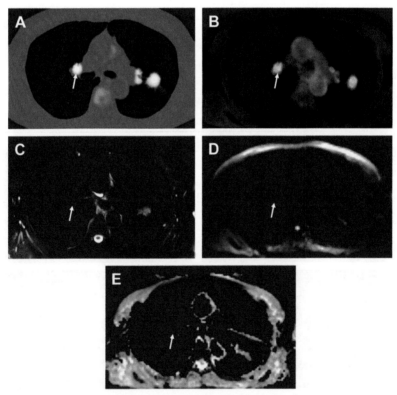

Fig. 4. Axial PET/CT image (*A*), PET/MR image (*B*), HASTE images (*C*), DWI at the b value of 800 (*D*), and apparent diffusion coefficient (ADC) map (*E*) in a 65-year-old man with T3N1M0 lung cancer in the left upper lobe. In the PET/CT system, the presumptive N staging of lung cancer was N3 because of high metabolic uptake in the right interlobar lymph node (*arrow*, maximum SUV, 15.8) (*A*). In the PET/MR system, the signal intensity of right interlobar lymph node (*arrow*) was equal to or slightly less than that of muscle on HASTE image (*C*). The node had no diffusion restriction on DWI (*D*) and ADC map (*E*). These features allowed for the correct exclusion of the possibility of nodal metastasis on PET/MR system, although the right interlobar lymph node had a maximum SUV of 6.3.

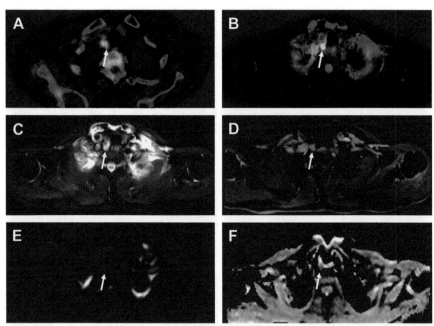

Fig. 5. Axial PET/CT image (*A*), PET/MR image (*B*), HASTE images (*C*), postcontrast VIBE) image (*D*), DWI at the b value of 800 (*E*), and ADC map (*F*) in a 77-year-old man with T2N0M0 lung cancer in the right upper lobe. The maximum SUV of the right upper paratracheal lymph node on PET/CT and PET/MR systems was 3.5, suggesting the possibility of nodal metastasis (*A, B; arrow*). This node (*C-F; arrow*) had a high signal intensity on HASTE image (*C*), enhancement on postcontrast VIBE image (*D*), and diffusion restriction on DWI (*E*) and ADC map (*F*). Right upper lobectomy with dissection of the mediastinal lymph node was performed. There was no evidence of metastasis in resected lymph nodes reflecting the limitation of PET/MR in this case.

metastases can easily be detected with the PET component of PET/CT as well as PET/MR systems (**Fig. 6**). Hence, the PET/MR imaging system is more beneficial than the PET/CT system in M staging only when oligometastatic lesions difficult to detect with the PET/CT system are identified on MR imaging. With the correct M staging of oligometastatic lesions, futile thoracotomy can be avoided and better overall survival can be achieved through metastasectomy in specific organs.[53]

Frequent sites of oligometastatic disease are similar to those of overt metastatic disease, including the brain, lung, bone, liver, and adrenal gland.[54] It is evident that the PET/MR imaging system is superior in detecting brain metastases to the PET/CT system. However, brain MR is a mandatory imaging examination in addition to PET/CT scanning in patients with clinical stage III or IV non-small-lung cancer.[42] Conversely, chest CT scan generally recommended in patients with lung cancer at initial diagnosis[42] can complement the disadvantage of the PET/MR imaging system in detecting small pulmonary metastasis from the viewpoint of clinical practice. Overall, it is uncertain that the PET/MR imaging system can offer

much additional value over the PET/CT system in detecting extrathoracic metastases of lung cancer other than brain metastases.

In regard to intrathoracic pleural metastasis, preliminary hybrid PET/MR imaging studies have rarely addressed this issue. One MR imaging study showed that DWI in conjunction with dynamic contrast-enhanced MR showed excellent diagnostic accuracy of greater than 90% in determining pleural metastasis and was able to properly diagnose undetermined cases of the PET/CT system.[55] Ohno and colleagues[27] also reported a representative case of pleural metastasis well visualized on co-registered PET/MR images but not detected on PET/CT (**Fig. 7**).

Finally, although it was not the main interest of this review, the multiparametric capability of the hybrid PET/MR imaging system can expand the comprehension of tumor characteristics.[56] Various kinds of MR sequences, including DWI, dynamic contrast-enhanced MR, blood oxygenation–level dependent MR, and MR spectroscopy can finely illustrate cellular proliferation, angiogenesis, hypoxia, and tissue metabolites of tumor tissue. The biologic characteristics of tumor tissue, such as altered metabolism, hypoxia, cellular proliferation,

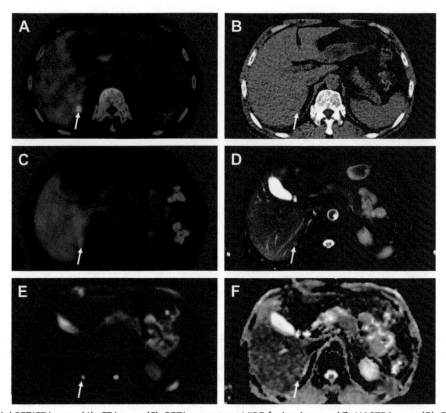

Fig. 6. Axial PET/CT image (*A*), CT image (*B*), PET/precontrast VIBE fusion images (*C*), HASTE image (*D*), DWI at the b value of 800 (*E*), and ADC map (*F*) in a 52-year-old man with lung cancer metastatic to the liver and bone. PET/CT image showed hepatic metastasis (*arrow*) with maximum SUV of 4.7 (*A*). This lesion could not be localized on CT image (*arrow*) (*B*). This hepatic metastasis (*C-F*; *arrow*) had a low signal intensity on precontrast VIBE (*C*), high signal intensity on HASTE image (*D*), and diffusion restriction on DWI (*E*) and ADC map (*F*). PET/MR imaging allowed better depiction of hepatic metastasis, although the detectability of hepatic and bony metastases was not different.

and apoptosis, can also be revealed by several radiotracers used in nuclear medicine, including ^{18}F-FDG, ^{18}F-fluorothymidine ^{15}O-labeled water, ^{18}F-fluoromisonidazole, ^{124}I-annexin V, and so on. Preclinical experiences regarding multiparametric imaging with the PET/MR system showed complexities and heterogeneities of tumor tissue and the surrounding microenvironment, which have been rarely illustrated with pre-existing imaging modalities used in clinical practice.[16,57,58] Thus, multiparametric interpretation along with accurate anatomic and temporal registration using the hybrid PET/MR imaging system is expected to allow the early prediction of cancer progression as well as response to anticancer agents, including targeted therapy, although it will take time to be implemented in lung cancer.

One final thing worth mentioning is the expectation regarding the role of PET/MR imaging in lung cancer. Various MR techniques are still being developed along with the introduction of new candidates for MR contrast and some of these MR techniques may overcome the current limitations of the PET/MR imaging system.[59,60]

SUMMARY

There have only been a few preliminary PET/MR imaging studies dealing with lung cancer; however, the results of most of these studies showed similar diagnostic performance with the PET/CT system, although it did not show superiority in terms of TNM and overall staging. In considering these findings, the implementation of PET/MR imaging in routine practice may be much delayed for chest disease considering the longer examination time and higher costs involved with PET/MR imaging, except for the pediatric population, which may benefit greatly from the lowered radiation exposure. To ensure the successful implementation of the PET/MR imaging system in clinical practice, optimized pulmonary MR sequences need to be

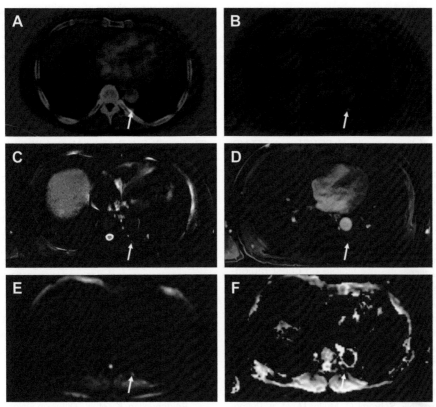

Fig. 7. Axial PET/CT image (*A*), PET/MR image (*B*), HASTE image (*C*), postcontrast VIBE image (*D*), DWI at the b value of 800 (*E*), and ADC map (*F*) in a 53-year-old man with lung cancer having pleural metastasis (*A-F; arrow*). No abnormality could be found in the pleura on PET/CT image (*A*). The PET/MR image showed a mild focal metabolic uptake in the pleura with maximum SUV of 2.0 (*B*). This pleural lesion had high signal intensity on HASTE image (*C*), focal enhancement on postcontrast VIBE image (*D*), and mild diffusion restriction on DWI (*E*) and ADC map (*F*) favoring pleural metastasis. Thoracoscopy revealed pleural seeding nodules without pleural effusion.

established for the PET/MR imaging system to fully use the advantages of MR imaging over CT.

REFERENCES

1. Antoch G, Vogt FM, Freudenberg LS, et al. Whole-body dual-modality PET/CT and whole-body MRI for tumor staging in oncology. JAMA 2003;290(24): 3199–206.

2. Bar-Shalom R, Yefremov N, Guralnik L, et al. Clinical performance of PET/CT in evaluation of cancer: additional value for diagnostic imaging and patient management. J Nucl Med 2003;44(8):1200–9.

3. Fischer B, Lassen U, Mortensen J, et al. Preoperative staging of lung cancer with combined PET-CT. N Engl J Med 2009;361(1):32–9.

4. De Wever W, Ceyssens S, Mortelmans L, et al. Additional value of PET-CT in the staging of lung cancer: comparison with CT alone, PET alone and visual correlation of PET and CT. Eur Radiol 2007;17(1):23–32.

5. Antoch G, Stattaus J, Nemat AT, et al. Non-small cell lung cancer: dual-modality PET/CT in preoperative staging. Radiology 2003;229(2):526–33.

6. Pichler BJ, Kolb A, Nagele T, et al. PET/MRI: paving the way for the next generation of clinical multimodality imaging applications. J Nucl Med 2010; 51(3):333–6.

7. Torigian DA, Zaidi H, Kwee TC, et al. PET/MR imaging: technical aspects and potential clinical applications. Radiology 2013;267(1):26–44.

8. Yoon SH, Goo JM, Lee SM, et al. Positron emission tomography/magnetic resonance imaging evaluation of lung cancer: current status and future prospects. J Thorac Imaging 2014;29(1):4–16.

9. Shan ZY, Mateja SJ, Reddick WE, et al. Retrospective evaluation of PET-MRI registration algorithms. J Digit Imaging 2011;24(3):485–93.

10. Slomka PJ, Baum RP. Multimodality image registration with software: state-of-the-art. Eur J Nucl Med Mol Imaging 2009;36(Suppl 1):S44–55.

11. Zaidi H, Del Guerra A. An outlook on future design of hybrid PET/MRI systems. Med Phys 2011;38(10): 5667–89.

12. Keereman V, Mollet P, Berker Y, et al. Challenges and current methods for attenuation correction in PET/MR. MAGMA 2013;26(1):81–98.

13. Martinez-Moller A, Souvatzoglou M, Delso G, et al. Tissue classification as a potential approach for attenuation correction in whole-body PET/MRI: evaluation with PET/CT data. J Nucl Med 2009;50(4):520–6.

14. Osman MM, Cohade C, Nakamoto Y, et al. Respiratory motion artifacts on PET emission images obtained using CT attenuation correction on PET-CT. Eur J Nucl Med Mol Imaging 2003;30(4):603–6.

15. Rakheja R, DeMello L, Chandarana H, et al. Comparison of the accuracy of PET/CT and PET/MRI spatial registration of multiple metastatic lesions. AJR Am J Roentgenol 2013;201(5):1120–3.

16. Schmidt H, Brendle C, Schraml C, et al. Correlation of simultaneously acquired diffusion-weighted imaging and 2-deoxy-[18F] fluoro-2-D-glucose positron emission tomography of pulmonary lesions in a dedicated whole-body magnetic resonance/positron emission tomography system. Invest Radiol 2013; 48(5):247–55.

17. Brendle CB, Schmidt H, Fleischer S, et al. Simultaneously acquired MR/PET images compared with sequential MR/PET and PET/CT: alignment quality. Radiology 2013;268(1):190–9.

18. Morikawa M, Demura Y, Ishizaki T, et al. The effectiveness of 18F-FDG PET/CT combined with STIR MRI for diagnosing nodal involvement in the thorax. J Nucl Med 2009;50(1):81–7.

19. Schwenzer NF, Schraml C, Muller M, et al. Pulmonary lesion assessment: comparison of whole-body hybrid MR/PET and PET/CT imaging–pilot study. Radiology 2012;264(2):551–8.

20. Chandarana H, Heacock L, Rakheja R, et al. Pulmonary nodules in patients with primary malignancy: comparison of hybrid PET/MR and PET/CT imaging. Radiology 2013;268(3):874–81.

21. Heusch P, Buchbender C, Kohler J, et al. Correlation of the apparent diffusion coefficient (ADC) with the standardized uptake value (SUV) in hybrid 18F-FDG PET/MRI in non-small cell lung cancer (NSCLC) lesions: initial results. Rofo 2013;185(11):1056–62.

22. Heusch P, Kohler J, Wittsack HJ, et al. Hybrid [(1)(8) F]-FDG PET/MRI including non-Gaussian diffusion-weighted imaging (DWI): preliminary results in non-small cell lung cancer (NSCLC). Eur J Radiol 2013; 82(11):2055–60.

23. Kohan AA, Kolthammer JA, Vercher-Conejero JL, et al. N staging of lung cancer patients with PET/MRI using a three-segment model attenuation correction algorithm: initial experience. Eur Radiol 2013;23(11):3161–9.

24. Stolzmann P, Veit-Haibach P, Chuck N, et al. Detection rate, location, and size of pulmonary nodules in trimodality PET/CT-MR: comparison of low-dose CT and Dixon-based MR imaging. Invest Radiol 2013; 48(5):241–6.

25. Yi CA, Lee KS, Lee HY, et al. Coregistered whole body magnetic resonance imaging-positron emission tomography (MRI-PET) versus PET-computed tomography plus brain MRI in staging resectable lung cancer: comparisons of clinical effectiveness in a randomized trial. Cancer 2013; 119(10):1784–91.

26. Heusch P, Buchbender C, Kohler J, et al. Thoracic staging in lung cancer: prospective comparison of 18F-FDG PET/MR imaging and 18F-FDG PET/CT. J Nucl Med 2014;55(3):373–8.

27. Ohno Y, Seki S, Nishio M, et al. Whole-body MRI vs. co-registered whole-body FDG-PET with MRI (PET/ MRI) vs. integrated FDG-PET/CT: capability of clinical stage and operability assessments in non-small cell carcinoma. Proc Intl Soc Mag Reson Med 2014;22. Joint Annual Meeting ISMRM-ESMRMB. Milan, Italy, May 10–16, 2014.

28. Rauscher I, Eiber M, Furst S, et al. PET/MR imaging in the detection and characterization of pulmonary lesions: technical and diagnostic evaluation in comparison to PET/CT. J Nucl Med 2014;55(5): 724–9.

29. Catalano OA, Rosen BR, Sahani DV, et al. Clinical impact of PET/MR imaging in patients with cancer undergoing same-day PET/CT: initial experience in 134 patients–a hypothesis-generating exploratory study. Radiology 2013;269(3):857–69.

30. Buchbender C, Hartung-Knemeyer V, Beiderwellen K, et al. Diffusion-weighted imaging as part of hybrid PET/MRI protocols for whole-body cancer staging: does it benefit lesion detection? Eur J Radiol 2013;82(5):877–82.

31. Tian JH, Fu LP, Yin DY, et al. Does the novel integrated PET/MRI offer the same diagnostic performance as PET/CT for oncological indications? PLoS One 2014;9(6):e90844.

32. Al-Nabhani KZ, Syed R, Michopoulou S, et al. Qualitative and quantitative comparison of PET/CT and PET/MR imaging in clinical practice. J Nucl Med 2014;55(1):88–94.

33. Schäfer JF, Gatidis S, Schmidt H, et al. Simultaneous whole-body PET/MR imaging in comparison to PET/ CT in pediatric oncology: initial results. Radiology 2014;273:220–31.

34. Padovani B, Mouroux J, Seksik L, et al. Chest wall invasion by bronchogenic carcinoma: evaluation with MR imaging. Radiology 1993;187(1):33–8.

35. Koyama H, Ohno Y, Seki S, et al. Magnetic resonance imaging for lung cancer. J Thorac Imaging 2013;28(3):138–50.

36. Hong YJ, Hur J, Lee HJ, et al. Respiratory dynamic magnetic resonance imaging for determining aortic invasion of thoracic neoplasms. J Thorac Cardiovasc Surg 2014;148(2):644–50.

37. Lee CH, Goo JM, Kim YT, et al. The clinical feasibility of using non-breath-hold real-time MR-echo imaging for the evaluation of mediastinal and chest wall tumor invasion. Korean J Radiol 2010;11(1):37–45.

38. Akata S, Kajiwara N, Park J, et al. Evaluation of chest wall invasion by lung cancer using respiratory dynamic MRI. J Med Imaging Radiat Oncol 2008; 52(1):36–9.

39. Chang S, Hong SR, Kim YJ, et al. Usefulness of thin-section single-shot turbo spin echo with half-fourier acquisition in evaluation of local invasion of lung cancer. J Magn Reson Imaging 2015;41(3):747–54.

40. Ohno Y, Adachi S, Motoyama A, et al. Multiphase ECG-triggered 3D contrast-enhanced MR angiography: utility for evaluation of hilar and mediastinal invasion of bronchogenic carcinoma. J Magn Reson Imaging 2001;13(2):215–24.

41. Heye T, Ley S, Heussel CP, et al. Detection and size of pulmonary lesions: how accurate is MRI? A prospective comparison of CT and MRI. Acta Radiol 2012;53(2):153–60.

42. Silvestri GA, Gonzalez AV, Jantz MA, et al. Methods for staging non-small cell lung cancer diagnosis and management of lung cancer, 3rd ed: American College of Chest Physicians evidence-based clinical practice guidelines. Chest 2013;143(5): E211–50.

43. Lv YL, Yuan DM, Wang K, et al. Diagnostic performance of integrated positron emission tomography/computed tomography for mediastinal lymph node staging in non-small cell lung cancer: a bivariate systematic review and meta-analysis. J Thorac Oncol 2011;6(8):1350–8.

44. Liao CY, Chen JH, Liang JA, et al. Meta-analysis study of lymph node staging by 18 F-FDG PET/CT scan in non-small cell lung cancer: comparison of TB and non-TB endemic regions. Eur J Radiol 2012;81(11):3518–23.

45. Ohno Y, Koyama H, Nogami M, et al. STIR turbo SE MR imaging vs. coregistered FDG-PET/CT: quantitative and qualitative assessment of N-stage in non-small-cell lung cancer patients. J Magn Reson Imaging 2007;26(4):1071–80.

46. Ohno Y, Koyama H, Yoshikawa T, et al. N stage disease in patients with non-small cell lung cancer: efficacy of quantitative and qualitative assessment with STIR turbo spin-echo imaging, diffusion-weighted MR imaging, and fluorodeoxyglucose PET/CT. Radiology 2011;261(2):605–15.

47. Wu LM, Xu JR, Gu HY, et al. Preoperative mediastinal and hilar nodal staging with diffusion-weighted magnetic resonance imaging and fluorodeoxyglucose positron emission tomography/computed tomography in patients with non-small-cell lung cancer: which is better? J Surg Res 2012;178(1):304–14.

48. Zhang R, Ying K, Shi L, et al. Combined endobronchial and endoscopic ultrasound-guided fine needle aspiration for mediastinal lymph node staging of lung cancer: a meta-analysis. Eur J Cancer 2013; 49(8):1860–7.

49. Moloney F, Ryan D, McCarthy L, et al. Increasing the accuracy of F-18-FDG PET/CT interpretation of "mildly positive" mediastinal nodes in the staging of non-small cell lung cancer. Eur J Radiol 2014; 83(5):843–7.

50. Toney LK, Vesselle HJ. Neural networks for nodal staging of non-small cell lung cancer with FDG PET and CT: importance of combining uptake values and sizes of nodes and primary tumor. Radiology 2014;270(1):91–8.

51. Rami-Porta R, Crowley JJ, Goldstraw P. The revised TNM staging system for lung cancer. Ann Thorac Cardiovasc Surg 2009;15(1):4–9.

52. Albain KS, Crowley JJ, LeBlanc M, et al. Survival determinants in extensive-stage non-small-cell lung cancer: the Southwest Oncology Group experience. J Clin Oncol 1991;9(9):1618–26.

53. Endo C, Hasumi T, Matsumura Y, et al. A prospective study of surgical procedures for patients with oligometastatic non-small cell lung cancer. Ann Thorac Surg 2014;98(1):258–64.

54. Quint LE, Tummala S, Brisson LJ, et al. Distribution of distant metastases from newly diagnosed non-small cell lung cancer. Ann Thorac Surg 1996; 62(1):246–50.

55. Coolen J, De Keyzer F, Nafteux P, et al. Malignant pleural disease: diagnosis by using diffusion-weighted and dynamic contrast-enhanced MR imaging-initial experience. Radiology 2012;263(3): 884–92.

56. Padhani AR, Miles KA. Multiparametric imaging of tumor response to therapy. Radiology 2010;256(2): 348–64.

57. Cho H, Ackerstaff E, Carlin S, et al. Noninvasive multimodality imaging of the tumor microenvironment: registered dynamic magnetic resonance imaging and positron emission tomography studies of a preclinical tumor model of tumor hypoxia. Neoplasia 2009;11(3):247–59, 2p following 259.

58. Schelhaas S, Wachsmuth L, Viel T, et al. Variability of proliferation and diffusion in different lung cancer models as measured by 3'-Deoxy-3'-18F-fluorothymidine PET and diffusion-weighted MR imaging. J Nucl Med 2014;55(6):983–8.

59. Johnson KM, Fain SB, Schiebler ML, et al. Optimized 3D ultrashort echo time pulmonary MRI. Magn Reson Med 2013;70(5):1241–50.

60. Klenk C, Gawande R, Uslu L, et al. Ionising radiation-free whole-body MRI versus (18)F-fluorodeoxyglucose PET/CT scans for children and young adults with cancer: a prospective, non-randomised, single-centre study. Lancet Oncol 2014;15(3):275–85.

Imaging Pulmonary Arterial Thromboembolism
Challenges and Opportunities

Sebastian Ley, MD[a,b],*

KEYWORDS

- Magnetic resonance angiography • Pulmonary arteries • Pulmonary perfusion
- Acute pulmonary embolism • Chronic thromboembolic pulmonary hypertension (CTEPH)

KEY POINTS

- Magnetic resonance (MR) angiography of the pulmonary arteries has proven clinical usefulness.
- Contrast-enhanced (CE) and non-CE angiographic techniques are widely available for high spatial and real-time imaging of the pulmonary arteries.
- Multiple-step protocols, such as MR perfusion followed by high–spatial resolution contrast-enhanced magnetic resonance angiography (CE-MRA), seem to be an optimal clinical approach for the assessment of different vascular diseases affecting the pulmonary arteries.

INTRODUCTION

Given the speed and robustness of modern multi-detector computed tomography (MDCT) scanners, this technique has become the noninvasive gold standard for imaging of the pulmonary arteries.[1,2] The advantages of MDCT are fast examination with high resolution and visualization of even subsegmental pulmonary arteries. The technique is usually available 24/7 and allows exclusion of other causes of chest pain in the same examination. As a drawback, the amount of functional information is usually limited.

Direct visualization of the pulmonary arteries can be done using invasive techniques such as digital subtraction angiography (DSA), which are nowadays reserved for special preoperative settings, such as chronic thromboembolic pulmonary hypertension (CTEPH) and settings in which an invasive mean pulmonary arterial pressure measurement is required. Computed tomography (CT) and DSA have the inherent problem of irradiation and the need for nephrotoxic contrast agents.

MR imaging has evolved as a competitive noninvasive imaging modality.[3,4] Over the past decades MR imaging has undergone significant technical improvements such as faster acquisitions, larger coverage, and faster reconstruction, leading to substantially improved patient acceptance of this modality. Furthermore, the availability of MR systems has improved over the past years. These factors have positively influenced development of MR applications in the chest. The implementation of MR angiography (MRA), lung perfusion imaging, and the assessment of right heart function seem to be promising techniques for a comprehensive evaluation in patients with either congenital or acquired pulmonary arterial pathologies.[5]

The author has nothing to disclose.
^a Diagnostic and Interventional Radiology, Chirurgische Klinik Dr Rinecker, Am Isarkanal 30, Munich 81379, Germany; ^b Department of Clinical Radiology, Ludwig Maximilians University, Marchioninistrasse 15, Munich 81377, Germany
* Diagnostic and Interventional Radiology, Chirurgische Klinik Dr Rinecker, Am Isarkanal 30, Munich 81379, Germany.
E-mail address: ley@gmx.net

Magn Reson Imaging Clin N Am 23 (2015) 261–271
http://dx.doi.org/10.1016/j.mric.2015.01.013

This review highlights the current state of various MRA techniques for the diagnosis of acute and chronic thromboembolic disease.

Technique

Different imaging strategies are available for imaging pulmonary arteries including CE and non-CE acquisitions. The most often used technique is high–spatial resolution CE-MRA.

Contrast-enhanced magnetic resonance angiography with high spatial resolution

CE-MRA consists of heavily T1-weighted gradient echo MR sequences after an intravenous injection of a paramagnetic MR contrast agent.[6] In general, 3-dimensional (3D) techniques with a relaxation time (TR) of less than 5 ms and an echo time (TE) of less than 2 ms are used for CE-MRA of the pulmonary arteries.[7] A short TR allows for short breath-hold acquisitions, and a short TE minimizes background signal and susceptibility artifacts. Nowadays, acquisition time has been shortened further using parallel imaging.[8] In parallel imaging, the image is reconstructed from an undersampled k-space in the phase-encoding direction and thus acquisition time decreases. With a typical acceleration factor of 2, every second line in k-space is skipped, which leads to reduction of scan time of approximately 50%.[9] This reduced acquisition time can also be traded for higher spatial resolution. The trade-off for the reduction of scan time or the higher spatial resolution is a decreased signal to noise ratio (SNR). It is inversely proportional to the square root of the acceleration factor times a geometry factor that is determined mainly by the coil design.[10] In the case of an acceleration factor of 2, the signal is at best 71% of the original signal.[10] Although an acceleration factor of 3 seems to be acceptable for the renal arteries,[11] an acceleration factor of 2 is usually recommended for the pulmonary arteries; this leads to high spatial resolution with a voxel size of 1.2 mm × 1.0 mm × 1.6 mm requiring a breath-hold of 20 to 30 seconds for acquisition. Artifacts in the center of the image can appear if acceleration factors of 2 are used in a coronal acquisition. To overcome this problem, patients are scanned with their arms above their heads, which could, however, cause discomfort in some patients.[8] The use of non-Cartesian, k-space filling techniques, such as radial and spiral image data acquisition, has also been proposed for use in the chest.[12,13] As breath-hold is crucial for image quality, the scan is generally acquired in the coronal orientation because the number of slices required for full coverage is lower than in other orientations (**Fig. 1**). This method requires a single injection of contrast. To improve spatial resolution and reduce the duration of the breath-hold, the sequential acquisition of 2 sagittal slabs covering the right and left lung separately has also been used successfully in patients with CTEPH.[14]

By combination of the latest technical developments, such as 32-channel chest coil, 3T MR imaging, high relaxivity contrast agent, and acceleration factor of 6, the acquisition of isotropic (1 × 1 × 1 mm^3) voxels covering the entire pulmonary circulation in 20 seconds is feasible.[15]

Contrast administration

For T1 shortening of the blood, a gadolinium (Gd) compound is injected in a peripheral vein as a bolus, preferably by an automated power injector. Mostly, standard-strength Gd compounds in a standard dose (0.1 mmol/kg body weight) are used for optimal opacification of the pulmonary

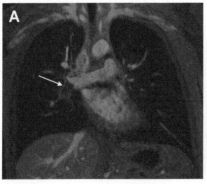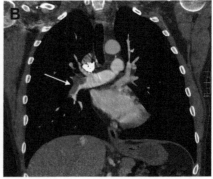

Fig. 1. (A) MR angiography in a 39-year-old man with central acute pulmonary embolism (*arrow*). The data set was acquired in a coronal orientation with a spatial resolution of 1.3 × 1.3 × 1.4 mm. Usually 2 to 3 angiographic phases are acquired even in patients with dyspnea. In this case, the second phase is shown demonstrating the thromboembolic material in the main right pulmonary artery. (B) Corresponding coronal reformatted CT angiography (4 days earlier) showed similar findings.

arteries. To guarantee an optimal bolus profile, the administration of the contrast agent with flow rates between 2 and 5 mL/s is mandatory. The bolus geometry is mainly determined by injection parameters; cardiac function is of minor importance.[16] An injection scheme with a flow rate of 2 mL/s results in a mean transit time of the contrast agent through the pulmonary circulation of 14 seconds, and it is reduced to 9 seconds using an injection speed of 4 mL/s. The administration of a saline flush, minimum 20 mL injected at the same flow rate, immediately afterward is strongly recommended to achieve a compact bolus profile. The saline chaser ensures that the whole amount of contrast medium contributes to vessel opacification. Adequate timing of the contrast agent together with an adapted flow rate is essential to achieve high contrast between pulmonary artery branches and surrounding structures. The Gd concentration should be optimal at the time of central k-space acquisition, as this determines the vascular signal intensity. Because a significant number of patients referred for MRA of the pulmonary arteries present with right heart compromise and/or pulmonary hypertension, the scan delay should be individually adjusted using a care bolus procedure or a test bolus examination. In general, arterial enhancement should dominate because overlay of pulmonary veins might otherwise impair the assessment of arteries.

Initially, MRA was seen as a promising tool for patients with renal insufficiency avoiding the nephrotoxicity of iodinated CT contrast media. However, a series of cases with nephrogenic systemic fibrosis came up around 2008. It was soon found that the prevalence was different with different Gd compounds.[17] Based on this, the Prospective Investigation of Pulmonary Embolism Diagnosis (PIOPED) study that was underway adopted a conservative approach and lowered the Gd dose from 0.2 mmol/kg to 0.1 mmol/kg (single dose). This lower dose of Gd was later even found to have superior image quality.[18,19]

In an animal model (rabbit) a blood pool contrast agent outperformed a standard Gd-DOTA (gadoteric acid) contrast media for detection of embolic vascular pathologies.[20] Given the primarily intravascular distribution of the contrast media, high-resolution MR angiographies could be obtained up to 15 minutes after injection.

Contrast-enhanced magnetic resonance angiography with high temporal resolution

Another approach is to optimize the MR sequence for high temporal resolution and to apply it as a multiphasic acquisition.[21,22] In time-resolved MRA, the scan time for the individual 3D data set

is reduced to less than 5 seconds. The rationale is 3-fold: first, patients with severe respiratory disease and limited breath-hold capabilities can be examined. Second, the arterial-venous discrimination is improved, allowing for characterization of vascular territories, especially in anomalies and shunts. Third, time-resolved multiphasic CE-MRA is independent from the bolus timing, because the contrast injection and the MR sequence are started simultaneously. Advanced time-resolved imaging techniques integrate a view-sharing approach to achieve a temporal resolution of 3.3 seconds for a 3D data set with a high spatial resolution of, for example, 1.3 × 1.8 × 3 mm^3.[23] Latest experimental approaches combine view sharing with spiral k-space filling, allowing for even higher–spatial resolution images with shorter acquisition times.[24] If the temporal resolution is substantially reduced further, that is, 1 second per 3D data set, the perfusion of the lung parenchyma can be assessed parallel to the central pulmonary arteries,[25] allowing for easy depiction of perfusion deficits due to vascular obstruction (**Fig. 2**).

Noncontrast-enhanced overlapping steady-state free precession sequences

Critically ill patients do not even tolerate a short breath-hold time of 5 to 10 seconds for CE-MRA. The same is true for CT angiography (CTA), and its imaging results might also be suboptimal in these scenarios. For these patients, free-breathing real-time imaging techniques based on steady-state free precession (SSFP), also called balanced fast-field echo or fast imaging using steady-state acquisition, are available.[26,27] The whole chest can be covered in all 3 orientations in less than 180 seconds with 50% overlapping of the slices due to an acquisition time per image of approximately 0.4 to 0.5 seconds (**Fig. 3**). This approach allows for a lobar and segmental evaluation of the pulmonary arteries. Real-time MR imaging showed high specificity (98%) and sensitivity (89%) in a study of patients with acute pulmonary embolism (PE), with 16-slice MDCT serving as the reference modality.[28]

Noncontrast-enhanced respiratory-gated steady-state free precession

One technique that may offer an alternative to breath-hold imaging is navigator-gated MR imaging, in which imaging is performed during free breathing. The navigator was first described in 1989 by Ehman and Felmlee,[29] and it has been used primarily to image blood vessels that are subject to respiratory and cardiac motion, particularly the coronary arteries.[30] However, this method

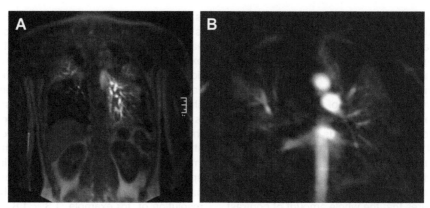

Fig. 2. Same patient as in **Fig. 1.** (*A*) Time-resolved data set (1.3 seconds per 3D data set) shows the perfusion defects and represents the functional impairment of the vascular obstruction. As expected from the angiographic study, the main loss of perfusion is located on the right. (*B*) Given the serial acquisition of multiple data sets a subtraction can be performed between data set without contrast media and one with the maximum enhancement of the pulmonary parenchymal phase. A subtraction image of the 3D data set is shown with a clear-cut wedge-shaped perfusion defect in the left upper lope and a patchy perfusion defect in the left lower lobe. These areas of vascular obstruction were not noted on the previous MRA or CT angiographic studies.

has rarely been used for pulmonary imaging.[31] With the advent of faster gradient systems and continued development of SSFP, it has become possible to perform rapid 3D imaging. The faster gradient systems allow for reduced repetition times, making SSFP practical. Further, the refocusing nature of SSFP, as opposed to the standard spoiled gradient echo technique, allows for both a higher flip angle and many more views per segment before significant signal decay.[32] In a study in healthy volunteers, a breath-hold SSFP sequence was compared with a navigator-gated SSFP. Both sequences resulted in comparable image quality with the same SNR level; however, no analysis was performed regarding vessel conspicuity on a segmental level. Image acquisition was approximately 29 seconds for the breath-hold and 180 seconds for the navigator technique.[33] Therefore, in critically ill patients, this technique may be worth trying as an alternative.

Besides respiratory artifacts, pulsation artifacts lead to impaired image quality. This drawback can be overcome by electrocardiography (ECG) and respiratory-triggered SSFP techniques (see **Fig. 3**).[34] In the aforementioned study (21 patients), this double-triggered sequence showed a sensitivity of 67% and a specificity of 100%.

3D gradient echo during recirculation phase
Image acquisition during the first pass of the contrast media through the pulmonary arteries is the mainstay of visualization of the pulmonary arteries. However, this approach is a one shot try and sometimes results in nonoptimal images. Given the excellent enhancement of the vasculature by the current contrast media, even late image acquisitions up to 10 minutes are possible. This method was used in the study by Kalb and colleagues,[34] whereby approximately 3 minutes after the first-pass angiography a late-phase

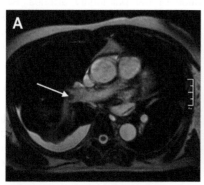
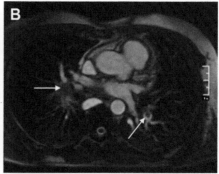

Fig. 3. (*A*) A 61-year-old man with an incidental finding of a central pulmonary embolism (*arrow*) on a nongated, free-breathing SSFP sequence. (*B*) Using an axial electrocardiography-gated, breath-hold SSFP sequence, the central pulmonary embolic material can be more easily depicted (*arrows*, same patient as in **Fig. 1**).

angiography data set was acquired. An axial breath-hold (15 seconds) 3D gradient echo (GRE) sequence was used with a spatial resolution of $1.3 \times 1.3 \times 2.8$ mm^3. This approach and sequence had the highest accuracy (compared with MRA and triggered SSFP) with a sensitivity of 73% (**Fig. 4**).[34]

The sequences described earlier can be used in various combinations to provide a stepwise approach to comprehensive assessment of pulmonary arteries and perfusion deficits. A combination of time-resolved angiography followed by high–spatial resolution angiography provides comprehensive assessment of perfusion defects and pulmonary arterial emboli. The authors' preferred institutional protocol is shown in **Table 1**.

ACUTE PULMONARY EMBOLISM

Most frequently, the pulmonary arteries are examined for clinically suspected PE, one of the most common medical problems in the Western world.[35] Owing to the robustness and speed of examination, pulmonary CTA is the recommended standard protocol of care in case of suspected PE[35] and might even be complemented by CT venography. Because of the inherent advantage of MR imaging with stepwise protocols and the possibility of functional evaluation of the burden on the right ventricle, MR imaging was used for diagnosis of PE since the early days (see **Figs. 1** and **2**). Comprehensive review of the recent literature using MR imaging for diagnosis of acute PE

has been published.[5,25] Therefore, in this review, only the latest studies with state-of-the-art scanner technology are discussed in detail.

In 2005, the diagnostic performance of MR imaging was evaluated in 89 patients with suspected PE using coronal-, axial-, and sagittal-orientated CE-MRA. The images were interpreted independently by 2 teams of radiologists. A heterogeneous combination of clinical probability, D-dimer testing, spiral CT, compression venous ultrasound imaging, and pulmonary DSA served as the gold standard.[36] The study cohort had a high prevalence of PE (71%), and depending on the team of readers, the sensitivity and specificity of CE-MRA ranged between 31% and 71% and 85% and 92%, respectively. Pleszewski and colleagues[37] reported a higher sensitivity and specificity of 82% and 100%, respectively, in 48 patients with suspected PE, with overall a slightly lower sensitivity of CE-MRA than CTA. These results are similar to another study using high–spatial resolution ($0.7 \times 1.2 \times 1.5$ mm) CE-MRA acquired in a 15-second breath-hold time performed in 62 patients with suspected PE. CE-MRA had a sensitivity of 81% and specificity of 100% when compared with CTA acquired with a 16-slice MDCT.[28] In contrast, a study from 2012 that used a state-of-the art MR scanner to acquire a $1.2 \times 1.2 \times 1.3$ mm^3 3D volume[34] only had a sensitivity of 55% and specificity of 99% compared with CTA. However, the time interval between CTA and MRA was 30 hours, and treatment was started after positive results on CTA scan. A technical failure rate of 14% was seen.

These more recent numbers from a single center are in keeping with the results from the PIOPED III study, with a sensitivity ranging between 45% and 100% (averaging 78%).[38]

In a different study, 8 patients with dyspnea with known or suspected PE were examined using a time-resolved CE-MRA with a scan time of less than 4 seconds per 3D data set. Pulmonary CE-MRA allowed for the assessment of the pulmonary arterial tree down to a subsegmental level and identified PE in all cases, which were subsequently confirmed. All patients could hold their breath for at least 8 seconds, during which a data set with an angiogram of the pulmonary arteries could be obtained.[21] In another study, conventional pulmonary DSA served as the gold standard in 48 patients with suspected acute PE. A time-resolved CE-MRA with parallel imaging (sensitivity encoding [SENSE]) resulted in a high sensitivity (92%) and specificity (94%) for the detection of PE.[39]

In 41 patients with suspected PE, perfusion MR imaging showed a high intermodality agreement with single-photon emission computed tomography

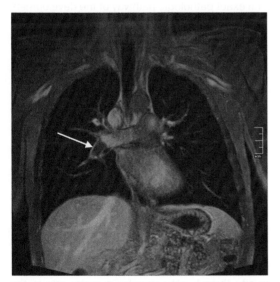

Fig. 4. After contrast administration, a T1w volume-interpolated breath-hold examination sequence (resolution $0.8 \times 0.8 \times 5$ mm^3) was acquired showing the central thromboembolic material (*arrow*).

Table 1
Proposed MR imaging protocol for patients with suspected pulmonary arterial thromboembolism

Rationale	Sequences
Initial overview of morphology	T2w HASTE transverse & coronal
Vascular imaging (noncontrast)	SSFP transverse & coronal
Contrast-enhanced vascular imaging and perfusion	FLASH 3D (time resolved), 0.1 mmol/kg
Postcontrast assessment (between time-resolved and high–spatial resolution angiography)	VIBE transverse & coronal
Contrast-enhanced vascular imaging	FLASH 3D (high spatial resolution), 0.1 mmol/kg

Abbreviation: FLASH, Fast Low-Angle Shot.

An initial overview of lung morphology is best done by T2w half-Fourier acquisition single-shot turbo spin echo (HASTE) imaging for detection of pleural effusions, pneumonia, and so on. For visualization of the pulmonary vasculature, steady-state free precession (SSFP) is easy to apply, as it can be acquired either free breathing or with breath-holds, depending on the patient. This sequence can even be acquired with ECG gating, increasing vessel visualization. This procedure is followed by a contrast-enhanced time-resolved angiographic technique and post-contrast T1w volume-interpolated breath-hold examination (VIBE) sequence. The last sequence is a high–spatial resolution angiographic data set.

for perfusion defects (kappa value per examination was 0.98).[40] The visualization of typically wedge-shaped parenchymal perfusion defects (see **Fig. 2**) allows for fast and reliable detection of vascular obstruction (even at a subsegmental level); however, direct visualization of the thrombotic material is often not possible. Perfusion MR imaging had the highest sensitivity in detection of PE in comparison with 3 different MR imaging techniques.[28] In clinical practice, however, pulmonary perfusion MR imaging and high-resolution CE-MRA are acquired in a combined protocol, which is more accurate than the individual examinations.[28,41,42] A combined protocol of pulmonary perfusion MR imaging and high-resolution CE-MRA provides a sensitivity and specificity for the detection of acute PE of more than 90% and agrees closely with CTA.[28] A combination of triggered SSFP sequences, CE-MRA, and late-enhancement 3D GRE outperformed the individual sequences in detection of acute PE, with a sensitivity of 84%.[34]

In a stepwise MR examination with SSFP, perfusion, and angiography, the perfusion sequence showed the highest sensitivity (lobar, 98%; segmental, 95%).[43] On the other hand, real-time SSFP and MRA showed the highest specificity (lobar, 90%–100%; segmental, 95%–97%). The combination of all MR sequences matched closely the results of MDCT (lobar: sensitivity 98%, specificity 100%; segmental: sensitivity 95%, specificity 97%).

As it has been shown that some patients with acute PE show incomplete thrombus resolution and development of chronic PE despite appropriate anticoagulation therapy, therapy response monitoring of these patients should be performed.[44] The combination of high diagnostic sensitivity with a radiation-free technique makes

perfusion MR imaging a highly appropriate tool for monitoring thrombus resolution during anticoagulation therapy.[45,46] In a follow-up study, 33 patients with acute PE were examined with pulmonary perfusion MR imaging initially and 1 week after initiation of therapy. A subgroup of 8 patients also underwent a second follow-up examination. Between examinations, pulmonary perfusion changed noticeably, that is, the time-to-peak enhancement decreased and the peak enhancement of the affected areas increased.[46]

CHRONIC THROMBOEMBOLIC PULMONARY HYPERTENSION

The exact pathologic pathway of the development of CTEPH is not yet fully understood.[47] In the THESEE (Tinzaparin ou Heparin Standard: Evaluation dans l'Embolie Pulmonaire Study) study a perfusion lung scan was performed in 157 patients, 8 days and 3 months after acute PE. After 3 months, a residual obstruction was found in 66% of patients and 10% had no resolution at all.[48] Similarly, Pengo and colleagues[49] found a cumulative incidence of symptomatic CTEPH of 3.8% after 2 years in patients with an acute episode of PE. Instead of thrombolysis, the thromboembolic material follows an aberrant path of organization and recanalization, leading to characteristic abnormalities such as intraluminal webs and bands, pouchlike endings of arteries, irregularities of the arterial wall, and stenotic lesions (**Figs. 5** and **6**).[50–52] This aberrant path of obstruction and reopening occurs in repeated cycles over many years. Other data suggest that in situ thrombosis may play a major role in the development of CTEPH.[53,54] In addition, small-vessel hypertensive arteriopathy, similar to that seen in other forms of pulmonary hypertension,

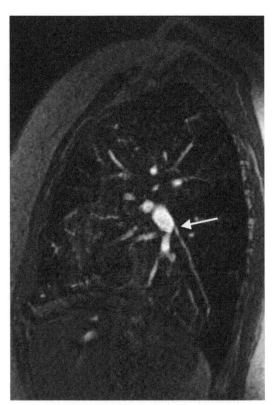

Fig. 5. MR angiography showing the typical abrupt changes in vessel diameter (*arrow*) seen in chronic pulmonary embolism. Subsequently, the perfusion in the lower lobe is reduced.

develops in small unobstructed vessels.[51,52] Patients become symptomatic if approximately 60% of the total diameter of the pulmonary arterial bed is obstructed. This obstruction leads to an increase in pulmonary arterial pressure and vascular resistance with subsequent cor pulmonale ending in right heart failure with a corresponding 5-year-survival rate of only 30%.[50–52] The primary treatment of CTEPH is surgical pulmonary endarterectomy (PEA), which leads to a permanent improvement in the pulmonary hemodynamics.[55–57] The technical feasibility and success of surgery mainly depend on the localization of the thromboembolic material; surgical candidates have organized thrombi not extending distal to the lobar arteries or the origin of the segmental vessels to develop a safe dissection plane for endarterectomy.[58]

On occasions, however, patients with CTEPH may have disease that is not accessible to surgery (distal obstructive changes), or the patients themselves may be unsuitable for surgery because of other significant comorbidities. In these situations, pulmonary arterial hypertension–specific drug treatment can reduce the symptoms.[59] In rare cases, balloon angioplasty may be considered. Lung (or heart–lung) transplantation can also be considered in selected cases in which PEA is not feasible or when significant pulmonary hypertension persists after PEA.[54]

MR imaging is especially well suited for diagnosis and follow-up of patients with CTEPH.[60] However, there are only few studies exploring the usefulness of CE-MRA in the diagnostic workup of CTEPH.[61] In a study with 34 patients, the depiction of typical findings for CTEPH was

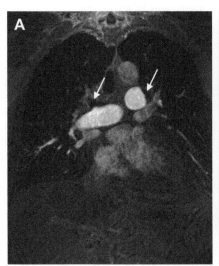
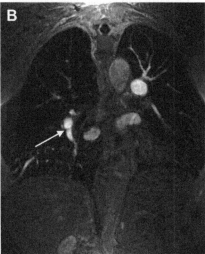

Fig. 6. (*A*) Arrows point to the wall adherent central thromboembolic material on coronal MRA. The right upper lobe pulmonary artery is completely obliterated. (*B*) MRA showing the typical intraluminal bandlike filling defect (*arrow*).

successfully done using CE-MRA.[62] The typical findings comprise wall-adherent thromboembolic material in the central parts of the pulmonary arteries down to the segmental level, intraluminal webs and bands, abnormal proximal-to-distal tapering, and abrupt vessel cutoffs (see **Figs. 5** and **6**). A thorough analysis of source images and the creation of multiplanar reformations are most important for the exact assessment of the morphologic findings. Maximum intensity projections on the other hand provide an overview and an impression of the arterial vascular tree that is comparable to those provided by the DSA images. In that study, pulmonary MRA depicted all patent vessel segments down to the level of segmental arteries (533/533 vessel segments) when compared with selective DSA. For subsegmental arteries, DSA detected significantly more patent vessel segments than MRA (733 vs 681). MRA was superior to DSA in delineating the exact central beginning of the thromboembolic material. In all cases, the most proximal site as assessed by MRA corresponded to the beginning of the dissection procedure during PEA. However, as all patients suffered from CTEPH and were candidates for surgery, there was no statement possible regarding the ability of CE-MRA in differentiating it from other causes of pulmonary hypertension. Postoperatively, CE-MRA enabled the delineation of reopened segmental arteries and a decrease in the diameter of the central pulmonary arteries. A complete normalization of pulmonary arterial vasculature was not documented in any case.

In a study of 29 patients with CTEPH and primary pulmonary hypertension (PPH), CE-MRA ($1.0 \times 0.7 \times 1.6$ mm^3) was compared with DSA and/or CTA.[41] CE-MRA had sensitivities between 83% and 86% for detection of complete vessel obstruction and free-floating thrombi and sensitivities between 50% and 71% for the depiction of older and/or organized thrombi, webs, and bands. The specificities ranged between 73% and 95% for nonobstructing findings and from 91% to 96% for occlusive findings, respectively. CE-MRA enabled correct differentiation of PPH and CTEPH in 24 of 29 patients (83%). As in acute PE, pulmonary perfusion MR can help in identification of the typical wedge-shaped perfusion defects; this was also performed in the aforementioned study,[41] and perfusion defects were classified either as patchy and/or diffuse (indicating PPH) or segmental and/or circumscribed (indicating CTEPH). Compared with perfusion scintigraphy as the standard of reference, MR imaging had an overall sensitivity of 77% in detecting perfusion defects on a per-patient basis. Compared with the final diagnosis, MR perfusion

imaging enabled a correct diagnosis of PPH or CTEPH in 20 (69%) of 29 patients. The combined interpretation of MR perfusion imaging and MRA led to a correct diagnosis of PPH or CTEPH in 26 (90%) of 29 patients when compared with the final reference diagnosis (combination of perfusion scintigraphy with DSA or CTA). In another series, MR perfusion was used to differentiate between patients with idiopathic pulmonary arterial hypertension (IPAH), CTEPH, and healthy volunteers.[42] Based on a per-segment analysis, patients with PPH showed patchy and/or diffuse reduction of perfusion in 71 (79%) of 90 segments, normal findings in 18 (20%) of 90 segments, and 1 focal defect (1%). Patients with CTEPH showed focal perfusion defects in 47 (52%), absent segmental perfusion in 23 (26%), and normal perfusion in 20 (22%) of 90 segments. On a per-patient basis, there was no difficulty in differentiating the 2 pathologic entities and in depicting the healthy volunteers. Semiquantitative analysis showed that healthy volunteers demonstrated a significantly shorter transit time of the contrast agent through the pulmonary circulation than patients with IPAH and CTEPH (14 ± 1 seconds vs 22 ± 4 seconds and 25 ± 11 seconds, respectively). No difference was found between both patient populations.

A more recent paper compared the diagnostic capabilities of DSA, ECG-gated MDCT, and MRA.[63] In this state-of-the-art comparison, ECG-gated MDCT showed the best results and outperformed MRA and DSA. The results (sensitivity and specificity) regarding CTEPH-related changes at the main/lobar and at the segmental levels were MD-CTA 100%/100% and 100%/99%; CE-MRA 83.1%/98.6% and 87.7%/98.1%; DSA 65.7%/100% and 75.8%/100%.

CHALLENGES AND OPPORTUNITIES

Over the past years, MR has been able to demonstrate high diagnostic performance for assessment of the pulmonary arteries. However, it is still mainly performed for planned examinations rather than being using in the acute clinical setting. In clinical practice, MR slots are usually booked ahead, with limited slots for emergent conditions such as suspected acute PE. In addition, MR examinations take longer than CT examinations, which implies that an emergency patient might have to wait some time before the scanner is available. Last but not the least, there are reservations about critically ill patients in the MR environment as surveillance of vital parameters can be more challenging and dedicated MR-compatible hardware has to be used. However, even in severely compromised patients (with central PE) MR examinations are possible and using a stepwise approach the diagnosis can almost always be established.[43]

Most emergency CT scans ordered for PE show negative results (82%).[64] These data were acquired in a large tertiary hospital with a high level of expertise among the emergency room (ER) physicians. The data clearly show that the clinical presentation of acute PE is variable and that there is a considerable need to exclude acute PE. However, the radiation dose is considerably high for a CTA study. Given these numbers, it might be worth reserving a few MR slots per day for those ER patients, especially young patients who would greatly benefit from a frequently used examination without radiation exposure. In the author's experience, even late pregnant patients tolerate MR examination when placed on their side. As application of Gd is discouraged in pregnant patients, application of the noncontrast part of the examination protocol (see **Table 1**) is advised. In this case, the SSFP sequences are acquired with breath-hold and additional sequences are obtained free-breathing with ECG gating. Most often, exclusion of central embolic disease is sufficient for further management of the patient. A standard CTA scan generally fails in assessing the functional burden of a vascular obstruction. This issue can be easily assessed by MR imaging.

In summary, the technology is there and the patients would benefit, but what is really needed is the implementation and widespread acceptance of this technology.

SUMMARY

MRA of the pulmonary arteries is a rapidly evolving technique with proven clinical usefulness. Multiple-step protocols, such as MR perfusion followed by high–spatial resolution MRA, seem to be a good approach for the assessment of different vascular diseases affecting the pulmonary arteries. In combination with other imaging sequences, MR imaging is one of the most comprehensive potential noninvasive imaging techniques available.

REFERENCES

1. Schoepf UJ, Costello P. CT angiography for diagnosis of pulmonary embolism: state of the art. Radiology 2004;230(2):329–37.
2. Bruzzi JF, Remy-Jardin M, Delhaye D, et al. When, why, and how to examine the heart during thoracic CT: part 2, clinical applications. AJR Am J Roentgenol 2006;186(2):333–41.
3. Ley S, Kauczor HU. MR imaging/magnetic resonance angiography of the pulmonary arteries and pulmonary thromboembolic disease. Magn Reson Imaging Clin N Am 2008;16(2):263–73.
4. Hochhegger B, Ley-Zaporozhan J, Marchiori E, et al. Magnetic resonance imaging findings in acute pulmonary embolism. Br J Radiol 2011;84(999):282–7.
5. Pedersen MR, Fisher MT, van Beek EJ. MR imaging of the pulmonary vasculature - an update. Eur Radiol 2006;16(6):1374–86.
6. Prince MR. Gadolinium-enhanced MR aortography. Radiology 1994;191:155–64.
7. Zhang H, Maki JH, Prince MR. 3D contrast-enhanced MR angiography. J Magn Reson Imaging 2007;25(1):13–25.
8. Oosterhof T, Mulder BJ. Magnetic resonance angiography for anatomical evaluation of the great arteries. Int J Cardiovasc Imaging 2005;21(2–3):323–4.
9. Sodickson DK, Griswold MA, Jakob PM, et al. Signal-to-noise ratio and signal-to-noise efficiency in SMASH imaging. Magn Reson Med 1999;41(5):1009–22.
10. Pruessmann KP, Weiger M, Scheidegger MB, et al. SENSE: sensitivity encoding for fast MRI. Magn Reson Med 1999;42(5):952–62.
11. Michaely HJ, Herrmann KA, Kramer H, et al. High-resolution renal MRA: comparison of image quality and vessel depiction with different parallel imaging acceleration factors. J Magn Reson Imaging 2006;24(1):95–100.
12. Yeh EN, Stuber M, McKenzie CA, et al. Inherently self-calibrating non-Cartesian parallel imaging. Magn Reson Med 2005;54(1):1–8.
13. Kressler B, Spincemaille P, Prince MR, et al. Reduction of reconstruction time for time-resolved spiral 3D contrast-enhanced magnetic resonance angiography using parallel computing. Magn Reson Med 2006;56(3):704–8.
14. Oberholzer K, Romaneehsen B, Kunz P, et al. Contrast-enhanced 3D MR angiography of the pulmonary arteries with integrated parallel acquisition technique (iPAT) in patients with chronic-thromboembolic pulmonary hypertension CTEPH - sagittal or coronal acquisition? Rofo 2004;176(4):605–9.
15. Nael K, Fenchel M, Krishnam M, et al. 3.0 Tesla high spatial resolution contrast-enhanced magnetic resonance angiography (CE-MRA) of the pulmonary circulation: initial experience with a 32-channel phased array coil using a high relaxivity contrast agent. Invest Radiol 2007;42(6):392–8.
16. Kreitner KF, Kunz RP, Weschler C, et al. Analysis of first-pass bolus geometry in contrast-enhanced MRA of thoracic vessels. Rofo 2005;177(5):646–54.
17. Thomsen HS, Marckmann P. Extracellular Gd-CA: differences in prevalence of NSF. Eur J Radiol 2008;66(2):180–3.
18. Rybicki FJ. MR pulmonary angiography: assessment of PIOPED III data. Int J Cardiovasc Imaging 2012;28(2):313–5.

19. Woodard PK, Chenevert TL, Sostman HD, et al. Signal quality of single dose gadobenate dimeglumine pulmonary MRA examinations exceeds quality of MRA performed with double dose gadopentetate dimeglumine. Int J Cardiovasc Imaging 2012;28(2): 295–301.

20. Keilholz SD, Bozlar U, Fujiwara N, et al. MR diagnosis of a pulmonary embolism: comparison of P792 and Gd-DOTA for first-pass perfusion MRI and contrast-enhanced 3D MRA in a rabbit model. Korean J Radiol 2009;10(5):447–54.

21. Goyen M, Laub G, Ladd ME, et al. Dynamic 3D MR angiography of the pulmonary arteries in under four seconds. J Magn Reson Imaging 2001;13(3):372–7.

22. Fink C, Ley S, Kroeker R, et al. Time-resolved contrast-enhanced three-dimensional magnetic resonance angiography of the chest: combination of parallel imaging with view sharing (TREAT). Invest Radiol 2005;40(1):40–8.

23. Ersoy H, Goldhaber SZ, Cai T, et al. Time-resolved MR angiography: a primary screening examination of patients with suspected pulmonary embolism and contraindications to administration of iodinated contrast material. AJR Am J Roentgenol 2007; 188(5):1246–54.

24. Du J, Bydder M. High-resolution time-resolved contrast-enhanced MR abdominal and pulmonary angiography using a spiral-TRICKS sequence. Magn Reson Med 2007;58(3):631–5.

25. Fink C, Ley S, Schoenberg SO, et al. Magnetic resonance imaging of acute pulmonary embolism. Eur Radiol 2007;17(10):2546–53.

26. Pereles FS, McCarthy RM, Baskaran V, et al. Thoracic aortic dissection and aneurysm: evaluation with nonenhanced true FISP MR angiography in less than 4 minutes. Radiology 2002;223(1):270–4.

27. Kluge A, Muller C, Hansel J, et al. Real-time MR with TrueFISP for the detection of acute pulmonary embolism: initial clinical experience. Eur Radiol 2004; 14(4):709–18.

28. Kluge A, Luboldt W, Bachmann G. Acute pulmonary embolism to the subsegmental level: diagnostic accuracy of three MRI techniques compared with 16-MDCT. AJR Am J Roentgenol 2006;187(1):W7–14.

29. Ehman RL, Felmlee JP. Adaptive technique for high-definition MR imaging of moving structures. Radiology 1989;173(1):255–63.

30. Spuentrup E, Bornert P, Botnar RM, et al. Navigator-gated free-breathing three-dimensional balanced fast field echo (TrueFISP) coronary magnetic resonance angiography. Invest Radiol 2002;37(11):637–42.

31. Wang Y, Rossman PJ, Grimm RC, et al. 3D MR angiography of pulmonary arteries using real-time navigator and magnetization preparation. Magn Reson Med 1996;36:579–87.

32. Deshpande VS, Shea SM, Laub G, et al. 3D magnetization-prepared true-FISP: a new technique for imaging coronary arteries. Magn Reson Med 2001;46(3):494–502.

33. Hui BK, Noga ML, Gan KD, et al. Navigator-gated three-dimensional MR angiography of the pulmonary arteries using steady-state free precession. J Magn Reson Imaging 2005;21(6):831–5.

34. Kalb B, Sharma P, Tigges S, et al. MR imaging of pulmonary embolism: diagnostic accuracy of contrast-enhanced 3D MR pulmonary angiography, contrast-enhanced low-flip angle 3D GRE, and non-enhanced free-induction FISP sequences. Radiology 2012;263(1):271–8.

35. Stein PD, Beemath A, Matta F, et al. Clinical characteristics of patients with acute pulmonary embolism: data from PIOPED II. Am J Med 2007;120(10): 871–9.

36. Blum A, Bellou A, Guillemin F, et al. Performance of magnetic resonance angiography in suspected acute pulmonary embolism. Thromb Haemost 2005;93(3):503–11.

37. Pleszewski B, Chartrand-Lefebvre C, Qanadli SD, et al. Gadolinium-enhanced pulmonary magnetic resonance angiography in the diagnosis of acute pulmonary embolism: a prospective study on 48 patients. Clin Imaging 2006;30(3):166–72.

38. Stein PD, Chenevert TL, Fowler SE, et al. Gadolinium-enhanced magnetic resonance angiography for pulmonary embolism: a multicenter prospective study (PIOPED III). Ann Intern Med 2010;152(7): 434–43.

39. Ohno Y, Higashino T, Takenaka D, et al. MR angiography with sensitivity encoding (SENSE) for suspected pulmonary embolism: comparison with MDCT and ventilation-perfusion scintigraphy. AJR Am J Roentgenol 2004;183(1):91–8.

40. Kluge A, Gerriets T, Stolz E, et al. Pulmonary perfusion in acute pulmonary embolism: agreement of MRI and SPECT for lobar, segmental and subsegmental perfusion defects. Acta Radiol 2006;47(9): 933–40.

41. Nikolaou K, Schoenberg SO, Attenberger U, et al. Pulmonary arterial hypertension: diagnosis with fast perfusion MR imaging and high-spatial-resolution MR angiography–preliminary experience. Radiology 2005;236(2):694–703.

42. Ley S, Fink C, Zaporozhan J, et al. Value of high spatial and high temporal resolution magnetic resonance angiography for differentiation between idiopathic and thromboembolic pulmonary hypertension: initial results. Eur Radiol 2005;15(11): 2256–63.

43. Hosch W, Schlieter M, Ley S, et al. Detection of acute pulmonary embolism: feasibility of diagnostic accuracy of MRI using a stepwise protocol. Emerg Radiol 2014;21(2):151–8.

44. Remy-Jardin M, Louvegny S, Remy J, et al. Acute central thromboembolic disease: posttherapeutic

follow-up with spiral CT angiography. Radiology 1997;203(1):173–80.

45. Fink C, Risse F, Semmler W, et al. MRI of pulmonary perfusion. Radiologe 2006;46(4):290–9.

46. Kluge A, Gerriets T, Lange U, et al. MRI for short-term follow-up of acute pulmonary embolism. Assessment of thrombus appearance and pulmonary perfusion: a feasibility study. Eur Radiol 2005; 15(9):1969–77.

47. Peacock A, Simonneau G, Rubin L. Controversies, uncertainties and future research on the treatment of chronic thromboembolic pulmonary hypertension. Proc Am Thorac Soc 2006;3(7):608–14.

48. Wartski M, Collignon MA. Incomplete recovery of lung perfusion after 3 months in patients with acute pulmonary embolism treated with antithrombotic agents. THESEE Study Group. Tinzaparin ou Heparin Standard: Evaluation dans l'Embolie Pulmonaire Study. J Nucl Med 2000;41(6):1043–8.

49. Pengo V, Lensing AW, Prins MH, et al. Incidence of chronic thromboembolic pulmonary hypertension after pulmonary embolism. N Engl J Med 2004; 350(22):2257–64.

50. Auger WR, Kerr KM, Kim NH, et al. Chronic thromboembolic pulmonary hypertension. Cardiol Clin 2004; 22(3):453–66, vii.

51. Dartevelle P, Fadel E, Mussot S, et al. Chronic thromboembolic pulmonary hypertension. Eur Respir J 2004;23(4):637–48.

52. Frazier AA, Galvin JR, Franks TJ, et al. From the archives of the AFIP: pulmonary vasculature: hypertension and infarction. Radiographics 2000;20: 491–524.

53. Egermayer P, Peacock AJ. Is pulmonary embolism a common cause of chronic pulmonary hypertension? Limitations of the embolic hypothesis. Eur Respir J 2000;15(3):440–8.

54. McNeil K, Dunning J. Chronic thromboembolic pulmonary hypertension (CTEPH). Heart 2007;93(9): 1152–8.

55. Kim NH. Assessment of operability in chronic thromboembolic pulmonary hypertension. Proc Am Thorac Soc 2006;3(7):584–8.

56. Madani MM, Jamieson SW. Technical advances of pulmonary endarterectomy for chronic thromboembolic pulmonary hypertension. Semin Thorac Cardiovasc Surg 2006;18(3):243–9.

57. Puis L, Vandezande E, Vercaemst L, et al. Pulmonary thromboendarterectomy for chronic thromboembolic pulmonary hypertension. Perfusion 2005; 20(2):101–8.

58. Jamieson SW, Kapelanski DP. Pulmonary endarterectomy. Curr Probl Surg 2000;37(3):165–252.

59. Hoeper MM, Kramm T, Wilkens H, et al. Bosentan therapy for inoperable chronic thromboembolic pulmonary hypertension. Chest 2005;128(4):2363–7.

60. Prince MR, Alderson PO, Sostman HD. Chronic pulmonary embolism: combining MR angiography with functional assessment. Radiology 2004;232(2): 325–6.

61. Wirth G, Bruggemann K, Bostel T, et al. Chronic thromboembolic pulmonary hypertension (CTEPH) - potential role of multidetector-row CT (MD-CT) and MR imaging in the diagnosis and differential diagnosis of the disease. Rofo 2014;186(8):751–61.

62. Kreitner KF, Ley S, Kauczor HU, et al. Chronic thromboembolic pulmonary hypertension: pre- and postoperative assessment with breath-hold MR imaging techniques. Radiology 2004;232(2):535–43.

63. Ley S, Ley-Zaporozhan J, Pitton MB, et al. Diagnostic performance of state-of-the-art imaging techniques for morphological assessment of vascular abnormalities in patients with chronic thromboembolic pulmonary hypertension (CTEPH). Eur Radiol 2012;2(3):607–16.

64. Chen YA, Gray BG, Bandiera G, et al. Variation in the utilization and positivity rates of CT pulmonary angiography among emergency physicians at a tertiary academic emergency department. Emerg Radiol 2014. [Epub ahead of print].

MR Imaging of the Thoracic Aorta

Jadranka Stojanovska, MD, MS*, Karen Rodriguez, Gisela C. Mueller, MD, MS, Prachi P. Agarwal, MD

KEYWORDS

- Thoracic aorta • MR imaging • Aortic pathology

KEY POINTS

- MR imaging allows for comprehensive evaluation of thoracic aorta without exposure to iodinated contrast or ionizing radiation.
- Basic knowledge of pulse sequences and common artifacts and ways to avoid them is essential for successful MR imaging of the aorta.
- Noncontrast magnetic resonance angiography (MRA) of the aorta can adequately answer clinical questions, even in scenarios where gadolinium administration is contraindicated.

INTRODUCTION

Invasive imaging preceded noninvasive cross-sectional imaging in evaluation of thoracic aorta. Recently, advances in CT and MR imaging have significantly improved knowledge, understanding, and management of thoracic aortic diseases. Iodinated contrast-enhanced (CE) CT is readily available, provides superior spatial resolution, and constitutes the cornerstone for pre- and post-operative evaluation of the thoracic aorta. MR imaging provides morphologic and functional information without utilization of iodinated contrast or radiation exposure. MR imaging is, therefore, preferred in younger patients in whom annual follow-ups are required.

This article discusses MR imaging techniques, protocols, imaging planes, and application of MR imaging in the assessment of common thoracic aortic pathologies, such as aneurysms, aortic dissection, penetrating ulcers, congenital anomalies, and postoperative complications. Imaging artifacts that potentially lead to misdiagnosis and ways of overcoming these artifacts also are discussed.

MR IMAGING TECHNIQUES

MR imaging of thoracic aorta is commonly used for interrogation of a variety of genetic, traumatic, atherosclerotic, inflammatory, and idiopathic disease processes. Although gadolinium-based contrast material is frequently used for thoracic aortic assessment, depending on the clinical scenario and patient specific factors, the clinical question about specific aortic pathology can be adequately answered even without gadolinium as needed. This section focuses on various MR sequences and their applications.

Black Blood Imaging

Black blood (BB) images of blood vessels are acquired with double-inversion recovery prepulse technique.[1] This flow-sensitive technique uses 2 180° inversion recovery prepulses to null the signal of flowing blood:

- The first prepulse is not slice selective and inverts the longitudinal magnetization vector (Mz) in the entire body.

Department of Radiology, University of Michigan Health System, 1500 East Medical Center Drive, Ann Arbor, MI 48109, USA
* Corresponding author. University of Michigan Health System, 1500 East Medical Center Drive, TC-B1–132, Ann Arbor, MI 48109.
E-mail address: jstoanov@med.umich.edu

Magn Reson Imaging Clin N Am 23 (2015) 273–291
http://dx.doi.org/10.1016/j.mric.2015.01.004

mri.theclinics.com

- The second prepulse is slice selective and inverts Mz back to its original orientation but only in the selected slice.

The excitation pulse is applied when Mz of blood that was initially outside the imaging slice has relaxed to zero, therefore not generating any signal. If there is flow, this blood from outside has replaced the blood in the imaging slice, resulting in nulled (dark) blood pool signal.

For routine BB imaging of the thoracic aorta, the authors use a vectorcardiogram (VCG)-gated proton density–weighted 2-D fast spin-echo (FSE) sequence with a slice thickness of 6 to 8 mm. The routine protocol includes a stack of 6- to 8-mm slices in the transverse plane of the chest and in the sagittal oblique (candy cane) view of the aortic arch. VCG gating increases imaging time but, however, significantly reduces motion artifact. Single-shot FSE (SSFSE) sequences are much faster than basic FSE sequences and allow for acquisition of the entire imaging stack in a single breath-hold. In the acute setting, it is recommended to acquire T1-weighted BB images with fat saturation, to increase the conspicuity of aortic wall hematoma.[2] T2-weighted BB imaging with fat saturation can demonstrate aortic wall or peri-aortic edema in inflammatory disorders.[3,4]

Despite being a robust and established technique, BB images are prone to artifact. Common issues are incomplete nulling of the blood pool, particularly if flow is aligned with the imaging plane, which is commonly encountered with imaging of the descending aorta in the candy cane plane and can be alleviated by decreasing the slice thickness of the second (slice-selective) inversion recovery prepulse (BB slice thickness) (**Fig. 1**). Another issue is incomplete visualization of the vessel wall, which can be resolved by increasing the BB slice thickness.

Bright Blood Imaging

VCG-gated cine acquisitions with 2-D steady state free precession (SSFP) sequences generate time-resolved images, which help not only depict the anatomy of thoracic aorta (**Fig. 2**) but also visualize flow jets, without use of gadolinium-based contrast material. Signal intensity of the blood pool on SSFP images is inherently high and relatively independent from inflow effects, which is explained by T2/T1-weighted image contrast, which is particularly high for blood and all fluids. 2-D SSFP cine imaging is used to evaluate aortic size, depict aneurysms, and demonstrate dissection flaps and any filling defects, such as

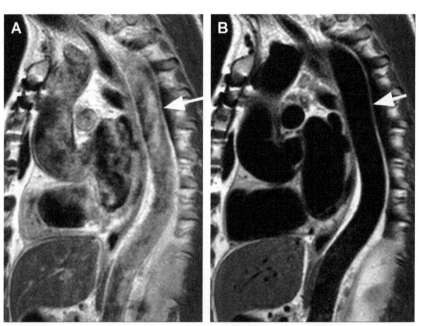

Fig. 1. A 45-year-old man with ascending aortic aneurysm. (*A*) Double-inversion BB image in sagittal oblique plane demonstrating high signal intensity within the blood in the thoracic aorta (*arrow*), due to inadequate nulling of the blood pool. (*B*) The same sequence was repeated after reducing the BB slice thickness. Note the homogeneous suppression of blood pool (*arrow*). As a rule of thumb, BB slice thickness has been suggested as 1 to 1.5 times the image slice thickness for in plane flow.

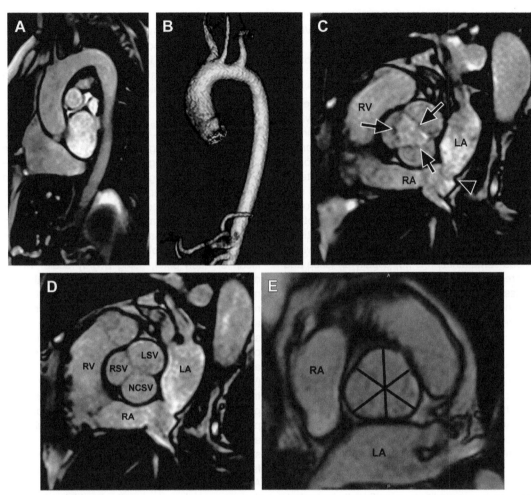

Fig. 2. Screening MR imaging of a 45-year-old man with family history of thoracic aortic aneurysm. (*A*) 2-D SSFP image in sagittal oblique plane and (*B*) volume-rendered image from first-pass gadolinium-enhanced 3-D MRA demonstrate normal morphologic appearance of thoracic aorta with 3-vessel branching. Normal tricuspid aortic valve is demonstrated on true short-axis 2-D SSFP cine images of the aortic root in (*C*) systole (arrows point to aortic cusps) and (*D*) diastole. Note typical position of noncoronary sinus (NCSV) adjacent to interatrial septum (*arrowhead*). (*E*) Demonstrates sinus to opposing commissure measurements of the aortic root obtained from a VCG- and respiratory navigator–gated 3-D SSFP image. Gadolinium-enhanced MRA is not VCG gated and not well suited for aortic root measurements. LA, left atrium; LSV, left sinus of Valsalva; RA, right atrium; RSV, right sinus of Valsalva; RV, right ventricle.

intraluminal thrombus. Cine 2-D SSFP is particularly useful for dynamic visualization of the aortic root, aortic valve morphology and motion (see **Fig. 2**), and aortic valve stenosis and regurgitation. The aortic root is best evaluated in multiple planes, including long-axis planes of the left ventricular outflow tract (LVOT) and a stack of consecutive true short-axis images of the aortic root from the aortic annulus to the sinoaortic junction (see **Fig. 2**). The remainder of the thoracic aorta is best evaluated with images in the transverse plane of the chest and in the sagittal oblique view of the aortic arch (see **Fig. 2**). The authors routinely

acquire cine images with 6- to 8-mm slice thickness and 25 to 30 reconstructed phases per heartbeat usually during breath-hold. Images can also be acquired during free breathing, by averaging multiple acquisitions.

Angiographic MR imaging of the vasculature without gadolinium is becoming increasingly popular and is indispensable in patients with renal failure in whom both iodinated and gadolinium-based contrast material are contraindicated precluding CE-CT and gadolinium-enhanced MRA. For noncontrast MRA of the thoracic aorta, traditional techniques, such as time-of-flight, have been replaced by newer methods. The most commonly used contemporary method is VCG- and respirator navigator–gated 3-D SSFP (see **Fig. 2**), allowing for near isotropic high spatial resolution imaging of the thoracic aorta and its branches, including the proximal coronary arteries, with minimal motion artifact. The inherent high fluid signal of the SSFP sequence provides excellent bright blood contrast, which is further improved by a T2 preparatory pulse to improve contrast between coronary arteries and myocardium.[5] Other advanced noncontrast MRA techniques, such as VCG-gated FSE and arterial spin labeling, aim to suppress venous and background signal and are most beneficial for imaging of the peripheral vasculature.[6] They are not routinely used for imaging of the thoracic aorta, where venous contamination is not usually an issue and suppression of background signal is often not necessary.

Both cine 2-D SSFP and 3-D SSFP sequences provide consistent image quality. When prescribing the VCG- and respirator navigator–gated 3-D SSFP, it is important to tailor the beginning and duration of the acquisition to the diastolic rest period, to avoid image blurring secondary to cardiac motion. This sequence can be affected by arrhythmia and erratic breathing, resulting in lengthy acquisitions, and suffers from low signal-to-noise ratio particularly at small voxel sizes. Despite being a noncontrast MRA technique, when this sequence is used after gadolinium administration, the signal-to-noise ratio and, therefore, image quality are significantly improved. SSFP sequences in general are susceptible to magnetic field inhomogeneity, particularly at higher field strength, which can result in off-resonance artifacts. Sternotomy wires are rarely problematic but embolization coils can render SSFP images nondiagnostic. Both cine 2-D SSFP and 3-D SSFP imaging are less useful for imaging of the aortic wall, which is better appreciated with BB or CE techniques.

Phase-Contrast Imaging

Phase-contrast imaging is used for quantitative flow velocity mapping, usually as part of a comprehensive MR imaging of the heart and aorta in patients with valvular or congenital heart disease. Phase contrast is achieved by applying bipolar gradients to generate phase shifts in moving protons, proportional to their velocity. Phase-contrast images display those phase shifts (velocities) for each pixel, using a gray scale, where midgray indicates zero velocity. Directional information is encoded in the color where white pixels represent velocities in the flow encoding direction and black pixels represent velocities in the opposite direction. An important consideration when performing phase-contrast imaging is setting an appropriate peak velocity encoding value (VENC). Ideally, VENC should be set slightly higher than the peak velocity being measured. Because peak velocities are not known a priori, a common pitfall is using a VENC that is too low, resulting in aliasing or velocity wraparound (**Fig. 3**). In this situation, the phase shift exceeds 180° and the faster flows are not appropriately represented. Although it is important to have a VENC higher than expected peak velocity, too high a VENC is not desirable because it results in less accurate measurements. For dynamic measurement of velocities during the cardiac cycle, the authors

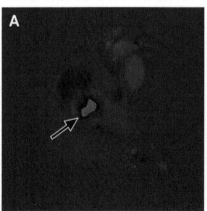
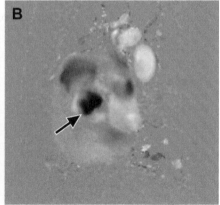

Fig. 3. A 56-year-old woman with atrial fibrillation and family history of thoracic aortic aneurysm. Phase-contrast images are shown through the aortic valve performed with different VENC values. (*A*) Shows aliasing (*arrow*) due to VENC (100 cm/s) set lower than the actual peak velocity. (*B*) This artifact resolves (*arrow*) after increasing the VENC (200 cm/s).

use a VCG-gated cine 2-D acquisition, with approximately 40 reconstructed phases per heartbeat. The most common application is measurement of through plane flow, which is obtained using commercial software by drawing regions of interest around vessel lumen and integrating flow perpendicular to the imaging plane over the duration of the cardiac cycle. Clinical uses are quantification of aortic valve regurgitation, determination of pulmonary to systemic flow ratio (Qp/Qs) in patients with shunts, and evaluation of aortic coarctation. For research purposes, measures of aortic stiffness, such as aortic pulse wave velocity, can be assessed.[7]

Advanced Applications

4-D flow MR imaging is a time-resolved 3-D phase-contrast acquisition that helps evaluate blood flow patterns. This technique is currently investigational and has been used in the thoracic aorta to study flow features in various settings, such as in patients with Marfan syndrome.[8]

Contrast-Enhanced Magnetic Resonance Angiography

CE-MRA acquires angiographic MR images of the thoracic aorta. CE-MRA is traditionally performed during first pass of a bolus of intravenously injected gadolinium-based contrast material. More recently, techniques to acquire high-quality CE-MRA during the equilibrium phase have become available (described later).

First-Pass Contrast-Enhanced Magnetic Resonance Angiography

First-pass CE-MRA, an established technique, is used for a broad range of clinical applications, including evaluation of aortic aneurysms, dissection, and postoperative anatomy. The strengths of this method are high signal-to-noise ratio and accurate depiction of the aortic lumen and its branches, including small vessels. A low-molecular extracellular gadolinium chelate is administrated intravenously using a power injector, with a dose of 0.1 mmol gadolinium/kg body weight. Images are acquired with a T1-weighted 3-D spoiled gradient-recalled echo (SPGR) sequence, usually during breath-hold. Exact timing of the acquisition to the short time period of maximum aortic enhancement is crucial and can be achieved either with test bolus or with monitoring of the contrast bolus. Isotropic 3-D SPGR acquisition allows for reformatting of source images in multiple planes, maximum intensity projections (MIPs), shaded surface display, and volume rendering (see **Fig. 2**; **Fig. 4**). First-pass CE-MRA is, however, not well suited for evaluation of the aortic root because of the short time window available for image acquisition, which precludes cardiac gating. Also, this technique is contraindicated in

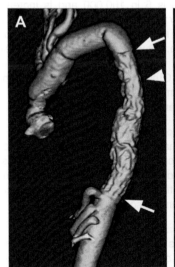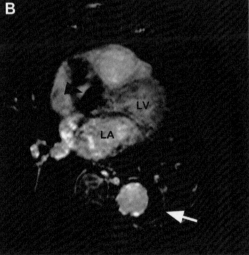

Fig. 4. A 40-year-old man with LDS, graft replacement of ascending aorta, arch, and proximal descending aorta and endograft in the mid-descending thoracic aorta. Patients with LDS have the smallest diameter threshold for aortic intervention. (*A*) Volume-rendered image from first-pass CE-MRA using gadofosveset provides overview of aortic morphology. Arrowhead indicates the position of endograft in descending thoracic aorta, with arrows pointing to proximal and distal ends of the endograft. (*B*) Axial reformatted image from MRA with gadofosveset in the equilibrium phase shows absence of endoleak in the excluded aneurysm sac (*arrow*). Position of the aortic valve prosthesis is shown by susceptibility artifact (*arrowhead*). LA, left atrium; LV, left ventricle.

patients with anaphylaxis to gadolinium and in patients with impaired renal function (an important risk factor for nephrogenic systemic fibrosis).

Contrast-Enhanced Magnetic Resonance Angiography with Gadolinium-Based Blood Pool Contrast Agents

Gadolinium-based contrast agents with increased T1 relaxivity and longer plasma half-life (blood pool agents) extend the time window for CE-MRA image acquisition. The first Food and Drug Administration–approved gadolinium-based blood pool agent is gadofosveset. Gadofosveset can be used for first-pass CE-MRA similar to conventional contrast agents (see **Fig. 4**). In addition, long duration of the equilibrium phase allows for delayed imaging with increased spatial resolution and with cardiac gating, which is particularly useful for imaging of the aortic root and coronary artery imaging. A VCG- and respiratory navigator–gated inversion recovery prepared 3-D SPGR sequence can be used to generate near isotropic angiographic images of the thoracic aorta and the coronary arteries, with high spatial resolution and minimal cardiac motion.[9,10] Gadofosveset-enhanced MRA during the equilibrium phase has been shown in some preliminary studies superior to first-pass CE-MRA and superior to CE CT in evaluation of endoleak in patients with aortic endografts (see **Fig. 4**).[11]

Recent Advances

Time-resolved CE-MRA demonstrates dynamic enhancement of blood vessels similar to conventional angiography. Images are acquired with a 3-D SPGR sequence, similar to conventional CE-MRA. Parallel imaging and keyhole data sampling are used for accelerated image acquisition necessary for the time-resolved scan. Time-resolved CE-MRA is an invaluable technique for comprehensive evaluation of the thoracic vasculature, including aorta and systemic venous and pulmonary vessels in patients with congenital heart disease.[12]

IMAGING PLANES

A comprehensive approach to evaluation of thoracic aorta includes obtaining 2-D sequences in specific planes that enable detailed assessment of the aorta as well as aortic valve and cardiac morphology and function, as necessary. A sagittal oblique plane parallel to the aortic arch, also called candy cane view, provides exquisite demonstration of the arch along with ascending and descending thoracic aorta in a single plane (see

Fig. 2), which is important when the clinical question entails assessment of aortic dissection and relationship of the arch vessels to the flap, aortic aneurysm, or other subtle arch abnormalities. The LVOT views (3-chamber and coronal oblique plane along the LVOT) (**Fig. 5**) provide information regarding aortic valve function, allow qualitative assessment of associated ventricular changes, and help plan phase-contrast imaging for the aortic valve. The true short-axis plane of the aortic valve is particularly helpful in determining the morphologic anatomy of the aortic valve (see **Fig. 5**) and in assessing patterns of commissural fusion in bicuspid valves.

AORTIC PATHOLOGY

A wide variety of aortic abnormalities can be assessed with MR imaging. This section focuses on MR assessment of aortic aneurysms (atherosclerotic, inflammatory or infectious, traumatic, post-dissection, and genetic), aortic dissection, penetrating atherosclerotic ulcers, congenital abnormalities (such as coarctation and aortic interruption), and postoperative imaging.

Aortic Aneurysm

Aortic aneurysm is defined as an abnormal enlargement of the aorta, with a diameter of 1.5 times or greater compared with the normal expected diameter for a given age and body type.[13,14] The incidence is 5 in 100,000 and is increasing as the elderly population continues to grow.[13] It is the thirteenth leading cause of death and is more common in men.[13] A wide variety of causes have been implicated, with the most common cause atherosclerosis. Other causes include aortitis (infectious or inflammatory), trauma, chronic aortic dissection, and genetic abnormalities.

Atherosclerotic
This may be associated with and exacerbated by other comorbidities, such as hypertension, smoking, advanced age, and hyperlipidemia. Atherosclerotic aneurysms are typically located in the arch and descending aorta.

Aortitis
Aortitis is defined as inflammation of the aorta, which can be infectious[15] or noninfectious, usually related to vasculitis or other rheumatologic conditions. Infectious aneurysms can be due to syphilis, bacterial infections, or tuberculosis and typically manifest as saccular aneurysms with wall thickening and adjacent infection/abscess.

The most common causes of noninfectious aortitis are large-vessel vasculitides, in particular giant

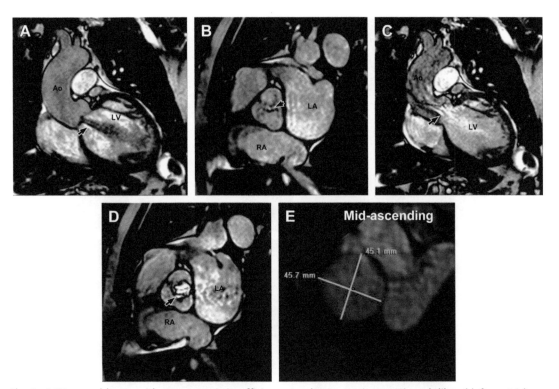

Fig. 5. A 61-year-old man with severe aortic insufficiency, moderate aortic stenosis and dilated left ventricle on echocardiography. (*A*) Diastolic 2-D SSFP image in a coronal oblique view of the LVOT demonstrates dephasing jet directed from the aortic valve into the left ventricle (*arrow*) consistent with aortic insufficiency. (*B*) Diastolic 2-D SSFP image in true short-axis plane through the aortic root demonstrates incomplete closure of the cusps (*arrow*). Restricted opening of unicommissural aortic valve with flow acceleration (*arrow*) consistent with aortic stenosis is shown on systolic 2-D SSFP images in (*C*) coronal and (*D*) axial oblique planes. (*D*) Note eccentric keyhole opening of the aortic valve consistent with unicommissural morphology. (*A*) Left ventricular dilatation is best seen on coronal oblique images through the LVOT. (*E*) Shows poststenotic dilatation of ascending aorta measuring 45 × 46 mm on reformatted image from gadolinium-enhanced 3-D MRA. Ao, aorta; LA, left atrium; LV, left ventricle; RA, right atrium.

cell arteritis and Takayasu arteritis.[15] Giant cell arteritis typically occurs in older patients, is more common in women, and is accompanied by shoulder and hip ache, jaw claudication, and markedly elevated inflammatory markers. These patients are at risk for thoracic aortic aneurysms particularly involving the ascending aorta. Takayasu arteritis, a granulomatous inflammation of the aorta and its main branches, typically occurs in young women (**Fig. 6**). The characteristic manifestation is arterial narrowing leading to symptoms, such as arm and leg claudication, although aneurysms can occur as well.

When aortitis is suspected, imaging of the aortic wall is necessary. Wall thickening and high signal intensity representing edema can be seen on T2-weighted fat-suppressed images.[3,4] CE-MRA not only provides luminal information, with delineation of areas of narrowing and aneurysmal dilatation,[16] but also information on disease activity by demonstrating wall enhancement (see **Fig. 6**). Aortitis

can be differentiated from an intramural hematoma (IMH) by its hypointense appearance on T1-weighted images[16] and enhancement after contrast. The MRA protocol, particularly for Takayasu disease, should extend the craniocaudal coverage to include the base of the neck and increase the transverse field of view to include the subclavian and axillary arteries.

Trauma

MR imaging is generally used in the follow-up of posttraumatic aneurysms. These aneurysms typically occur at the isthmus, ascending aorta, root, and diaphragmatic hiatus. Apart from blunt trauma, iatrogenic trauma is another cause of aortic aneurysms.

Chronic aortic dissection

A chronic aortic dissection with a persistent false lumen predisposes to aneurysmal dilatation. A partially thrombosed false lumen has been shown

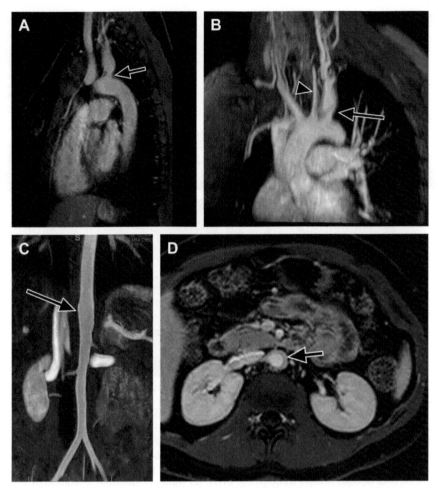

Fig. 6. A 43-year-old woman with history of Takayasu arteritis. (*A*) Gadolinium-enhanced MR image and (*B*) coronal MIP image of the thorax show narrowing of the proximal left subclavian artery (*arrow*) with poststenotic dilation. (*B*) Also demonstrates diffuse narrowing of the left carotid artery (*arrowhead*). (*C*) Coronal gadolinium-enhanced 3-D MRA image demonstrates mild dilation of the proximal abdominal aorta (*arrow*). (*D*) Gadolinium-enhanced axial 2-D SPGR image shows enhancing circumferential wall thickening and mild luminal narrowing of the aorta at the level of the kidneys (*arrow*).

to correlate with a faster regional aortic growth rate compared with a completely patent or completely thrombosed false lumen.[17]

Genetic abnormalities

Multiple genetic conditions and syndromes can predispose to aortic aneurysms. These include Marfan syndrome, Ehlers-Danlos syndrome, bicuspid aortic valve (BAV), Turner syndrome (TS), Loeys-Dietz syndrome (LDS), and familial nonsyndromic thoracic aortic aneurysms.

Genetic abnormalities tend to have a more aggressive growth rate and are prone to earlier complications, therefore requiring a lower threshold for intervention. The most well-known abnormality in this group is Marfan syndrome (**Fig. 7**), which is characterized on imaging by annuloaortic ectasia

producing a pear-shaped appearance of the dilated root and ascending aorta with effaced sinotubular junction. Such an appearance can also be seen with Ehlers-Danlos syndrome or may be idiopathic.

BAV (see **Fig. 7**) is also associated with aortic wall weakening, medial degeneration, and subsequent aneurysm formation, typically involving the root to the proximal arch. This can occur in 1% to 2 % of general population or in up to 30% of patients with TS.[18] In recent literature, TS even in absence of BAV has been shown to be associated with aortic complications, such as dissection and dilatation.

LDS is an autosomal dominant disease with 2 distinct subtypes: type I is characterized by arterial tortuosity and aneurysms, hypertelorism, and bifid uvula/cleft palate, whereas type II refers to a less

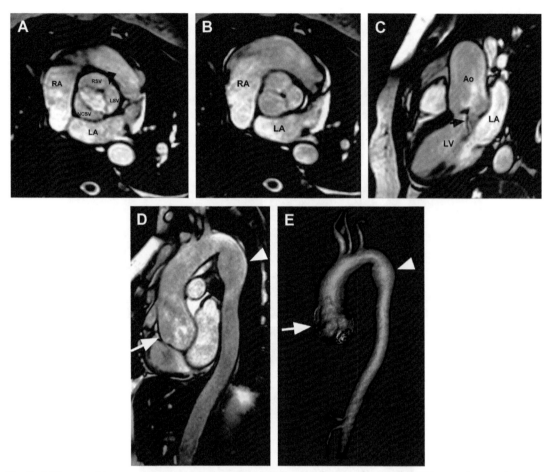

Fig. 7. A 51-year-old woman with Marfan syndrome, BAV, and aortic aneurysm. 2-D SSFP images in true short-axis plane of the aortic root in (*A*) systole and (*B*) diastole demonstrate a functional BAV with fusion of the intercoronary commissure (*arrowhead*). (*C*) Note aortic insufficiency (*arrow*) seen on the 2-D SSFP image in LVOT view. There is a dilated aortic root with effacement of sinotubular junction (*arrow*) on SSFP image in candy cane plane (*D*) and on the volume-rendered image from the CE-MRA (*E*). (*D, E*) There is also focal ectasia (*arrowhead*) of proximal descending thoracic aorta. Ao, aorta; LA, left atrium; LSV, left sinus of Valsalva; NCSV, noncoronary sinus of Valsalva; RA, right atrium; RSV, right sinus of Valsalva.

severe form including bifid uvula (but no other craniofacial manifestations) and less pronounced vascular abnormalities.[19] The most common site of vascular involvement is the aortic root with aneurysms at this site in 98% of these patients (**Fig. 8**).[19] Thoracic aortic dissections are the most common cause of death in this patient population. Given the high risk of complications, aortic aneurysms in LDS have one of the smallest thresholds for operative intervention.

Management of aortic aneurysms

The natural history of aneurysms is variable, with a rate of enlargement of approximately 0.1 cm per year for atherosclerotic ascending aortic aneurysms. Accelerated growth rates and complications often occur with genetic abnormalities, such as Marfan syndrome and BAV, where the aneurysm may grow at 0.2 cm per year.[20] In accordance with the law of Laplace, larger aneurysms grow faster, thereby increasing the risk of complications. The decision to operate is made on a patient-by-patient basis, weighing the risks and benefits. Operative mortality is not negligible, but surgical intervention is mandated when the risk of waiting outweighs the risk of the operation.[14] Based on the annual risk of complications relative to size,[14] current guidelines suggest surgical or endovascular intervention in patients with no genetic abnormality when the ascending aorta is greater than 5.5 cm, when the descending aorta is greater than 6.0 cm, or if there is a rapid increase in size (>0.5 cm/y).[20,21] The threshold to intervene is lower for individuals with a genetic basis for

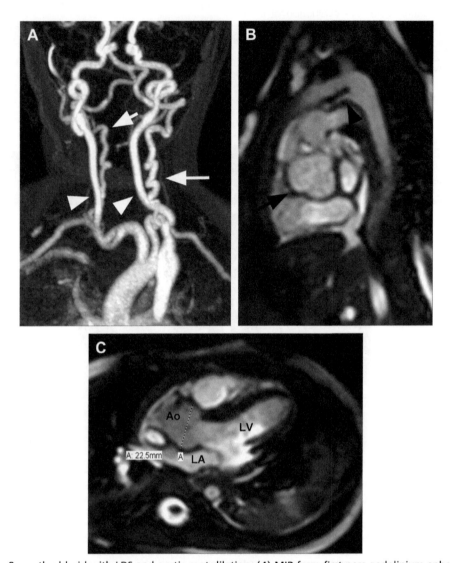

Fig. 8. An 8-month-old girl with LDS and aortic root dilation. (*A*) MIP from first-pass gadolinium-enhanced 3-D MRA demonstrates tortuous carotid (*arrowheads*) and vertebral (*arrows*) arteries. Severe aortic root dilatation is appreciated on 2-D SSFP images in (*B*) the true short-axis plane of the aortic root (*arrow*) and (*C*) the LVOT plane. (*B*) The patient also had a small patent ductus arteriosus (*black arrowhead*). Ao, aorta; LA, left atrium; LV, left ventricle.

ascending aneurysm (such as Marfan syndrome and BAV) and is usually 5 cm for the ascending aorta, unless a family history of aortic dissection is present when the threshold is lowered to 4.5 cm. Patients with LDS have the lowest threshold of 4.2 cm on transesophageal echocardiogram (using internal diameter) and 4.4 to 4.6 cm on MR imaging[22] (using external diameter incorporating the aortic wall) (see **Fig. 4**).

Imaging surveillance guidelines for aortic aneurysms recommend baseline study followed by 6-month follow-up and annual studies for stable ascending aortic aneurysms measuring less than

4.5 cm. More frequent (biannual) follow-up may be performed for aneurysms that are growing rapidly or measure 4.5 cm or greater. For LDS, MR imaging coverage should include cerebrovascular circulation to the pelvis.[22] In view of the need for regular surveillance, MR imaging has a distinct advantage over CT in terms of avoidance of ionizing radiation in this young patient population.

Imaging goals are accurate assessment of aortic diameters, morphology (fusiform vs saccular), extent of aneurysm, and involvement of branch vessels. These goals are accomplished using a combination of BB imaging, 2-D SSFP and 3-D

SSFP sequences, and gadolinium-enhanced MRA. MR imaging provides an insight to the cause of an aneurysm by allowing assessment of aortic wall thickening and enhancement in aortitis, periaortic abscesses in cases of infectious aneurysms, and concomitant assessment of aortic valve morphology and function. Aortic diameter measurements are made perpendicular to the flow incorporating the aortic wall using multiplanar reconstructions of 3-D data sets.[3,23] Although gadolinium-enhanced MRA is commonly used for aortic dimensions, root measurement is best performed on an ECG-gated sequence, such as 3-D SSFP, given the presence of significant motion at this level on nongated MRA images. It is important to consistently use the same technique of measurement, MR imaging sequence, and anatomic site for follow-up studies.

Aortic Dissection

CT and MR imaging are both extremely accurate in the assessment of acute aortic syndrome (AAS), although the choice of modality is dictated primarily by access and availability of the imaging technique. In general, CT is preferred due to its ready availability (especially in an emergent setting) and short examination time. Based on the International Registry of Acute Aortic Dissection, CT was used in 61% of cases of all types of AAS compared with MR imaging, which was used in less than 5%.[24] MR imaging is typically done in cases of diagnostic uncertainty or when iodinated contrast is contraindicated. Noncontrast MR imaging, if needed, can be performed and provides more comprehensive assessment than noncontrast CT.

Typical and atypical aortic dissection
Sudden, severe sharp tearing or ripping pain characterizes aortic dissection, a life-treating condition with an early mortality of 1% to 2% per hour. Imaging has improved the accuracy of diagnosing AAS in emergency departments.[25] Incidence is estimated at 5 to 30 per million per year.[26] Typical dissection begins with an intimal tear, followed by separation of the layers within the wall and propagation of false passage within the media and elevation of intimal flap. On the other hand, IMH is considered a variant or precursor to dissection with rupture of vasa vasorum within the media and formation of hematoma. Hypertension, advanced age, male gender, genetic factors associated with wall weakening (eg, Marfan syndrome or BAV), prior cardiac surgery, trauma, and less commonly, cocaine use and inflammatory conditions are risk factors for developing aortic dissection. The Stanford classification divides dissections into type A (with involvement of the ascending aorta) and type B (without ascending aortic involvement) to address therapeutic and prognostic differences.[2] Type A requires urgent surgery whereas medical therapy or stent grafting is often used for type B dissections. Management of IMH is similar to that of classic dissection, with ascending aortic involvement conferring a worse prognosis. Imaging goals for dissection include confirmation of the diagnosis, determination of the extent of dissection with tear localization, ascending aortic involvement, presence of aortic insufficiency, hemopericardium, mediastinal hematoma, and branch vessel involvement. Special attention should be paid to involvement of coronary arterial ostia and/or aortic valve, particularly in type A dissections.

If MR imaging is performed in a clinical scenario where gadolinium is contraindicated; evaluation includes a combination of T1-weighted BB imaging, 2-D cine SSFP sequences in axial and candy cane planes, and 3-D SSFP sequence. These allow evaluation of the presence of dissection, morphology and extent of the dissection flap, and presence of hematoma and hemopericardium. Presence of aortic regurgitation and coronary ostial involvement can be determined using 2-D SSFP and 3-D SSFP sequences, respectively. In cases of IMH, T1-weighted BB images demonstrate intermediate or high signal intensity in the aortic wall, which is better assessed and differentiated from adjacent mediastinal fat by using fat suppression technique. The signal intensity of the thickened aortic wall depends on the age of hematoma, with oxyhemoglobin producing intermediate signal and methemoglobin producing high signal intensity on T1-weighted imaging. BB sequence alone, however, may fail in distinguishing IMH from slow-flowing blood, which also produces intermediate to high signal intensity.[2] Hence, this should be correlated with additional sequences, such as SSFP and CE-MRA, when possible.

Pre- and postcontrast SPGR sequence is useful in identifying IMH as a crescentic high signal intensity of the aortic wall, which does not enhance after contrast. 3-D MRA with multiplanar reconstruction (Fig. 9) nicely depicts the dissection by highlighting the intimal flap, evaluating the true and false lumina, and most importantly, evaluating the patency of branch vessels. Also, it helps in resolving any artifacts or questionable abnormalities seen on other sequences. A time-resolved MRA provides additional information about the dynamics of true and false luminal enhancement. Depending on a patient's clinical stability, if needed, additional sequences, such as phase-contrast imaging, can include quantification of

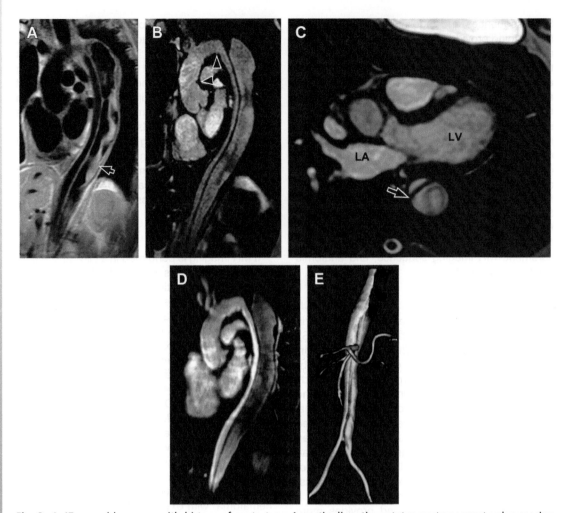

Fig. 9. A 47-year-old woman with history of acute type A aortic dissection; status postemergent valve-sparing aortic root, ascending aorta, and proximal aortic arch repair. (*A*) BB and (*B*) 2-D SSFP images in candy cane view demonstrate graft of ascending aorta and proximal arch (*arrowheads*) and dissection flap in native descending thoracoabdominal aorta. (*A*) Increased signal intensity in false lumen (*arrow*) of descending aorta on BB image is secondary to sluggish flow in the imaging plane. (*C*) Demonstrates appearance of dissection flap (*arrow*) on 2-D SSFP image in descending aorta. Dissection flap is also appreciated on gadolinium-enhanced 3-D MRA of the chest in candy cane view (*D*) and volume-rendered reconstruction of abdominal aorta from gadolinium-enhanced 3-D MRA (*E*). LA, left atrium; LV, left ventricle.

aortic regurgitation and the amount of relative flow between the true and false lumens.

Flow velocity data using time-resolved 3-D phase-contrast MR imaging can estimate wall shear stress as well as pulse wave velocities to serve as potential markers in follow-up scans.[2]

Penetrating Ulcer

Penetrating ulcer is defined as an ulceration that has eroded the inner elastic layer of the aortic wall, often associated with hematoma within the media (IMH). It is most commonly found in patients with severe systemic atherosclerosis. This entity can be depicted as luminal outpouchings on CE-MRA at the level of the ulcer often with accompanying adjacent IMH.

Congenital Aortic Anomalies

Various congenital aortic abnormalities can occur, such as coarctation, interrupted aortic arch, and aortic arch abnormalities, including vascular rings.

Coarctation

Coarctation of the aorta consists of focal narrowing and typically occurs distal to the origin of left subclavian artery.[27–29] Although traditionally classified as preductal (infantile), and postductal (adult) type, it is now believed that the time of onset of symptoms is more closely related to the presence of associated abnormalities and the severity of narrowing rather than the location. Surgical management involves a variety of approaches, with the most common resection and end-to-end anastomosis. Other options include aortoplasty (using prosthetic material or subclavian artery) and bypass grafting with a conduit insertion. Recently, balloon dilatation with stent insertion has been used to treat both coarctation and recoarctation as an alternative to surgery (**Fig. 10**).

MR imaging provides comprehensive morphologic and functional assessment of coarctation

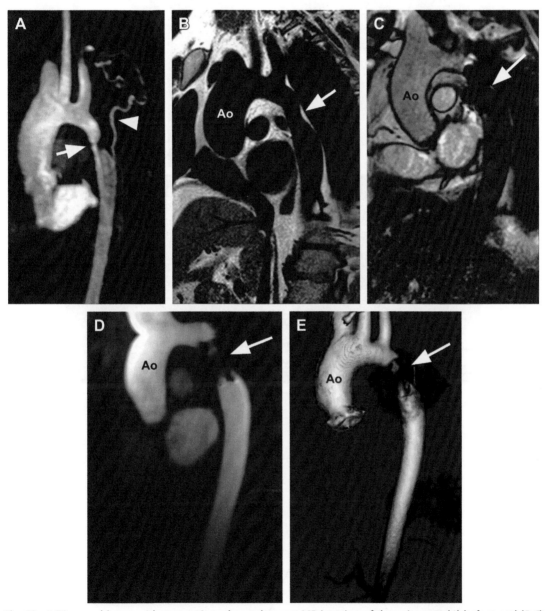

Fig. 10. A 54-year-old man with coarctation who underwent MR imaging of thoracic aorta (*A*) before and (*B–E*) after stent placement across the coarctation. (*A*) 3-D CE-MRA images demonstrate narrowing (*arrow*) of the proximal descending aorta with collateral vessels (*arrowhead*) and mild poststenotic dilatation. (*B*) Proton density–weighted BB image in candy cane plane of the thoracic aorta post–stent placement across the coarctation demonstrates mild residual narrowing (*arrow*). There is no significant artifact on (*B*) BB image compared with (*C*) 2-D SSFP (*arrow*), (*D*) MIP from gadolinium-enhanced 3-D MRA (*arrow*), and (*E*) volume-rendered reconstruction of 3-D MRA (*arrow*), which are more prone to susceptibility artifact from the stent. Ao, aorta.

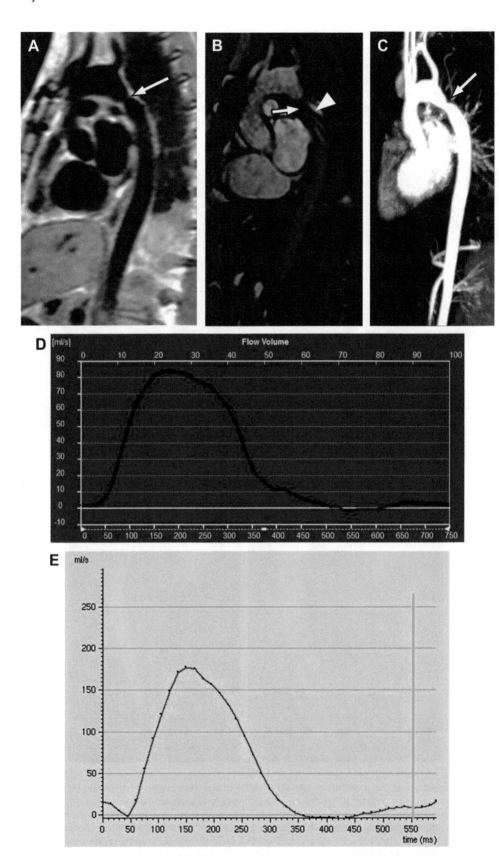

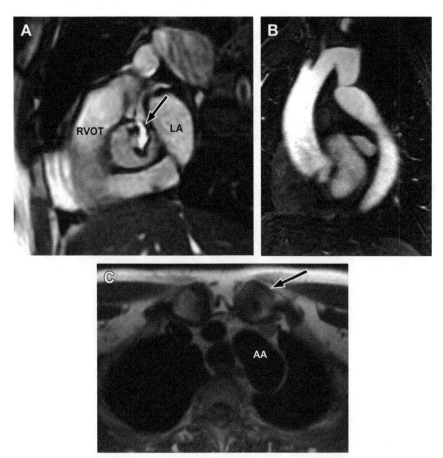

Fig. 12. A 47-year-old man with aortic stenosis. (*A*) Restricted opening of a unicommisural aortic valve (*arrow*) is seen on 2-D SSFP image in the true short-axis plane of the aortic root. (*B*) MIP from gadolinium-enhanced 3-D MRA demonstrates elongated high-riding arch with kink at level of the isthmus compatible with pseudocoarctation. There were no collaterals and there was no significant gradient. (*C*) The axial BB image shows high-riding (cervical) aortic arch (AA) at the level of the jugular fossa. (*C*) Arrow indicates medial left clavicle. LA, left atrium; RVOT, right ventricular outflow tract.

as well as evaluation of associated abnormalities, in particular BAV and tubular and isthmic hypoplasia. Gadolinium-enhanced MRA with its 3-D capability provides excellent anatomic depiction of aortic anatomy. It is important to precisely measure the minimum aortic diameter, assess relationship of narrowing with the arch vessels, and evaluate collateral vessels (**Fig. 11**). In patients with aortic stents, a BB 2-D FSE sequence should be part of the protocol because these sequences are less degraded by susceptibility artifact than SSFP techniques (see **Fig. 10**). A sagittal oblique plane is best suited for depiction of the arch and proximal descending thoracic anatomy. Phase-contrast imaging allows quantification of pressure gradient (by measuring peak velocity and using the modified Bernoulli equation) as well as estimation of collateral flow, which is accomplished by measuring flow immediately distal to coarctation and at the level of the diaphragmatic hiatus. In

Fig. 11. A 14-year-old boy with history of prior coarctation repair. (*A*) BB image, (*B*) 2-D SSFP image, and (*C*) MIP of 3-D CE-MRA in candy cane view demonstrate discrete narrowing (*arrow*) distal to left subclavian artery. Also, note the dephasing jet (*arrowhead*) extending distally from the area of narrowing on the 2-D SSFP image (*B*), compatible with restenosis post–coarctation repair. Assessment of flow pattern obtained from phase-contrast imaging in descending aorta at level of diaphragmatic hiatus shows abnormal prolonged deceleration slope suggesting proximal obstruction (*D*). For comparison, normal flow pattern in descending aorta at level of diaphragm is demonstrated in a different patient (*E*).

cases of collaterals, the more distal aortic flow is higher and the difference between the 2 measurements provides an estimate of collateral flow. Although estimation of pressure gradient is feasible on MR imaging, it is well known that MR imaging does not perform well in cases of turbulent flow, resulting in poor correlation with transcatheter peak gradient measurements.[27] Hence, other measures to predict hemodynamic severity of coarctation (corresponding to transcatheter systolic pressure gradient $\geq$20 mm Hg) have been evaluated. One recent study demonstrated that indexed minimal cross-sectional area less than 0.33 cm^2/m^2 and heart rate–corrected flow deceleration time in descending aorta of greater than or equal to 0.30 s$^{-0.5}$ are independent predictors of gradient greater than or equal to 20 mm Hg (see **Fig. 11**).[28]

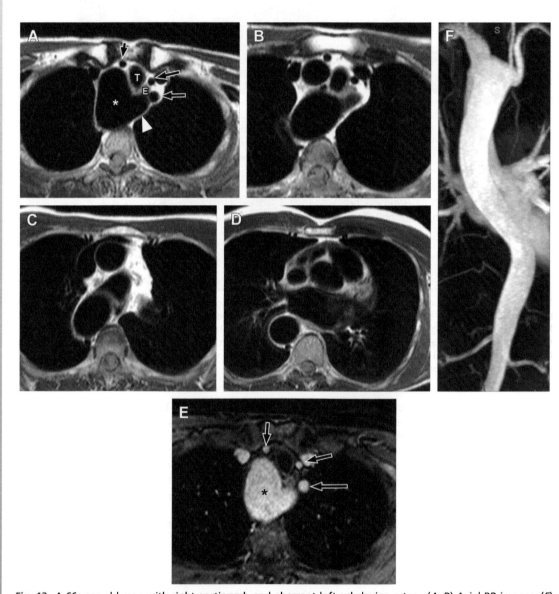

Fig. 13. A 66-year-old man with right aortic arch and aberrant left subclavian artery. (*A–D*) Axial BB images, (*E*) axial gadolinium-enhanced 3-D MRA, and (*F*) MIP from gadolinium-enhanced 3-D MRA demonstrate a right-sided aortic arch (*asterisk*) with aberrant left subclavian artery. The dilated retroesophageal origin of the left subclavian artery as the last branch from the right aortic arch is referred to as *diverticulum of Kommerell* (*arrowhead*). Esophagus is indicated by E and trachea by T, with arrows pointing to the arch vessels. This abnormality constitutes a vascular ring, with esophagus and trachea running between right artic arch, aberrant left subclavian artery (posterior), and ligamentum arteriosum (to the left and anterior).

In contrast to coarctation, pseudocoarctation is characterized by a kink in the distal arch without hemodynamically significant pressure gradient or collaterals (**Fig. 12**).[30]

Aortic interruption

Aortic interruption is a complete discontinuity of the aortic lumen and is categorized into 4 types based on the site of aortic interruption. Type B (interruption between left carotid and left subclavian artery) is the most common subtype. Patent ductus arteriosus provides distal aortic flow. There may be other associated congenital cardiac abnormalities as well.

Arch anomalies

Arch anomalies encompass a range of developmental anomalies. Causes of vascular ring include double aortic arch, right arch with aberrant left subclavian artery and left ligamentum (**Fig. 13**), right arch with mirror image branching and retroesophageal ligamentum, and circumaortic arch. Apart from gadolinium-enhanced MRA, which provides anatomic assessment of the ring, axial and coronal oblique BB images (oriented along the airways) help assess the impact on the tracheobronchial tree. A 3-D SSFP sequence is also helpful and provides information on both airways and vascular ring and can be viewed in any desired plane.

Postoperative Aorta

Continuing care of patients after aortic surgery is essential and may require lifelong follow-up. The aorta and the aortic arch may require surgery for a variety of reasons (discussed previously). Routine follow-up for complications is necessary and best achieved by noninvasive imaging, such as CT and MR imaging (**Figs. 14** and **15**). Metallic surgical clips, stents, and prosthesis, however, are associated with susceptibility artifacts on MR imaging, which degrade image quality. The extent of artifact depends on the location and type of implant/prosthesis (see **Figs. 4** and **14**).[31] As discussed previously, BB imaging can be particularly helpful in these scenarios. Another emerging application is assessment after endovascular aneurysm repair, which is becoming a common aortic procedure requiring surveillance imaging. Endoleaks are the most common complication and, although commonly assessed with CT, are beginning to be evaluated with MR imaging as well (particularly in the abdominal aorta). MR imaging is useful in evaluating postoperative aortic morphology, monitoring the aortic diameter, evaluating the integrity of proximal

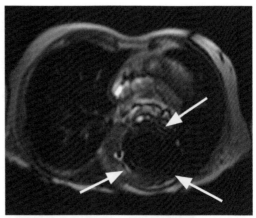

Fig. 14. A 69-year-old man post–endograft repair of a saccular aneurysm of distal aortic arch. Survey, axial image demonstrates significant susceptibility artifact (*arrows*) in descending thoracic aorta from thoracic endograft that rendered the study nondiagnostic. The type of endovascular stent can determine the extent of artifact. In this case, the endograft (Zenith, Cook, Bloomington, Indiana) with stainless steel component was MR conditional but associated with severe artifacts. In contrast, the nitinol-based endograft (Telent, Medtronic, Santa Rosa, California) depicted in **Fig. 4** shows minimal artifacts.

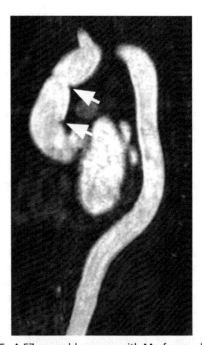

Fig. 15. A 57-year-old woman with Marfan syndrome, aortic valve replacement, and graft replacement of ascending aorta. 3-D gadolinium-enhanced MRA demonstrates normal postoperative appearance of the aorta with graft replacement of the ascending aorta (*arrows*).

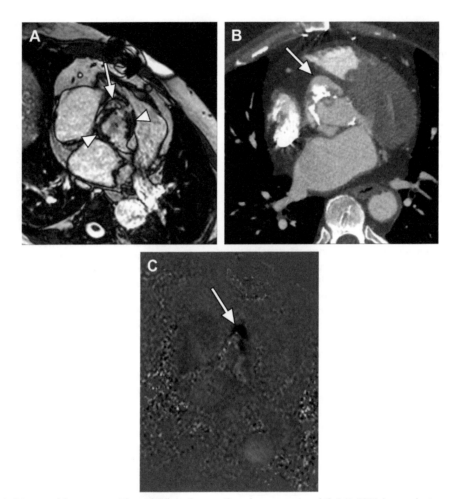

Fig. 16. A 54-year-old woman with multiple prior aortic valve surgeries. (A) 2-D SSFP image in true short-axis plane of the aortic root shows paravalvular leak (*arrow*) anterior to the low signal intensity corresponding to calcifications and postsurgical changes in the aortic root (*arrowheads*). (B) Corresponding axial CT image confirms the paravalvular leak (*arrow*). (C) Phase-contrast image in true axial plane of the aortic root during diastole shows flow through the paravalvular region (*arrow*). The patient had known severe aortic regurgitation on echocardiography.

and distal anastomotic sites, and detecting complications (**Fig. 16**).

SUMMARY

MR imaging allows holistic aortic evaluation, encompassing morphologic and functional assessment of thoracic aorta and aortic valve. The shortcomings of long scanning time and decreased spatial resolution relative to CT are overcome by absence of ionizing radiation and avoidance of nephrotoxic iodinated contrast. These factors make MR imaging the preferred method of evaluation in young individuals, particularly when serial follow-ups are needed. MR imaging protocol needs to be tailored depending on clinical scenario and specific clinical question.

REFERENCES

1. Simonetti OP, Finn JP, White RD, et al. "Black blood" T2-weighted inversion-recovery MR imaging of the heart. Radiology 1996;199(1):49–57.
2. Holloway BJ, Rosewarne D, Jones RG. Imaging of thoracic aortic disease. Br J Radiol 2011;84(Spec No 3):S338–54.
3. Rajiah P. CT and MRI in the evaluation of thoracic aortic diseases. Int J Vasc Med 2013;2013:797189.
4. Katabathina VS, Restrepo CS. Infectious and noninfectious aortitis: cross-sectional imaging findings. Semin Ultrasound CT MR 2012;33(3):207–21.
5. Shea SM, Deshpande VS, Chung YC, et al. Three-dimensional true-FISP imaging of the coronary arteries: improved contrast with T2-preparation. J Magn Reson Imaging 2002;15(5):597–602.

6. Miyazaki M, Akahane M. Non-contrast enhanced MR angiography: established techniques. J Magn Reson Imaging 2012;35(1):1–19.

7. Joly L, Perret-Guillaume C, Kearney-Schwartz A, et al. Pulse wave velocity assessment by external noninvasive devices and phase-contrast magnetic resonance imaging in the obese. Hypertension 2009;54(2):421–6.

8. Geiger J, Markl M, Herzer L, et al. Aortic flow patterns in patients with Marfan syndrome assessed by flow-sensitive four-dimensional MRI. J Magn Reson Imaging 2012;35(3):594–600.

9. Naehle CP, Kaestner M, Muller A, et al. First-pass and steady-state MR angiography of thoracic vasculature in children and adolescents. JACC Cardiovasc Imaging 2010;3(5):504–13.

10. Stuber M, Botnar RM, Danias PG, et al. Contrast agent-enhanced, free-breathing, three-dimensional coronary magnetic resonance angiography. J Magn Reson Imaging 1999;10(5):790–9.

11. Wieners G, Meyer F, Halloul Z, et al. Detection of type II endoleak after endovascular aortic repair: comparison between magnetic resonance angiography and blood-pool contrast agent and dual-phase computed tomography angiography. Cardiovasc Intervent Radiol 2010;33(6):1135–42.

12. Goo HW, Yang DH, Park IS, et al. Time-resolved three-dimensional contrast-enhanced magnetic resonance angiography in patients who have undergone a Fontan operation or bidirectional cavopulmonary connection: initial experience. J Magn Reson Imaging 2007;25(4):727–36.

13. Carpenter SW, Kodolitsch YV, Debus ES, et al. Acute aortic syndromes: definition, prognosis and treatment options. J Cardiovasc Surg 2014;55(2 Suppl 1):133–44.

14. Elefteriades JA. Natural history of thoracic aortic aneurysms: indications for surgery, and surgical versus nonsurgical risks. Ann Thorac Surg 2002; 74(5):S1877–80 [discussion: S1892–8].

15. Restrepo CS, Ocazionez D, Suri R, et al. Aortitis: imaging spectrum of the infectious and inflammatory conditions of the aorta. Radiographics 2011;31(2): 435–51.

16. Hartlage GR, Palios J, Barron BJ, et al. Multimodality imaging of aortitis. JACC Cardiovasc Imaging 2014; 7(6):605–19.

17. Tsai MT, Wu HY, Roan JN, et al. Effect of false lumen partial thrombosis on repaired acute type A aortic dissection. J Thorac Cardiovasc Surg 2014;148(5): 2140–6.e3.

18. Sachdev V, Matura LA, Sidenko S, et al. Aortic valve disease in turner syndrome. J Am Coll Cardiol 2008; 51(19):1904–9.

19. Johnson PT, Chen JK, Loeys BL, et al. Loeys-Dietz syndrome: MDCT angiography findings. AJR Am J Roentgenol 2007;189(1):W29–35.

20. Booher AM, Eagle KA. Diagnosis and management issues in thoracic aortic aneurysm. Am Heart J 2011;162(1):38–46.e1.

21. Svensson LG, Adams DH, Bonow RO, et al. Aortic valve and ascending aorta guidelines for management and quality measures. Ann Thorac Surg 2013;95(Suppl 6):S1–66.

22. Hiratzka LF, Bakris GL, Beckman JA, et al. 2010 ACCF/AHA/AATS/ACR/ASA/SCA/SCAI/SIR/STS/SVM guidelines for the diagnosis and management of patients with thoracic aortic disease. A report of the American college of cardiology foundation/American heart association task force on practice guidelines, American association for thoracic surgery, American college of radiology, american stroke association, society of cardiovascular anesthesiologists, society for cardiovascular angiography and interventions, society of interventional radiology, society of thoracic surgeons, and society for vascular medicine. J Am Coll Cardiol 2010;55(14): e27–129.

23. Evangelista A. Imaging aortic aneurysmal disease. Heart 2014;100(12):909–15.

24. Tsai TT, Nienaber CA, Eagle KA. Acute aortic syndromes. Circulation 2005;112(24):3802–13.

25. Evangelista A, Carro A, Moral S, et al. Imaging modalities for the early diagnosis of acute aortic syndrome. Nat Rev Cardiol 2013;10(8):477–86.

26. Baliga RR, Nienaber CA, Bossone E, et al. The role of imaging in aortic dissection and related syndromes. JACC Cardiovasc Imaging 2014;7(4):406–24.

27. Muzzarelli S, Ordovas KG, Hope MD, et al. Diagnostic value of the flow profile in the distal descending aorta by phase-contrast magnetic resonance for predicting severe coarctation of the aorta. J Magn Reson Imaging 2011;33(6):1440–6.

28. Muzzarelli S, Meadows AK, Ordovas KG, et al. Prediction of hemodynamic severity of coarctation by magnetic resonance imaging. Am J Cardiol 2011; 108(9):1335–40.

29. Lee EY, Siegel MJ, Hildebolt CF, et al. MDCT evaluation of thoracic aortic anomalies in pediatric patients and young adults: comparison of axial, multiplanar, and 3D images. AJR Am J Roentgenol 2004; 182(3):777–84.

30. Bluemke DA. Pseudocoarctation of the aorta. Cardiol J 2007;14(2):205–6.

31. Albayati MA, Clough R. Optimising pre and post operative imaging for thoracic aortic pathology. J Cardiovasc Surg 2014;55:529–41.

MR Imaging of Thoracic Veins

Gisela C. Mueller, MD, MS[a,*], Jimmy C. Lu, MD[b,c], Maryam Ghadimi Mahani, MD[d], Adam L. Dorfman, MD[b,c], Prachi P. Agarwal, MD[e]

KEYWORDS

- MR imaging • MR angiography • Systemic veins • Pulmonary veins • Cardinal venous system

KEY POINTS

- Anatomic and functional evaluation of the thoracic venous vasculature is achieved with intravenous gadolinium enhanced MRA, "noncontrast" MR techniques and phase contrast imaging.
- Congenital anomalies of systemic and pulmonary veins can be explained by disturbances at specific stages of the development of the primordial heart and venous systems.
- Acquired abnormalities are most frequently iatrogenic or related to cancer, and infrequently caused by inflammatory disorders.

INTRODUCTION

This article discusses the normal anatomy and development of the thoracic systemic and pulmonary veins, their common variants, developmental and acquired abnormalities, and MR imaging methods for their evaluation.

NORMAL ANATOMY AND DEVELOPMENT
Systemic Veins and Coronary Sinus

In the 3-week-old embryo, development of systemic thoracic veins starts with appearance of paired umbilical and vitelline veins, forming the sinus venosus.[1] Anterior and posterior cardinal veins appear in the fourth week. They drain deoxygenated blood from the cranial and caudal portion of the embryo into the sinus venosus via the right and left common cardinal veins (**Fig. 1**A). At this stage, the sinus venosus empties into a common atrium.

During the following weeks, a bridging vein develops between the anterior cardinal veins (see **Fig. 1**B), which eventually becomes the left brachiocephalic vein (LBCV; see **Fig. 1**C). During further development, there is regression of the left anterior cardinal vein, and the right common and anterior cardinal veins form the superior vena cava (SVC), and right brachiocephalic vein (see **Fig. 1**C). The azygos and hemiazygos system develops from the embryologic supracardinal veins, except the arch of the azygos vein, which is formed by the right posterior cardinal vein (see **Fig. 1**B). The suprahepatic inferior vena cava (IVC) is formed by the right vitelline vein, which also contributes to development of the hepatic veins, whereas the left vitelline vein, right umbilical vein, and suprahepatic left umbilical veins regress (see **Fig. 1**B). The right horn of the sinus venosus is absorbed into the developing right atrium and eventually forms the majority of the mature right atrium, except the right atrial appendage, which is

The authors have nothing to disclose.
[a] Department of Radiology, University of Michigan, Ann Arbor, MI 48109-2713, USA; [b] Department of Pediatrics, University of Michigan Congenital Heart Center, C.S. Mott Children's Hospital, University of Michigan, 1540 East Hospital Drive, Ann Arbor, MI 48109-4204, USA; [c] Department of Radiology, University of Michigan Congenital Heart Center, C.S. Mott Children's Hospital, University of Michigan, 1540 East Hospital Drive, Ann Arbor, MI 48109-4204, USA; [d] Department of Radiology, C.S. Mott Children's Hospital, University of Michigan, Floor 3 Recp A Room 3660A, 1540 East Hospital Drive SPC 4252, Ann Arbor, MI 48109, USA; [e] Department of Radiology, Cardiovascular Center, University of Michigan, Floor 5 Room 5383, 1500 East Medical Center Drive SPC 5868, Ann Arbor, MI 48109, USA
* Corresponding author. 11700 W Charleston Blvd Ste, 170-34, Las Vegas, NV 89135.
E-mail address: giselach@icloud.com

Magn Reson Imaging Clin N Am 23 (2015) 293–307
http://dx.doi.org/10.1016/j.mric.2015.01.001
1064-9689/15/$ – see front matter © 2015 Elsevier Inc. All rights reserved.

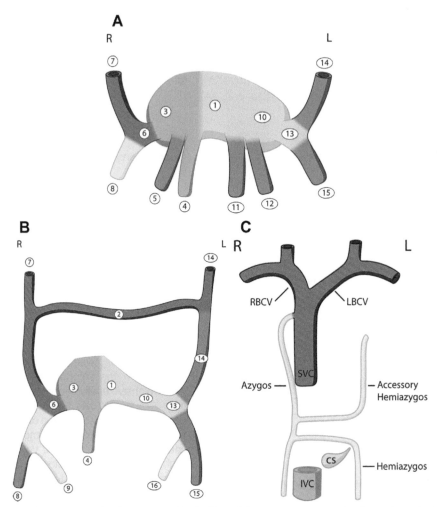

Fig. 1. Systemic thoracic vein development. Veins indicated in gray are present in the embryo but eventually degenerate. Structures indicated in orange contribute to the right atrium and suprahepatic inferior vena cava. Structures indicated in green contribute to coronary venous system. Veins indicated in purple develop into the superior vena cava and brachiocephalic veins. Veins indicated in yellow contribute to azygos/hemiazygos system. (*A*) Systemic vein development at the end of first month. (*B*) Systemic vein development at the end of the second month. (*C*) Mature venous system. (*A*, *B*) Unpaired veins: (1) transverse portion of sinus venosus, (2) bridging vein between left and right anterior cardinal vein. Right-sided veins: (3) right horn of sinus venosus, (4) right vitelline vein, (5) right umbilical vein, (6) right common cardinal vein, (7) right anterior cardinal vein, (8) right posterior cardinal vein, (9) right supracardinal vein. Left-sided veins: (10) left horn of sinus venosus, (11) left vitelline vein, (12) left umbilical vein, (13) left common cardinal vein, (14) left anterior cardinal vein, (15) left posterior cardinal vein, and (16) left supracardinal vein.

the remnant of the primitive right atrium. Transverse portion and left horn of sinus venosus forms the coronary sinus (CS) and the left common cardinal vein develops into the oblique vein of Marshal, a coronary vein running between the left atrial appendage and the left pulmonary veins.

The brachiocephalic veins drain deoxygenated blood from the subclavian and internal jugular veins. The LBCV courses to the right, crosses the midline anterior to the innominate artery, and merges with the right brachiocephalic vein to form the SVC, finally draining into the right atrium.

There is no valve within the SVC or between the SVC and the right atrium. Near the superior cavoatrial junction is the location of the sinoatrial node.

The azygos system consists of the azygos, hemiazygos, accessory hemiazygos, and left superior intercostal veins (**Fig. 2**). It drains blood from inferior body, diaphragm, chest wall, tracheobronchial tree, esophagus, and pericardium. The azygos vein courses in the right posterior mediastinum and arches over the right main bronchus, to drain into the SVC just anterior to the right tracheobronchial angle. The hemiazygos vein courses in the

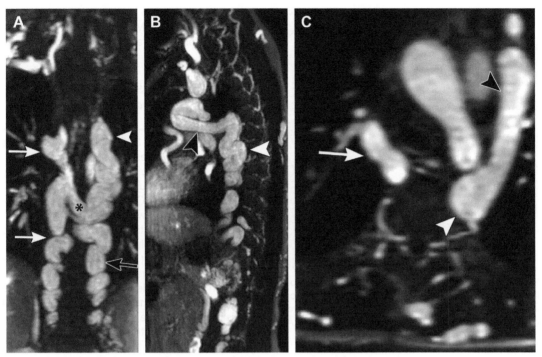

Fig. 2. A 12-year-old boy with a history of prune belly syndrome and acquired chronic obliteration of the superior vena cava and brachiocephalic veins. Multiplanar reconstructions from gadolinium enhanced 3-dimensional MR angiography are shown. (*A*) Coronal image demonstrates dilated and tortuous azygos (*white arrow*), hemiazygos (*black arrow*), and accessory hemiazygos (*white arrowhead*) veins functioning as collaterals. Asterisk indicates the hemiazygos vein crossing the midline, and draining into the azygos vein. (*B*) Sagittal-oblique image demonstrates dilated left superior intercostal vein (*black arrowhead*) and accessory hemiazygos vein (*white arrowhead*). (*C*) Transverse image at the level of the aortic arch demonstrates dilated left superior intercostal vein (*black arrowhead*), accessory hemiazygos vein (*white arrowhead*), and azygos arch (*white arrow*).

left posterior mediastinum, and crosses the midline at the level of T8–9, to drain into the azygos vein (see **Figs. 1**C, **2**A). The accessory hemiazygos vein courses in the left posterior mediastinum, and crosses the midline at the level of T7–8, to drain into the azygos vein. The accessory hemiazygos vein communicates with the left superior intercostal vein, which drains blood from the left second to fourth posterior intercostal veins into the LBCV (see **Fig. 2**B, C).

The IVC above the confluence with the hepatic veins courses through the "caval opening," an opening in the central tendon of the diaphragm, into the thoracic cavity. The supradiaphragmatic portion of the IVC is considered "intrapericardial" because it is covered anteriorly and laterally by pericardium. In the fetal heart, the Eustachian valve at the junction of the IVC with the right atrium directs the blood flow from the IVC toward the foramen ovale and the left atrium. It regresses after birth to a variable extent, and remnants of the Eustachian valve frequently remain as a small crescentic fold at the anterior aspect of the IVC ostium.

The CS drains the majority of deoxygenated blood from myocardium and is located in the posterior portion of the atrioventricular groove (**Fig. 3**). A variably sized Thebesian valve at its opening is encountered in the majority of pathology specimens.[2]

Pulmonary Veins

Oxygenated blood from the lungs is drained by pulmonary veins into the left atrium. Early development of pulmonary veins is separate from the heart. In the human embryo, lung buds develop after the third week as an outpouching of the foregut. The developing lungs are surrounded by splanchnic mesenchyme, and the pulmonary veins develop as part of the splanchnic venous system, which drains into the cardinal, and umbilicovitelline venous systems.[3] Independently, an outpouching from the primitive left atrium, the primordial common pulmonary vein, develops. The splanchnic pulmonary veins eventually connect with the common pulmonary vein, which starts to drain blood from the primitive lungs. Subsequently, the connections of the splanchnic

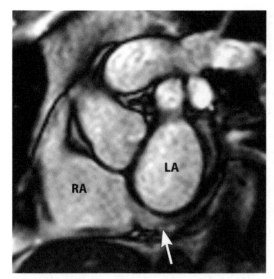

Fig. 3. Two-dimensional steady-state free precession image from vectorcardiogram-gated cine acquisition in the short axis plane of the heart demonstrates normal coronary sinus (*arrow*). LA, left atrium; RA, right atrium.

fibrillation and need to be described in the report of the pulmonary vein MR angiography (MRA) performed before left atrial or pulmonary vein ablation.

MR IMAGING TECHNIQUES
Gadolinium Enhanced 3-Dimensional MR Angiography

Gadolinium enhanced 3-dimensional (3D) MRA is an off-label, however, established and robust technique for evaluation of systemic and pulmonary veins. Images are acquired with a T1 weighted 3D spoiled gradient echo (GRE) sequence, usually during breath-hold, and without cardiac gating. For pulmonary vein evaluation, we acquire the images during intravenous bolus injection of 0.15 mmol/kg gadolinium contrast material, injected at a rate of 2 mL/s, and image acquisition is timed for enhancement of the left atrium. Systemic veins can be imaged using the same injection, by repeat acquisition during the early equilibrium phase, when gadolinium contrast material has reached the venous compartment, but has not distributed into the extracellular space. As an alternative, dedicated 3D MRA of the SVC and its tributaries can be performed directly, during bilateral or unilateral upper extremity vein injection of a 20:1 dilution of normal saline and gadolinium contrast material.[4] This method generates images that are relatively free of arterial contamination.

Image interpretation benefits from postprocessing, such as reformatting of the 3D dataset in multiple planes (see **Fig. 2**), maximum intensity projections, and volume rendering (see **Fig. 4**). Gadolinium-enhanced MRA is contraindicated in patients with prior anaphylactic reaction to gadolinium contrast material. Because of the risk of nephrogenic systemic fibrosis, gadolinium injection is also contraindicated in patients with advanced renal failure and in dialysis patients.

pulmonary veins with the primordial systemic veins regress. During further development, the common pulmonary vein and, to a variable degree, its central branches are incorporated into the left atrium, forming its posterior portion and resulting in the pulmonary veins connecting individually with the mature left atrium.

Most commonly, there are 2 right and 2 left pulmonary veins (**Fig. 4**A). However, variations are very common, specifically an additional right middle pulmonary vein (see **Fig. 4**B) and a common trunk of the left pulmonary veins (see **Fig. 4**C). Normal variants of the pulmonary veins are important in patients who undergo invasive electrophysiologic procedures for the treatment of atrial

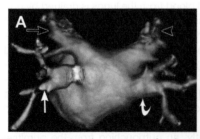
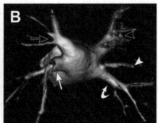
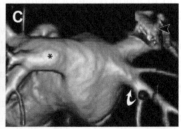

Fig. 4. Normal and variations of pulmonary venous anatomy. Posterior views of volume rendered images from gadolinium enhanced 3-dimensional MR angiography are shown. (*A*) Standard pulmonary venous anatomy, with right superior pulmonary vein (*black arrowhead*), right inferior pulmonary vein (*white curved arrow*), left superior pulmonary vein (*black arrow*), and left inferior pulmonary vein (*white arrow*). (*B*) A right middle pulmonary vein (*white arrowhead*) drains separately into the left atrium, near the right inferior pulmonary vein ostium. (*C*) Common trunk of left pulmonary veins (*asterisk*).

"Noncontrast" MR imaging Techniques

MR techniques for evaluation of the vasculature without gadolinium administration are broadly categorized into white blood, black blood, and phase contrast acquisitions.

Bright blood imaging

Bright blood imaging was originally performed with spoiled GRE sequences. A time of flight acquisition utilizes a spoiled GRE sequence with a high flip angle and a short repetition time. To evaluate the SVC for thrombus, a stack of consecutive 2D time of flight images in the transverse plane of the chest can be acquired (Fig. 5A, B).

Currently, for imaging of the vasculature without gadolinium, GRE sequences have been largely replaced by 2-dimensional (2D) and 3D steady-state free precession (SSFP) acquisitions. SSFP is less sensitive to flow, but provides excellent contrast between fluid and soft tissue: the signal depends on the ratio of T2/T1, which is particularly high for fluids including blood. Two-dimensional SSFP images of the thoracic vasculature can be acquired with or without cardiac gating, during breath-hold or during free breathing. A vectorcardiogram (VCG)-gated 2D SSFP cine acquisition with about 20 to 30 reconstructed phases per heart beat and a slice thickness of 6 to 8 mm depicts accurately systemic and pulmonary veins, and also provides excellent visualization of the CS (see Fig. 3). The 3D SSFP technique is described in detail elsewhere in this article.

Black blood imaging

Black blood images of blood vessels are acquired with double inversion recovery prepulse

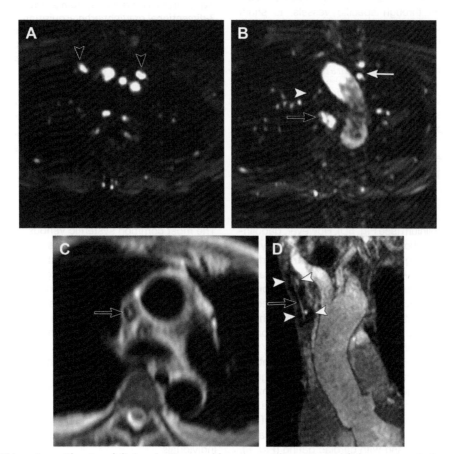

Fig. 5. MR imaging without gadolinium in 78-year-old woman with acute renal failure and central venous catheter in the superior vena cava (SVC). (A, B) Transverse time of flight images demonstrate patent right brachiocephalic and left internal jugular veins (*black arrowheads*). Note mildly prominent azygos (*black arrow*) and left superior intercostal (*white arrow*) veins with no appreciable SVC (*white arrowhead* indicates expected location of SVC). (C) Transverse vectorcardiogram (VCG)-gated black blood image demonstrates catheter (*black arrow*) but no appreciable flow in small caliber SVC. (D) Coronal maximum intensity projection of VCG and respiratory navigator gated 3-dimensional steady-state free precession demonstrates catheter in SVC (*black arrow*) with adjacent thrombus (*white arrowheads*).

technique, a flow-sensitive method to null the signal of flowing blood. For routine black blood imaging of systemic and pulmonary veins, we use a VCG-gated proton density weighted 2D fast spin echo sequence with a slice thickness of 6 to 8 mm. The slice thickness can be decreased to as low as 2 mm when imaging small children. As a minimum, we acquire a stack of consecutive slices in the transverse plane of the chest, with additional imaging planes as necessary (see **Fig. 5**C).

Phase contrast imaging

Phase contrast sequences measure flow velocity and provide information about direction of flow. Flow volume per minute is calculated from flow velocity and cross-sectional vessel area using dedicated postprocessing software. The main application of phase contrast imaging, apart from flow quantification through specific vessels, is shunt quantification by comparing flow volumes per minute in pulmonary (Qp) and systemic (Qs) circulations.

Vectorcardiogram- and respiratory-gated 3-dimensional acquisitions

These acquisitions are advantageous for motion artifact–free imaging of small vessels. They acquire near isotropic 3D images with high spatial resolution during free breathing. Cardiac and respiratory motion compensation is achieved by simultaneous VCG gating and tracking of diaphragmatic motion (respiratory navigator technique). A VCG- and respiratory navigator-gated 3D SSFP sequence with a voxel size of about 1.2 to 1.6 mm can be used without gadolinium (see **Fig. 5**D). However, gadolinium administration improves image quality by increasing the signal-to-noise ratio, particularly at small voxel sizes. Also available with the respiratory navigator technique are VCG-gated 3D inversion recovery GRE sequences. They can be utilized to acquire T1 weighted, gadolinium-enhanced, high-resolution images of the pulmonary and coronary veins and are particularly suited to be used with new gadolinium-based "blood pool" contrast agents. Intravenously injected blood pool agents have a much longer plasma half-time than conventional contrast agents, which quickly distribute into the extracellular space. The long duration of the equilibrium phase allows for imaging with increased spatial resolution, and with cardiac gating (**Fig. 6**). Gadofosveset is the first gadolinium-based blood pool agent to be approved by the US Food and Drug Administration. It requires the same safety precautions as conventional gadolinium-based contrast agents and should be avoided in patients with acute kidney injury or a glomerular filtration rate of less than 30 mL/min/1.73 m^2.

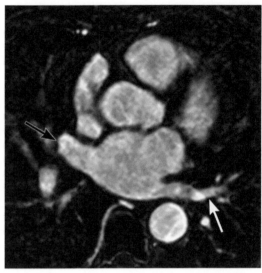

Fig. 6. Transverse reformat from an inversion recovery 3-dimensional gradient echo acquisition 5 minutes after intravenous injection of gadofosveset. The study was performed for pulmonary venous assessment and shows the right superior (*black arrow*) and left inferior (*white arrow*) pulmonary veins.

Image interpretation of all 3D acquisitions is enhanced by postprocessing, including reformatting of the 3D dataset in multiple planes, and maximum intensity projections (see **Fig. 5**D).

ANATOMIC VARIANTS AND CONGENITAL ANOMALIES
Systemic Veins and Coronary Sinus

The most common systemic venous variant in the chest is a left SVC, which has an incidence of about 0.3% in the general population,[5] and more than 5% in patients with congenital heart disease.[5–7] A left SVC is the abnormal persistence of the left anterior cardinal vein (see **Fig. 1**). It starts at the junction of the left internal jugular and left subclavian veins, and courses in the mediastinum lateral to the aortic arch (**Fig. 7**). Most commonly, the left SVC drains into an enlarged CS, via the vein of Marshall, a remnant of the left common cardinal vein (see **Fig. 1**A, B). The right SVC may be present (bilateral SVC) or absent. Similarly, the brachiocephalic ("bridging") vein may be present, or may be diminutive or absent in these individuals.

An incidental left SVC in adults is a harmless normal variant most of the time, without the need for a dedicated cardiac evaluation in a low-risk population without suspicion for congenital heart disease. However, a left SVC can complicate central venous catheter placement, cardiac device implantation, and invasive cardiac procedures. A

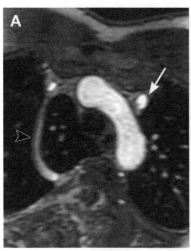
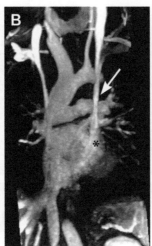
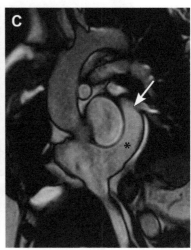

Fig. 7. A 13-year-old boy with persistent left superior vena cava (SVC). Transverse (*A*) and coronal reformat (*B*) of 3-dimensional gadolinium-enhanced MR angiography shows a persistent left SVC (*white arrow*) coursing lateral to aortic arch and draining into the coronary sinus (*asterisk*). Incidentally, there is an azygos lobe, as indicated by lateral course of azygos vein (*arrowhead*). Short axis 2-dimensional steady-state free precession image (*C*) at the base of the heart demonstrates a dilated coronary sinus (*asterisk*). The left brachiocephalic vein was congenitally absent. *White arrow* indicates left SVC near junction with CS.

left SVC has also been associated with arrhythmias.[8] The incidence of left SVC is increased in populations with congenital heart disease, syndromes, and genetic anomalies and is considered a marker of such if detected in a "high-risk" population.[8] Rarely, a left SVC drains into the left atrium, either directly or via a defect in the roof of the CS ("unroofed CS" [URCS]), leading to a right to left shunt with potential cerebral complications (stroke, brain abscess).[8,9] A left SVC draining directly into the left atrium connects with the left superior aspect of the left atrium, between the left atrial appendage and the left pulmonary veins.[9] Combination of a left SVC draining directly into the left atrium with absence of the CS and atrial septal defect (ASD) has been described and is referred to as Raghib anomaly.[9]

If a left SVC is found on MR imaging, the following findings should be evaluated and mentioned in the report:

- Right SVC: presence or absence; if present: comment on size.
- Left brachiocephalic "bridging" vein: presence or absence; if present: comment on size.
- Left SVC: drainage (CS or left atrium).
- CS: comment on size (normal or dilated); roof of CS: intact or evidence for "unroofed" CS; rare: absence of CS.
- Any evidence for ASD and any other findings suspicious for congenital heart disease. Those findings include unexplained dilatation of right atrium or right ventricle.

Anomalies of the right SVC are usually associated with additional congenital defects and include absence of the SVC (**Fig. 8**) or congenital stenosis, aneurysm, and abnormal drainage. Direct drainage of the right SVC into the roof of the left atrium,[10,11] and dual drainage of the right SVC into both right and left atrium,[12] results in a right-to-left shunt. In superior sinus venosus defects (**Fig. 9**), there is lack of infolding of the right atrial wall between the SVC and the right pulmonary veins, resulting in abnormal communication between the right and left atrium with overriding SVC.[13] This communication is associated frequently with abnormal drainage of right pulmonary veins through the defect or true anomalous connection with pulmonary veins separately connecting to the systemic veins.

Anomalies of the LBCV include absence and retroaortic course (**Fig. 10**).

Anomalies of the IVC include anomalous insertion (abnormally high into right atrium, into the CS, or into the left atrium), aneurysm, and interruption of the intrahepatic segment with azygos or hemiazygos continuation. Anomalous insertion is rare and occurs exclusively in patients with additional congenital anomalies (**Fig. 11**). Aneurysm of the suprahepatic IVC is exceedingly rare, but can be found as an isolated finding in otherwise healthy individuals. Interruption of the retrohepatic segment of the IVC with venous drainage via the azygos/hemiazygos system can be isolated, but is associated commonly with congenital anomalies (see **Fig. 8**).

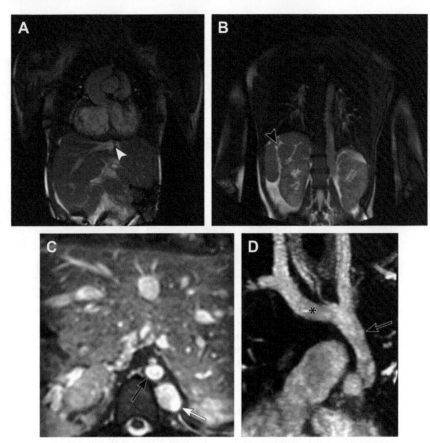

Fig. 8. A 17-year-old girl with a history of surgical repair of endocardial cushion defect and heterotaxy syndrome (left-sided isomerism). (*A, B*) Coronal localizer images demonstrate midline heart and liver, with midline confluence of the hepatic veins (*white arrowhead* in *A*), and polysplenia in right upper abdomen (*black arrowhead* in *B*). (*C*) Transverse reformatted 3-dimensional (3D) steady-state free precession image demonstrates continuation of the abdominal venous drainage via a large left-sided azygos vein (*white arrow*). The suprarenal inferior vena cava was absent. Black arrow shows descending aorta. (*D*) Coronal maximum intensity projections of 3D MR angiography demonstrates left superior vena cava (SVC; *black arrow*), and left brachiocephalic vein (*asterisk*). The right SVC is absent.

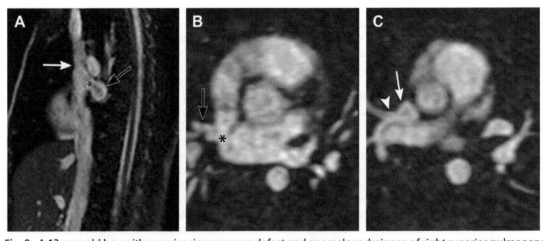

Fig. 9. A 13-year-old boy with superior sinus venosus defect and anomalous drainage of right superior pulmonary vein to superior vena cava (SVC). A 2-dimensional steady-state free precession (*A*) and maximum intensity projections of gadolinium enhanced 3-dimensional (3D) MR angiography (MRA; *B*) in the sagittal oblique plane and axial plane respectively demonstrate defect (*asterisk*) in the common wall between the SVC (*white arrow*) and right superior pulmonary vein (*black arrow*), leading to anomalous drainage of the right superior pulmonary vein. A transverse image from gadolinium enhanced 3D MRA more cranially (*C*) demonstrates an additional accessory right upper lobe pulmonary vein (*arrowhead*) draining a portion of the right upper lobe, which has a true anomalous connection with the SVC (*white arrow*).

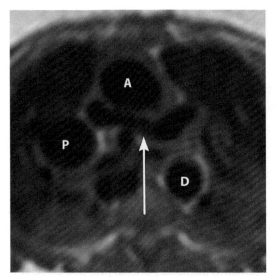

Fig. 10. A 4-month-old girl with repaired tetralogy of Fallot. Transverse black blood image demonstrates retroaortic left brachiocephalic vein (*arrow*). A, ascending aorta; D, descending aorta; P, aneurysmal right pulmonary artery.

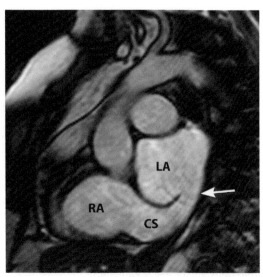

Fig. 12. Two-dimensional steady-state free precession image from vectorcardiogram-gated cine acquisition in the short axis plane of the heart demonstrates communication between the left atrium (LA) and the coronary sinus (CS) through a defect in the roof of the CS (*arrow*); right atrium (RA). Compare this with normal coronary sinus anatomy (see **Fig. 3**).

Anomalies of the CS include URCS, absence, and congenital occlusion. URCS refers to a direct connection between the CS and the left atrium (**Fig. 12**). This anomaly can be isolated, causing a

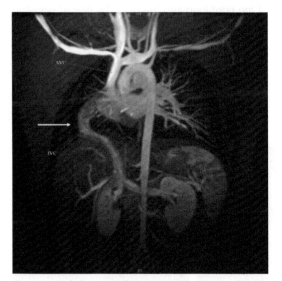

Fig. 11. Gadolinium-enhanced MR angiography image demonstrates abnormal high insertion of the inferior vena cava (*arrow*) into the right atrium simulating a scimitar vein. Pulmonary venous connections were normal. There was dextroposition of the right heart and a lobar sequestration. (*From* Aggarwal S, Joshi A, Bolger-Theut S, et al. Meandering inferior vena cava in a child with pseudo-scimitar syndrome. Ann Thorac Surg 2011;92(4):1528, with permission.)

left-to-right shunt that is physiologically similar to an ASD. URCS can also be associated with other congenital cardiac anomalies, particularly a left SVC.[14] When associated with a left SVC, URCS predisposes to cerebral complications owing to right-to-left shunt. Absence of the CS is rare and is seen typically in heterotaxy. Congenital occlusion of the CS by the Thebesian valve can potentially complicate CS cannulation for electrophysiologic procedures, however, is currently not evaluated by MR imaging.

PULMONARY VEINS
Anomalous Pulmonary Venous Connection

This abnormality ensues from disturbance of development of the primordial common pulmonary vein and its connection with the splanchnic pulmonary veins, when the anastomoses between primordial splanchnic and systemic venous systems are still open. As a result, all (total anomalous pulmonary venous connection) or several (partial anomalous pulmonary venous connection) pulmonary veins connect with the systemic venous system instead of the left atrium.

Partial anomalous pulmonary venous connection can be an isolated finding in otherwise healthy adults (0.1% of contrast-enhanced CTs[15]). This anomaly results in a left-to-right shunt and is an

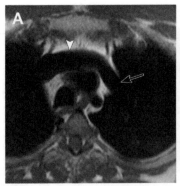
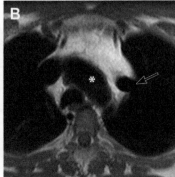
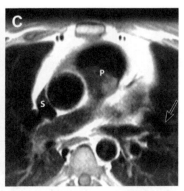

Fig. 13. A 41-year-old man with anomalous drainage of left superior pulmonary vein into left brachiocephalic vein (LBCV). Transverse vectorcardiogram-gated black blood images (*A–C*) show the course of the left superior pulmonary vein (*arrow*) lateral to the aortic arch (*asterisk*) and connecting with LBCV (white *arrowhead*). P, pulmonary trunk; S, superior vena cava.

important differential diagnosis to consider in patients with unexplained dilatation of the right cardiac chambers. Most common are anomalous drainage of a right superior pulmonary vein into the SVC (see **Fig. 9**C), and drainage of the left superior pulmonary vein into the LBCV, via a vertical vein (**Fig. 13**). The left vertical vein often courses lateral to the aortic arch, in a location similar to a left SVC; however, in contrast with a left SVC, the flow is directed cranially and there is no communication with the CS. Anomalous pulmonary venous drainage can be associated with other congenital cardiac anomalies, especially a sinus venosus defect. Patients are best evaluated with a comprehensive cardiac MR imaging examination to exclude associated abnormalities and to determine whether the shunt is significant hemodynamically. Apart from anatomic imaging consisting of MRA and cine imaging in various planes, shunt quantification can be done by estimating pulmonary arterial (Qp) and aortic flow (Qs) using phase contrast imaging. Important items of the cardiac MR imaging report are:

- Evidence of associated congenital cardiac anomalies;
- Evaluation of right and left ventricular volumes and function; and
- Ratio of pulmonary (Qp) to systemic flow (Qs).

Scimitar syndrome is an uncommon form of partial anomalous pulmonary venous connection, defined by partial or complete venous drainage of the right lung into the IVC. The name "scimitar" is derived from the shape of the anomalous pulmonary vein, which resembles a curved blade. Scimitar syndrome (**Fig. 14**) is associated commonly with additional abnormalities, such as:

- Hypoplasia of the right lung and the right pulmonary artery with dextroposition of the heart;

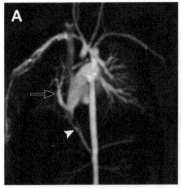
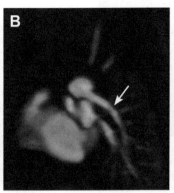
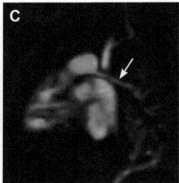

Fig. 14. A 5-day-old boy with scimitar syndrome. (*A*) Coronal maximum intensity projections (MIP) of gadolinium-enhanced, 3-dimensional MR angiography demonstrates anomalous right pulmonary vein (*arrow*) draining right lung into supradiaphragmatic inferior vena cava. An artery arising from the abdominal aorta (*arrowhead*) provides supply to right lower lobe. (*B*, *C*) sagittal-oblique maximum intensity projections demonstrate a normal-sized left pulmonary artery (*arrow* in *B*) and a diminutive right pulmonary artery (*arrow* in *C*).

- Systemic arterial supply to the right lung (sequestration); and
- ASD.[16]

In surgical candidates, it is important to determine whether the connection of the anomalous pulmonary vein with the IVC is intrapericardial (above the diaphragm), or infradiaphragmatic, and to determine the relationship of the vein to the atrial septum and any ASD, for potential surgical baffling. Flow velocity mapping of the right and left pulmonary arteries can be performed to evaluate for any differences in pulmonary artery flow between the right and the left lungs.

In total anomalous pulmonary venous connection, the entire venous return from the lungs drains into a systemic vein or the right atrium, where it mixes with deoxygenated blood returning from the body. Most commonly, there is an ASD through which a variable proportion of the returning mixed oxygenated/deoxygenated blood enters the systemic circulation.[17] Patients with total anomalous pulmonary venous connection are cyanotic and diagnosis is almost always made in infancy or childhood. Total anomalous pulmonary venous connection has been classified according to the anatomic location of the anomalous venous connection[17]:

- Supracardiac into SVC or brachiocephalic vein;
- Cardiac into right atrium or CS;
- Infracardiac into IVC, hepatic, or portal vein; and
- Mixed with more than one type of connection.

Anomalous connections between the pulmonary and systemic veins can be obstructive or nonobstructive. An anomalous infradiaphragmatic pulmonary venous connection is almost always obstructive. Obstruction is also more likely with increasing length of the abnormal connecting vein.

Cor triatriatum and congenital pulmonary vein stenosis

Cor triatriatum results from stenosis at the interface of the primordial common pulmonary vein and the primitive left atrium. As a result, the mature left atrium is subdivided by a membrane into an anterior chamber (from the primitive left atrium), and a posterior chamber (from the primordial common pulmonary vein). The posterior chamber receives the pulmonary veins. The anterior chamber includes the left atrial appendage and communicates with the mitral valve.[17] This abnormality can be isolated and asymptomatic if there is a wide communication between the anterior and posterior chambers. However, left heart obstruction can result from a small or absent communication. Cor triatriatum can be associated with other congenital heart defects.

Congenital pulmonary vein stenosis results from abnormal incorporation of the primordial common pulmonary vein and its branches into the developing left atrium.[17] Stenosis can be focal or diffuse, and affect a variable number of pulmonary veins. Severe cases manifest in infancy as unilateral or bilateral pulmonary edema. Mild forms are asymptomatic and may be detected in adulthood.[18]

Left-to-Right Shunts Between the Left Atrium and Systemic Veins

A levoatriocardinal vein is an anomalous communication between the left atrium or a pulmonary vein with a systemic vein. In congenital heart disease with left heart obstruction, the levoatriocardinal vein decompresses (drains blood away from) the left atrium, resulting in a left-to-right shunt.[19] The communication is usually with the SVC or the brachiocephalic vein. Although most commonly seen with left heart obstruction (particularly hypoplastic left heart syndrome), it can be encountered rarely

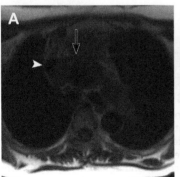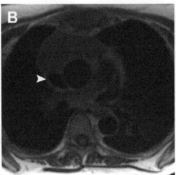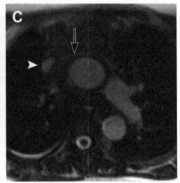

Fig. 15. A 57-year-old woman with anterior mediastinal mass, pathologically proven poorly differentiated carcinoma of lung primary. Vectorcardiogram-gated transverse black blood (*A, B*) and 2-dimensional steady-state free precession images (*C*) demonstrate encasement and narrowing of left brachiocephalic vein (*black arrow*) by anterior mediastinal mass and patent superior vena cava (*white arrowhead*).

in an otherwise normal heart. Flow in the levoatrio-cardinal vein can be bidirectional, and can be source of paradoxical embolus.

ACQUIRED DISEASE
Systemic Veins and Coronary Sinus

Most acquired obstructions of the SVC or brachio-cephalic veins are caused by indwelling catheters (see **Fig. 5**) or malignancy (**Fig. 15**).[20,21] Less common causes are radiation fibrosis, fibrosing media-stinitis, and postoperative strictures, which occur for example in heart transplant recipients and in patients with repaired congenital heart disease. Thrombosis of the subclavian and axillary veins associated with strenuous exercise has been described as Paget–von Schroetter syndrome and occurs in otherwise healthy individuals.[22]

Malignant obstruction of the SVC or brachioce-phalic veins is caused by encasement or invasion by adjacent tumors, such as lung cancer (most common), sarcoma, thymoma, or metastases (see **Fig. 15**). In contrast, malignant obstruction of the supradiaphragmatic IVC is caused more commonly by intraluminal extension of tumor thrombus, which is particularly common in renal cell cancer (**Fig. 16**), hepatocellular carcinoma, and adrenal neoplasms. The IVC tumor thrombus from renal cell cancer is amenable to surgical treatment and is evaluated commonly with MR imaging

before resection. Accurate determination of tumor thrombus extent into the supradiaphragmatic IVC is important because it alters the surgical approach.[23] Other, less common causes of malignant obstruction of the supradiaphragmatic IVC are direct extension of right atrial tumors and the rare primary leiomyosarcoma of the IVC.

Acquired dilatation of systemic veins is usually secondary to collateral flow. Chronic thrombosis

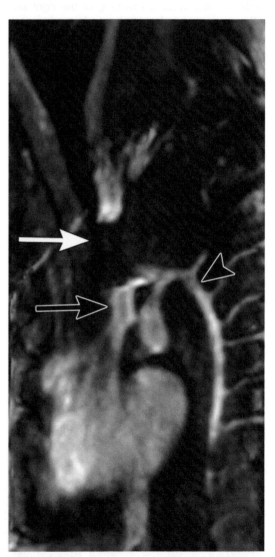

Fig. 17. Gadolinium-enhanced MR angiography to evaluate for patency of a 10-mm-wide and 26-mm-long stainless steel stent in the upper superior vena cava (SVC). Note susceptibility artifact in upper SVC (*white arrow*) corresponding with the stent. The azygos vein (*arrowhead*) is normal in size and the lower SVC (*black arrow*) is patent. Note the absence of collateral veins. The susceptibility artifact should not be mistaken for stent occlusion. Catheter angiography demonstrated a widely patent stent.

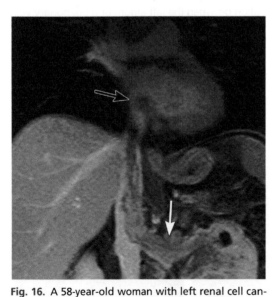

Fig. 16. A 58-year-old woman with left renal cancer and tumor thrombus. Coronal 2-dimensional spoiled gradient echo image after gadolinium administration demonstrates extension of tumor thrombus through the left renal vein (*white arrow*) to the supra-diaphragmatic inferior vena cava and right atrium (*black arrow*). There is heterogeneous enhancement with expansion of left renal vein.

often results in partial or complete obliteration of the affected vein, with development of dilated collateral veins. Typical collateral pathways for obstructed systemic thoracic veins are the internal mammary veins, azygos, hemiazygos, and accessory hemiazygos veins, and the superior intercostal vein (see **Fig. 2**). Dilated collateral veins can be demonstrated with both gadolinium enhanced and noncontrast MR imaging techniques. The presence or absence of dilated collateral veins is an important secondary imaging finding to whether an apparent venous obstruction is real or not. Artifactual filling defects can occur on MR images, for example, secondary to mixing of gadolinium enhanced and unenhanced blood, susceptibility artifact from concentrated gadolinium or intravascular stents, too early acquisition of MRA images, and incomplete nulling of black blood images.

MR imaging is not the preferred method to evaluate for patency of endovascular stents. Stents cause susceptibility artifact to a varying degree, which mainly depends on the material of the stent, the position of the stent within the main magnetic field, the strength of the magnetic field, the type of MR sequence, and certain sequence parameters, such as flip angle.[24] Stainless steel stents cause more susceptibility artifact than, for example, nitinol, tantalum, or platinum stents.[24] Stents oriented perpendicular to the main magnetic field, for example, stents in brachiocephalic or subclavian veins, are more prone to artifact than stents aligned with the main magnetic field, like SVC stents. Certain noncontrast MR sequences such as time of flight or SSFP sequences are more susceptible to artifact than gadolinium-enhanced

MRA; however, even gadolinium-enhanced MRA is limited.[25] A false-positive diagnosis of stent occlusion or overestimation of in-stent stenosis secondary to artifact has been described in the arterial system,[25,26] and occurs in the venous system as well (**Fig. 17**). The following is recommended if MR evaluation of stent patency is performed:

- Determination of the stent material (stainless steel or other), and orientation of the stent in the magnetic field, to anticipate the severity of the artifact.
- A black blood 2D fast spin echo sequence should be part of the protocol; fast spin echo sequences are degraded less by susceptibility artifact than GRE or SSFP techniques.
- Gadolinium-enhanced 3D MRA is recommended if no contraindication exists.
- In case of apparent stent occlusion on MR images: evaluation for presence of collateral vessels; absence of collateral vessels contradicts significant stenosis or occlusion.

Growth of primary and secondary cardiac tumors into the CS can occur (**Fig. 18**). Potential iatrogenic causes of coronary vein occlusion include cannulation of the CS for ablation of ventricular arrhythmia and thrombosis secondary to lead placement for biventricular pacing.[27]

Pulmonary Veins

Acquired pulmonary vein dilatation/varix is seen in patients with mitral valve disease. Acquired pulmonary vein narrowing or occlusion can be caused by tumors or benign entities. Encasement

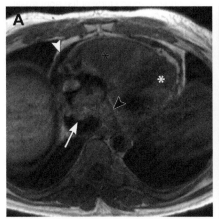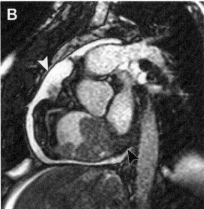

Fig. 18. Cardiac melanoma metastases. Vectorcardiogram-gated transverse T1 weighted black blood image (*A*) and 2-dimensional steady-state free precession image in the short axis plane of the heart (*B*) show lobulated metastases in right atrium, supradiaphragmatic inferior vena cava (*white arrow* in *A*) and coronary sinus (*black arrowhead* in *A*, *B*). There were also tumor metastases in the right (*black asterisk* in *A*) and left (*white asterisk* in *A*) ventricles and a small pericardial effusion (*white arrowhead*). The tumor shows intermediate signal intensity on the T1 weighted image (*A*). Compare (*B*) with normal coronary sinus anatomy (see **Fig. 3**).

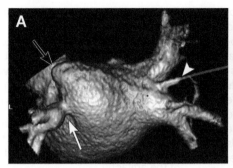
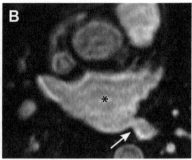

Fig. 19. Gadolinium-enhanced 3-dimensional MR angiography of the pulmonary veins after pulmonary vein ablation for atrial fibrillation. (*A*) Volume-rendered image, posterior view, demonstrating circumferential narrowing of the left inferior pulmonary vein (*white arrow*) and abrupt cutoff of the left superior pulmonary vein (*black arrow*), consistent with occlusion. There was a separate right middle pulmonary vein (*arrowhead*). (*B*) Transverse maximum intensity projection demonstrates narrowing of left inferior pulmonary vein (*white arrow*). Asterisk indicates the left atrium.

of a pulmonary vein by central lung cancer is seen frequently on staging CT and not usually evaluated with MR imaging. Less common is intraluminal extension of a pulmonary malignancy through a pulmonary vein into the left atrium.[28] Benign acquired etiologies of pulmonary vein narrowing are frequently iatrogenic, such as after pulmonary vein ablation or surgery. Other causes include radiation fibrosis and fibrosing mediastinitis. Pulmonary vein narrowing can be evaluated with noncontrast MR imaging techniques, specifically 2D SSFP cine imaging or, more accurately, with gadolinium-enhanced 3D MRA of the pulmonary veins (**Fig. 19**).

SUMMARY

Anatomic and functional evaluation of the thoracic venous vasculature is achieved with intravenous gadolinium enhanced MRA, "noncontrast" MR techniques (such as black blood, time of flight, and SSFP acquisitions) and phase contrast imaging. The protocol should be tailored based on the specific clinical questions. Congenital anomalies of systemic and pulmonary veins can be explained by disturbances at specific stages of the development of the primordial heart and venous systems. Acquired abnormalities are most frequently iatrogenic or related to cancer, and infrequently caused by inflammatory disorders.

REFERENCES

1. Lopez L, Huhta JC. Systemic venous anomalies. echocardiography in pediatric and congenital heart disease. Hoboken (NJ): Wiley-Blackwell; 2009. p. 143–57.

2. Noheria A, DeSimone CV, Lachman N, et al. Anatomy of the coronary sinus and epicardial coronary venous system in 620 hearts: an electrophysiology perspective. J Cardiovasc Electrophysiol 2013; 24(1):1–6.

3. Geva T, Stella K. Anomalies of the pulmonary veins. In: Allen HD, Shaddy RE, Feltes TF, editors. Moss and Adams' heart disease in infants, children, and adolescents: including the fetus and young adults. 7th edition. Philadelphia (PA): Lippincott Williams and Wilkins; 2008. p. 762–92.

4. Zhang H, Maki JH, Prince MR. 3D contrast-enhanced MR angiography. J Magn Reson Imaging 2007;25(1):13–25.

5. Cha EM, Khoury GH. Persistent left superior vena cava. Radiologic and clinical significance. Radiology 1972;103(2):375–81.

6. Parikh SR, Prasad K, Iyer RN, et al. Prospective angiographic study of the abnormalities of systemic venous connections in congenital and acquired heart disease. Cathet Cardiovasc Diagn 1996; 38(4):379–86.

7. Campbell M, Deuchar DC. The left-sided superior vena cava. Br Heart J 1954;16(4):423–39.

8. Irwin RB, Greaves M, Schmitt M. Left superior vena cava: revisited. Eur Heart J Cardiovasc Imaging 2012;13(4):284–91.

9. Raghib G, Ruttenberg HD, Anderson RC, et al. Termination of left superior vena cava in left atrium, atrial septal defect, and absence of coronary sinus; a developmental complex. Circulation 1965;31:906–18.

10. Gaynor JW, Weinberg PM, Spray TL. Congenital heart surgery nomenclature and database project: systemic venous anomalies. Ann Thorac Surg 2000;69(4 Suppl):S70–6.

11. Oppido G, Pace Napoleone C, Turci S, et al. Right superior vena cava draining in the left atrium: anatomical, embryological, and surgical considerations. Ann Thorac Surg 2006;81(6):2313–5.

12. Shapiro EP, Al-Sadir J, Campbell NP, et al. Drainage of right superior vena cava into both atria. Review of the literature and description of a case presenting with polycythemia and paradoxical embolization. Circulation 1981;63(3):712–7.

13. Li J, Al Zaghal AM, Anderson RH. The nature of the superior sinus venosus defect. Clin Anat 1998;11(5): 349–52.

14. Shah SS, Teague SD, Lu JC, et al. Imaging of the coronary sinus: normal anatomy and congenital abnormalities. Radiographics 2012;32(4): 991–1008.

15. Ho ML, Bhalla S, Bierhals A, et al. MDCT of partial anomalous pulmonary venous return (PAPVR) in adults. J Thorac Imaging 2009;24(2):89–95.

16. Vida VL, Padalino MA, Boccuzzo G, et al. Scimitar syndrome: a European Congenital Heart Surgeons Association (ECHSA) multicentric study. Circulation 2010;122(12):1159–66.

17. Herlong JR, Jaggers JJ, Ungerleider RM. Congenital heart surgery nomenclature and database project: pulmonary venous anomalies. Ann Thorac Surg 2000;69(4 Suppl):S56–69.

18. Tan J, Rivandi AH, Sawhney N, et al. Congenital narrowing of a pulmonary vein: slit-like pulmonary vein ostium. Pacing Clin Electrophysiol 2013;36(5): e150–2.

19. Bernstein HS, Moore P, Stanger P, et al. The levoatriocardinal vein: morphology and echocardiographic identification of the pulmonary-systemic connection. J Am Coll Cardiol 1995; 26(4):995–1001.

20. Sheikh MA, Fernandez BB Jr, Gray BH, et al. Endovascular stenting of nonmalignant superior vena cava syndrome. Catheter Cardiovasc Interv 2005; 65(3):405–11.

21. del Rio Sola ML, Fuente Garrido R, Gutierrez Alonso V, et al. Endovascular treatment of superior vena cava syndrome caused by malignant disease. J Vasc Surg 2014;59(6):1705–6.

22. Drakos N, Gausche-Hill M. A case report: a young waiter with Paget-Schroetter syndrome. J Emerg Med 2013;44(3):e291–4.

23. Ciancio G, Shirodkar SP, Soloway MS, et al. Renal carcinoma with supradiaphragmatic tumor thrombus: avoiding sternotomy and cardiopulmonary bypass. Ann Thorac Surg 2010;89(2):505–10.

24. Hagspiel KD, Leung DA, Nandalur KR, et al. Contrast-enhanced MR angiography at 1.5 T after implantation of platinum stents: in vitro and in vivo comparison with conventional stent designs. AJR Am J Roentgenol 2005;184(1):288–94.

25. Hamer OW, Finkenzeller T, Borisch I, et al. In vivo evaluation of patency and in-stent stenoses after implantation of nitinol stents in iliac arteries using MR angiography. AJR Am J Roentgenol 2005;185(5):1282–8.

26. Rizzo JA, Dodge A, White P, et al. Magnetic resonance angiography in the evaluation of carotid stent patency. Perspect Vasc Surg Endovasc Ther 2010; 22(4):261–3.

27. Luckie M, Goode GK, Brack MJ. Coronary sinus thrombus complicating left ventricular lead revision. Europace 2012;14(6):864.

28. Koo BC, Woldenberg LS, Kim KT. Pulmonary vein tumor thrombosis and left atrial extension in lung carcinoma. J Comput Tomogr 1984;8(4):331–6.

State-of-the-art Magnetic Resonance Imaging in Vascular Thoracic Outlet Syndrome

Ayaz Aghayev, MD*, Frank J. Rybicki, MD, PhD

KEYWORDS

- Vascular thoracic outlet syndrome • MR imaging • Contrast-enhanced 3D MR angiography

KEY POINTS

- The use of contrast-enhanced 3D MRA using provocative arm positioning provides comprehensive information on arterial and venous compression by surrounding organs.
- Equilibrium phase images increase detection venous abnormalities when enhancement is not adequate on the venous phase of contrast-enhanced 3D MRA.
- Contrast-enhanced 3D MRA with equilibrium phase images is a valuable tool, however should be used as complementary tests in diagnosis of vascular thoracic outlet syndrome.

INTRODUCTION

Thoracic outlet syndrome (TOS) is a constellation of symptoms caused by impingement of the subclavian vessels and brachial plexus during their passage from the thoracic cavity to the axilla. TOS has been classified into several types, including neurogenic TOS (nTOS), arterial TOS (aTOS), and venous TOS (vTOS).[1] The true incidence of TOS is controversial, and has been reported to range from 0.3% to 8%.[2] nTOS accounts for almost 90% of cases of TOS, whereas less than 10% of patients have only vascular or combined symptoms.[1,3–7] The female/male ratio for nTOS is 3.5:1 and there is no sex predilection for the arterial type.[4,8,9] vTOS is traditionally considered to be male predominant; however, the largest study reported a similar proportion of men and women.[10]

Underlying causes for compression are congenital or acquired factors, such as cervical rib, long C7 transverse process, exostosis, hypertrophic callus, congenital fibromuscular anomalies, posture, repetitive movements, and posttraumatic fibrosis of the scalene muscle.[1,11,12] aTOS is almost always associated with bone abnormalities, such as cervical rib, callus, or exostosis,[1,8] whereas venous disorder is caused by repetitive injury to the subclavian vein by the first rib, clavicle, subclavius muscle, anterior scalene muscle, and costoclavicular ligament.[13] Both vTOS and aTOS usually develop in young, healthy patients with few if any comorbid conditions.[8,13]

The symptoms caused by arterial compression are pain, claudication, pallor, and coldness; however, pain and edema can be seen with vTOS.[1] Edema of the upper extremity is the hallmark for venous compression, especially when it is associated with thrombosis (effort thrombosis, which is also known as Paget-Schroetter syndrome).[13] Pain is the most common feature in aTOS,

Disclosures: The authors have nothing to disclose.
Department of Radiology, Brigham and Women's Hospital, Harvard Medical School, 75 Francis Street, Boston, MA 02115, USA
* Corresponding author.
E-mail address: aaghayev@partners.org

Magn Reson Imaging Clin N Am 23 (2015) 309–320
http://dx.doi.org/10.1016/j.mric.2015.01.009
1064-9689/15/$ – see front matter Published by Elsevier Inc.

although some patients with venous compression experience paresthesia caused by swelling rather than nerve compression.[1,5] Although rare, potential severe complications have been reported, including venous gangrene of the hand, pulmonary embolism as a result of venous compression or digital ischemia, and stroke associated with aTOS (**Table 1**).[3,4,6,7,14,15]

TOS can be diagnosed with history and a physical examination that includes provocative tests. However, imaging is required to identify vascular abnormalities. Conventional digital subtraction angiography (DSA) has been considered the reference standard for diagnosis of vascular TOS.[16] However, DSA has potential risks, including nephrotoxicity from iodinated contrast agent, arterial puncture site complications, ionizing radiation, and rarely stroke. Also, it requires separate procedures for arteries and veins; therefore, DSA is reserved for minimally invasive interventions and preoperative evaluation of the vessel anatomy to determine surgical approach or bypass graft planning. Computed tomography angiography (CTA) can be used as an alternative to DSA to reveal vascular anatomy and disorders using multiplanar reformatted techniques and maximal intensity projections (MIPs).[17] However, similar to DSA, it requires iodinated contrast agent and considerable irradiation, particularly with multiphase acquisitions during the arm abduction and rest positions. Also, bolus injection at a high rate results in a streak artifact from contrast material

in the superior vena cava, which may obscure disorders in these regions.

Contrast-enhanced three-dimensional (3D) magnetic resonance angiography (MRA) with provocative arm positioning has emerged as the primary imaging tool to evaluate patients with TOS.[18–22] Contrast-enhanced 3D MRA is a noninvasive, user-independent imaging modality that does not affect renal function[23] when used in the recommended amount in patients who have normal renal function (glomerular filtration rate >30 mL/min). For vascular TOS assessment, flow-based bright-blood MR venography (MRV) including time of flight (TOF) has been used.[24] However, it is limited to a two-dimensional implementation because of signal saturation of slow flow. TOF is also more time consuming and images may be impaired by breathing artifacts.[25,26]

This article reviews the anatomy of the thoracic outlet, MR imaging techniques for evaluation of vascular TOS, and imaging features of vascular TOS.

ANATOMY

The thoracic outlet is an area located between thorax, shoulder, and under the clavicle.[27] Subclavian vessels course through several narrow passageways in the thoracic outlet (**Fig. 1**). First, the scalene triangle (interscalene triangle) is delineated by the anterior scalene muscle anteriorly, middle scalene muscle posteriorly, and the medial surface of the first rib inferiorly. The interscalene

---

Table 1
Vascular TOS: contrast-enhanced 3D MRA protocols for 1.5-T and 3-T MR imaging scanners

	aTOS	vTOS
Sex	Female/male equally	
Age (y)	20–30	20–35
Risk factors	Bone abnormalities (cervical rib and articulating with the first rib as a pseudoarthrosis; anomalous first rib; long C7 transverse process) Congenital fibrocartilaginous bands associated with the anterior scalene muscle Hypertrophic callus from healed clavicle or first rib fracture Vigorous exercise or activity involving affecting extremity Repetitive injury contributed by first rib, clavicle, subclavius muscle, and fibrous costoclavicular ligament leads to perivenous fibrosis and endothelial injury Posture	
Sign and symptoms	Pain Claudication Pallor Coldness	Paresthesia Hand swelling caused by edema Feeling of tightness worsens with exertion Venous engorgement with collateralization
Potential severe complications	Digital ischemia Stroke	Venous gangrene of the hand Pulmonary embolism

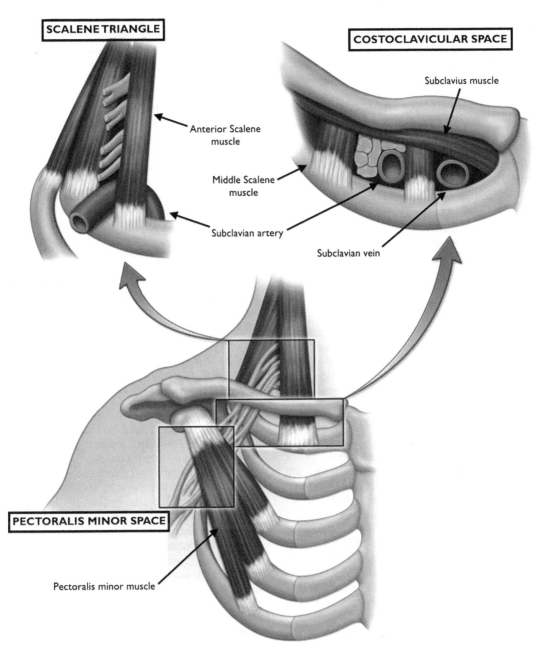

SCALENE TRIANGLE

Anterior Scalene
muscle

Middle Scalene
muscle

Subclavian artery

COSTOCLAVICULAR SPACE

Subclavius muscle

Subclavian vein

PECTORALIS MINOR SPACE

Pectoralis minor muscle

Fig. 1. Three potential spaces of the thoracic outlet that can cause vascular compression: scalene triangle, costo-clavicular space, and pectoralis minor space. (*From* Klaassen Z, Sorenson E, Tubbs RS, et al. Thoracic outlet syndrome: a neurological and vascular disorder. Clin Anat 2014;27(5):724–32; with permission.)

triangle contains the subclavian artery and brachial plexus. Second, the costoclavicular space is bordered by the clavicle superiorly, the subclavius muscle and costoclavicular ligament anteriorly, and by the first rib and anterior scalene muscle posteriorly. This space contains the sub-clavian vein. Third, the retropectoralis minor space (subcoracoid space) is limited by the pectoralis mi-nor anteriorly, subscapularis muscle superiorly,

and chest wall inferiorly and posteriorly. This space contains the neurovascular bundle.

MAGNETIC RESONANCE IMAGING AND PROTOCOLS

Contrast-enhanced 3D MRA, equilibrium phase venography, and T2-weighted images with com-bination of provocative maneuvers including both arm abduction and adduction are used to assess vascular abnormalities in patients with TOS.[18–20] Multiphase acquisition of contrast-enhanced 3D images yields arterial and venous phase images; in addition, equilibrium phase acquisition improves detection of venous abnormalities such as stenosis and the presence of thrombus. Equilibrium phase images are also helpful for identifying extrinsic masses compressing the vascular structures. For better characterization of extra-anatomic structures such as soft tissue masses, T2-weighted sequences should be acquired.[18]

Patient Preparation and Positioning

A 20-gauge peripheral intravenous line should be obtained in the forearm or antecubital fossa, before placing the patient on the table in a supine position. Multichannel phased-array coils provide better signal and excellent coverage. Patients should be instructed to hold their breath during the image acquisitions. All sequences should be acquired during 150° to 160° of bilateral arm abduction with head and neck in the neutral position and repeated during arm adduction position with additional contrast administration.

Magnetic Resonance Protocols and Image Acquisition

MRA examination can be performed on a 1.5-T or 3-T scanner; therefore imaging parameters should be adjusted accordingly. Before injecting contrast agent, T2-weighted sequences (HASTE [Half-Fourier acquisition single-shot turbo spin-echo]) and precontrast mask images should be obtained. For contrast-enhanced MRA, 20 mL of intravenous extracellular contrast agent (ECA) such as gadobenate dimeglumine (0.5 mol/L; MultiHance, Bracco Diagnostics) can be used with a 20-mL saline flush at a rate of 2 mL/s during abduction positioning. In addition, 15 mL of ECA should be administered for the same contrast-enhanced sequences in the rest position; that is, with the arms next to the torso. The timing of the MRA acquisition can be determined by fluoroscopic real-time monitoring or by using a test bolus, or via automatic triggering at contrast agent arrival.[28] For each arm positioning, 2 sets of coronal oblique 3D slabs should be acquired. Recently a blood-pool agent (BPA), gadofosveset trisodium (gadofosveset) was approved by the US Food and Drug Administration for MRA in the United States and single-injection BPA MRA has been shown to have diagnostic image quality and high vessel contrast, similar to double-injection imaging.[19] The gadolinium-based

contrast agents shorten T1 relaxation time of the blood and signal of the vascular contrast is independent of flow dynamics. 3D gradient echo (GRE) sequences with ultrashort recovery time (TR) and echo time (TE) are performed to obtain fast imaging speed and a large field of view with high spatial resolution in a single held breath. For optimal contrast enhancement, the center of k-space should be obtained when the contrast agent concentration is at its peak in the vessel of interest. Equilibrium phase imaging should be initiated around 5 minutes after injection with both axial and coronal orientations during breath holding. This sequence also produces T1-weighted 3D images using interpolation and/or partial Fourier technique. Typically, the less symptomatic arm is used for injection and contrast-enhanced imaging (3D MRA and volume interpolated gradient echo) is performed in abduction first, with identical sequences repeated in adduction. The detailed pulse sequences and their imaging parameters are described in **Table 2**.

IMAGING ANALYSIS AND NORMAL MAGNETIC RESONANCE ANGIOGRAPHY FINDINGS

Interpretation focuses on structures that deviate from normal (**Fig. 2**) and typically begins with multiplanar T2-weighted images, particularly in the sagittal plane, which provides a better understanding of anatomy and structures in the vicinity of the vessels at the thoracic outlet.[29,30] Normal vessels within all 3 critical spaces are embedded in fat, and are well delineated from neighboring bones and musculature on T2-weighted sequences (**Fig. 3**). Multiphase contrast-enhanced 3D MRA images are subsequently analyzed with multiplanar reformats in any desired plane.[18–20] The nearly isotropic voxel diameter of the 3D data eradicates stair-step artifacts during reconstruction. The next step is evaluation of the axial and coronal planes of contrast-enhanced equilibrium phase images. These images better depict the veins, especially when venous enhancement is not adequate on the venous phase of the 3D contrast-enhanced MRA/MRV sequences (**Fig. 4**).[18]

DISORDERS
Arterial Thoracic Outlet Syndrome

Although aTOS is the least common type, it is caused by compression of the subclavian artery and must be suspected in all patients with upper limb ischemia.[1,31] The subclavian artery passes through interscalene triangle and becomes an axillary artery after it reaches the subcoracoid

Table 2
Contrast-enhanced 3D MRA protocols for vascular TOS in 1.5-T and 3-T MR imaging scanners

Scanner	Pulse Sequences	Slice Thickness	TR/TE	Matrix	Flip Angle (°)	Bandwidth (Hz/Pixel)
1.5 T	HASTE	6	1000/91	256 × 160	180	710
	3D contrast-enhanced MRA	1.5	3/1.1	288 × 192	35	450
	Equilibrium volume interpolated GRE (coronal)	3	2.8/1.4	256 × 192	10	920
	Equilibrium volume interpolated GRE (axial)	3	2.8/1.1	320 × 192	10	600
3 T	HASTE	5.5	1200/101	320 × 224	150	780
	3D contrast-enhanced MRA	1.6	2.8/1.1	384 × 362	24	650
	Equilibrium volume interpolated GRE (coronal)	4	3.3/1.3	320 × 256	10	505
	Equilibrium volume interpolated GRE (axial)	4	4.4/1.8	320 × 168	10	505

space.[27] Chronic compression and repetitive trauma of the subclavian artery in any of these spaces can damage the wall and induce focal stenosis.[32] Subclavian trauma is usually caused by a cervical rib in the general population and muscular hypertrophy in competitive athletes.[8,9,17]

The first phase of contrast-enhanced 3D MRA delineates the arteries and associated abnormalities. Some venous contamination in the central thoracic and neck veins is inevitable, although the impact is typically much less than with CTA and the arteries should not be obscured. With contrast-enhanced 3D MRA images, degree of compression is classified as the percentage of the vessel diameter reduction (mild, <50%; moderate, 50%–75%; and severe, >75%) during hyperabduction of the arms and any degree of arterial compression should be considered significant (**Figs. 5–7**). Individual stenoses can have poststenotic aneurysmal

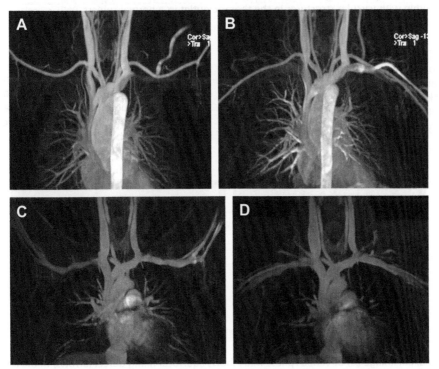

Fig. 2. Coronal MIP images of arterial (*A, B*) and venous (*C, D*) phase MR angiography during arm abduction (*A, C*) and at rest (*B, D*) in normal subject.

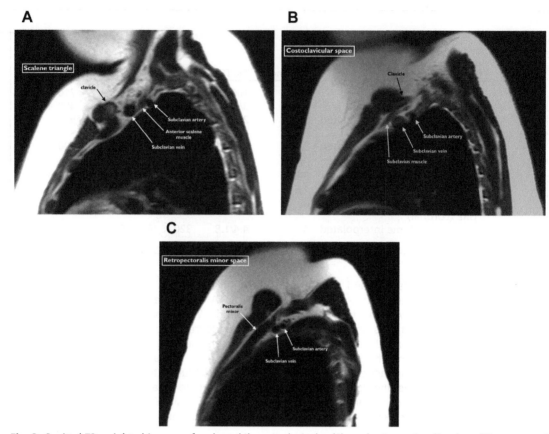

Fig. 3. Sagittal T2-weighted images of scalene (*A*), costoclavicular (*B*), and retropectoralis minor (*C*) spaces and their relationship with vascular structures in the thoracic outlet in a normal subject.

dilatation (**Fig. 8**) with mural thrombus formation.[33] Approximately half of patients with aTOS develop subclavian artery aneurysms.[4,32] The pathophysiology can eventually progress to focal arterial occlusion or distal embolization of thrombus from aneurysms.[9,33]

Venous Thoracic Outlet Syndrome

vTOS is a condition that results in stenosis of the axillary-subclavian vein caused by compression by extrinsic structures; patients typically present with intermittent or positional arm swelling.[1] The axillary and subclavian veins drain the upper

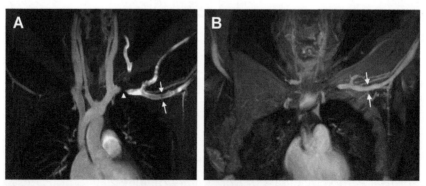

Fig. 4. Coronal MIP image (*A*) of venous phase MRA shows equivocal filling defect (*arrows*) in the left subclavian vein in a patient with severe stenosis (*arrowhead*); however, on equilibrium phase images (*B*), the vein opacifies homogeneously (*arrows*).

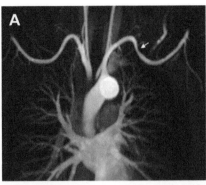
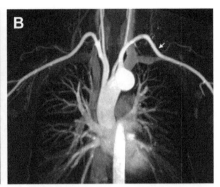

Fig. 5. A 48-year-old woman with left-sided arm pain and paresthesia: coronal MIP image (A) of arterial phase MRA during arm abduction shows moderate stenosis (arrow) of left subclavian artery within the costoclavicular space, which resolves on the arm rest image (B).

extremity by passing through the subcoracoid and costoclavicular space before entering the thorax.[27] Compression and recurrent venous injury are from the first rib, the clavicle, and the costoclavicular ligaments at the costoclavicular space.[30] The degree of venous compression during hyperabduction is interpreted using the same scale as for the arteries, and any lesion with more than 50% subclavian vein compression should be considered significant (Figs. 9 and 10).[18] Our experience corroborates reports that asymptomatic patients and volunteers may have compression during hyperabduction, and therefore contrast-enhanced 3D MRV alone cannot definitively diagnose TOS.[30,34,35]

Paget-Schroetter Syndrome

Paget-Schroetter syndrome, or effort thrombosis of the subclavian/axillary vein, usually occurs because of repetitive upper extremity activity in the presence of space-occupying structures in the thoracic outlet. It is usually seen in the dominant arm with excessive overhead activity.

Almost all patients have subclavian vein compression in the costoclavicular junction from an abnormal insertion of the costoclavicular ligament, although hypertrophied scalene muscle and/or callus formation from prior fracture can play a role.[27,36] A recent study suggested that effort thrombosis depends on the distance between the clavicle and the first rib, and thus risk factors for deep venous thrombosis are less important.[37] Thrombus is assessed with contrast-enhanced 3D MRV at equilibrium to minimize false-positive findings from turbulent flow (Fig. 11).[18,38] Contrast-enhanced MRV is as effective as conventional venography in identifying deep venous thrombosis[25,39,40] and there is no role for catheterization unless an intervention is anticipated.

Management and Recurrent Thoracic Outlet Syndrome

Initial treatment of most patients with TOS is conservative management, including modification of lifestyle by avoiding provocative activities,

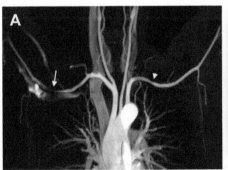
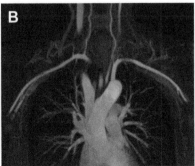

Fig. 6. A 54-year-old woman with bilateral arm pain and right-sided pallor: coronal MIP image (A) shows moderate stenosis in the right axillary artery (arrow) in the retropectoralis minor space and mild stenosis of the left subclavian artery (arrowhead) during hyperabduction. Both these stenoses resolve in the rest position (B).

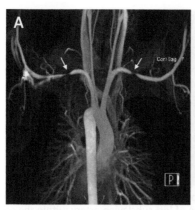
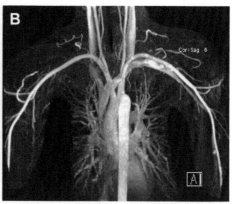

Fig. 7. A 38-year-old man with swelling and cyanosis in the bilateral upper extremities after recently increasing his upper body exercise regimen for weight training. Coronal MIP image (*A*) during abduction shows severe stenosis (*arrow*) of the subclavian arteries with resolution in the rest (*B*) position. A, anterior; P, posterior.

physical therapy, or anesthetic and steroid injection.[41] However 30% to 40% of these patients undergo surgical intervention to decompress the thoracic outlet. The reference-standard treatment is considered to be first rib resection and scalenectomy.[42] Also, patients with Paget-Schroetter syndrome require immediate care and some investigators advocate prompt surgery rather than conservative treatment with thrombolysis.[43] However, patients may have recurrent symptoms even after surgical decompression; these cases should be evaluated for residual first rib (**Fig. 12**) and/or adherent residual scalene muscle.[44]

PEARLS, PITFALLS, AND VARIANTS

Contrast-enhanced 3D MRA/MRV with equilibrium images is first-line imaging to evaluate patients with suspected TOS. The following pearls and pitfalls are reviewed to optimize the acquisition and image quality. The cornerstone of the study is hyperabduction and its comparison with the arms-down images. All sequences should be repeated for both positions, including contrast injections for MRA, although a double injection can be avoided with gadofosveset.[19] Susceptibility artifacts can be seen from high concentrations of contrast agent in the subclavian/axillary veins during the first phase; the artifact will resolve on the following phases. Also, intravenous line placement and contrast injection can be performed contralateral to the symptomatic arm.

Because of the previously noted inadequate spatial resolution of the T2-weighted images, assessment of anomalous ligaments or fibrous bands causing neurovascular compression can be difficult. Therefore, when this is suspected, focused higher resolution images with multiple weightings can be acquired.

WHAT THE REFERRING PHYSICIAN NEEDS TO KNOW

Few patients with TOS present with vascular symptoms, and MRA/MRV can identify those patients who are most likely to benefit from

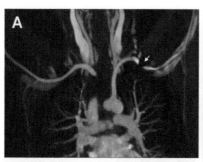
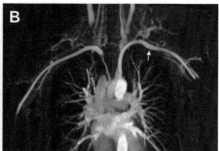

Fig. 8. A 40-year-old woman with neck and finger pain: coronal MIP image (*A*) during abduction shows severe stenosis (*arrow*) of the left subclavian artery caused by clavicle compression and resolution of the stenosis in the arm rest (*B*) position. Mild fusiform aneurysmal dilatation of the vessel is noted at the level of compression in the rest position (*arrow*).

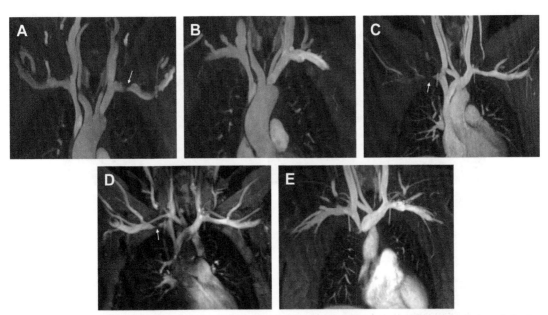

Fig. 9. A 45-year-old woman with shoulder pain: coronal MIP image (*A*) of venous phase MRA during abduction revealed moderate stenosis (*arrow*) of the left subclavian vein and complete resolution in the arm rest position (*B*). A 36-year-old woman with right upper extremity pain and neuropraxia who was referred for concern of TOS. Coronal MIP image (*C*) of venous phase MRA during abduction shows severe stenosis of the right subclavian vein in the costoclavicular junction. On the equilibrium phase image (*D*), there is better opacification of the vein with persistent severe. Rest position image (*E*) shows normal venous structure.

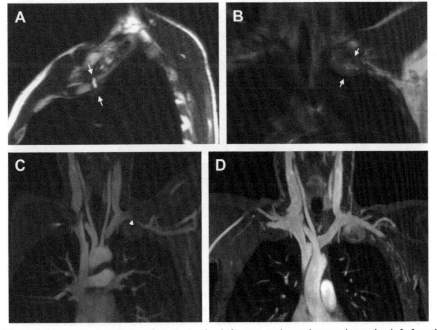

Fig. 10. A 32-year-old man presented with pain in the left arm and numbness along the left fourth and fifth digits. Sagittal and coronal T2-weighted images (*A*, *B*) revealed exostosis of the first rib from pseudoarthrosis (*arrows*) and associated severe stenosis of the right subclavian vein (*arrowhead*) during abduction (*C*) and resolution in the arm rest position (*D*).

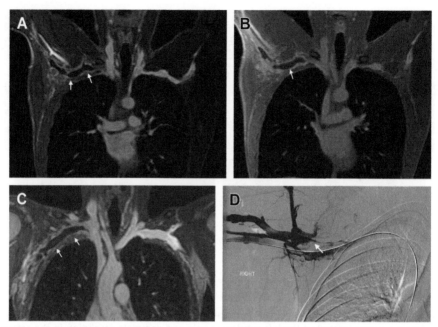

Fig. 11. A 34-year-old man with acute-onset right upper extremity pain and swelling. Coronal MIP image (*A*) of venous phase MRA during abduction shows complete thrombosis (*arrow*) of the right subclavian vein, which is also shown on equilibrium phase images (*arrows*) during abduction (*B*) and in the rest position (*C*). The patient underwent conventional angiography (*D*) for thrombolysis, which confirmed right subclavian vein occlusion (*arrow*).

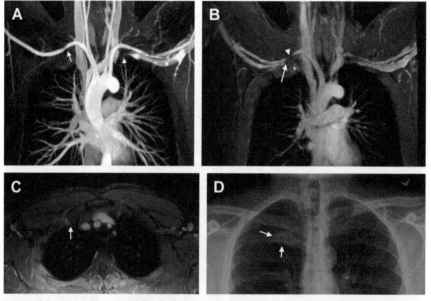

Fig. 12. A 45-year-old man status post right first rib resection presented with upper extremity pain and edema. Coronal MIP image (*A*) of the venous phase MRA during abduction revealed mild stenosis (*arrow*) in the right subclavian artery and severe stenosis in the left subclavian vein (*arrowhead*). Coronal equilibrium image (*B*) again shows mild stenosis of the right subclavian artery (*arrowhead*), severe stenosis of the right subclavian vein (*arrow*), and focal expansion of the residual first rib (*asterisk*). Axial equilibrium image (*C*) revealed residual right first rib with postoperative changes and enhancement (*arrow*). Chest radiograph (*D*) confirms residual right first rib (*arrows*), which is the cause of recurrent vascular TOS.

surgery to prevent serious complications, such as venous gangrene, pulmonary embolism, and digital ischemia. Thus, the ideal radiology report should include the following points:

1. Affected vessel during hyperabduction or rest position
2. Degree of luminal narrowing both for artery and vein: mild (<50%), moderate (50%–75%), and severe (>75%)
3. Location and potential cause for compression
4. Associated complications: occlusion, thrombosis, and poststenotic aneurysmal dilatation
5. Other incidental or associated findings

SUMMARY

Contrast-enhanced 3D MRA/MRV with provocative arm positioning enables assessment of arteries as well as veins of both arms and associated complications during 1 session, without radiation exposure. In addition to venous phase MRA, equilibrium phase images successfully identify venous thrombosis (Paget-Schroetter syndrome) and extravascular soft tissue masses in combination with T2-weighted images.

REFERENCES

1. Sanders RJ, Hammond SL, Rao NM. Diagnosis of thoracic outlet syndrome. J Vasc Surg 2007;46: 601–4.
2. Davidović LB, Kostic DM, Jakovljevic NS, et al. Vascular thoracic outlet syndrome. World J Surg 2003;27:545–50.
3. Cooke RA. Thoracic outlet syndrome—aspects of diagnosis in the differential diagnosis of hand-arm vibration syndrome. Occup Med (Lond) 2003;53: 331–6.
4. Davidović LB, Končar IB, Pejkić SD, et al. Arterial complications of thoracic outlet syndrome. Am Surg 2009;75:235–9.
5. Hood DB, Kuehne J, Yellin AE, et al. Vascular complications of thoracic outlet syndrome. Am Surg 1997;63:913–7.
6. Sanders RJ, Haug C. Review of arterial thoracic outlet syndrome with a report of five new instances. Surg Gynecol Obstet 1991;173:415–25.
7. Sheth RN, Belzberg AJ. Diagnosis and treatment of thoracic outlet syndrome. Neurosurg Clin N Am 2001;12:295–309.
8. Criado E, Berguer R, Greenfield L. The spectrum of arterial compression at the thoracic outlet. J Vasc Surg 2010;52:406–11.
9. Nehler MR. Upper extremity ischemia from subclavian artery aneurysm caused by bony abnormalities of the thoracic outlet. Arch Surg 1997;132:527.
10. Urschel HC, Razzuk MA. Paget-Schroetter syndrome: what is the best management? Ann Thorac Surg 2000;69:1663–8 [discussion: 1668–9].
11. Huang JH, Zager EL. Thoracic outlet syndrome. Neurosurgery 2004;55:897–903.
12. Nichols AW. Diagnosis and management of thoracic outlet syndrome. Curr Sports Med Rep 2009;8:240–9.
13. Hughes ES. Venous obstruction in the upper extremity; Paget-Schroetter's syndrome; a review of 320 cases. Surg Gynecol Obstet 1949;88(2):89–127.
14. Azakie A, McElhinney DB, Thompson RW, et al. Surgical management of subclavian-vein effort thrombosis as a result of thoracic outlet compression. J Vasc Surg 1998;28:777–86.
15. Angle N, Gelabert HA, Farooq MM, et al. Safety and efficacy of early surgical decompression of the thoracic outlet for Paget-Schroetter syndrome. Ann Vasc Surg 2001;15:37–42.
16. Cronenwett JL, Johnston KW. Rutherford's vascular surgery. Ann Vasc Surg 2014;28:114–932. Elsevier Health Sciences.
17. Demondion X, Herbinet P, Jan S. Imaging assessment of thoracic outlet syndrome. Radiographics 2006;26:1735–50.
18. Ersoy H, Steigner ML, Coyner KB, et al. Vascular thoracic outlet syndrome: protocol design and diagnostic value of contrast-enhanced 3D MR angiography and equilibrium phase imaging on 1.5- and 3-T MRI scanners. AJR Am J Roentgenol 2012;198: 1180–7.
19. Lim RP, Bruno M, Rosenkrantz AB, et al. Comparison of blood pool and extracellular gadolinium chelate for functional MR evaluation of vascular thoracic outlet syndrome. Eur J Radiol 2014;83(7):1209–15.
20. Charon JP, Milne W, Sheppard DG, et al. Evaluation of MR angiographic technique in the assessment of thoracic outlet syndrome. Clin Radiol 2004;59: 588–95.
21. Dymarkowski S, Bosmans H, Marchal G, et al. Three-dimensional MR angiography in the evaluation of thoracic outlet syndrome. AJR Am J Roentgenol 1999;173:1005–8.
22. Hagspiel KD, Spinosa DJ, Angle JF, et al. Diagnosis of vascular compression at the thoracic outlet using gadolinium-enhanced high-resolution ultrafast MR angiography in abduction and adduction. Cardiovasc Intervent Radiol 2000;23:152–4.
23. Ersoy H, Rybicki FJ. Biochemical safety profiles of gadolinium-based extracellular contrast agents and nephrogenic systemic fibrosis. J Magn Reson Imaging 2007;26:1190–7.
24. Esposito MD, Arrington JA, Blackshear MN, et al. Thoracic outlet syndrome in a throwing athlete diagnosed with MRI and MRA. J Magn Reson Imaging 1997;7:598–9.
25. Vogt FM, Herborn CU, Goyen M. MR venography. Magn Reson Imaging Clin N Am 2005;13:113–29, vi.

26. Spritzer CE. Progress in MR imaging of the venous system. Perspect Vasc Surg Endovasc Ther 2009; 21:105–16.

27. Urschel HC Jr. Anatomy of the thoracic outlet. Thorac Surg Clin 2007;17:511–20.

28. Ivancevic MK, Geerts L, Weadock WJ, et al. Technical principles of MR angiography methods. Magn Reson Imaging Clin N Am 2009;17:1–11.

29. Demondion X, Boutry N, Drizenko A, et al. Thoracic outlet: anatomic correlation with MR imaging. AJR Am J Roentgenol 2000;175:417–22.

30. Demondion X, Bacqueville E, Paul C, et al. Thoracic outlet: assessment with MR imaging in asymptomatic and symptomatic populations. Radiology 2003; 227:461–8.

31. Patton GM. Arterial thoracic outlet syndrome. Hand Clin 2004;20:107–11, viii.

32. Cormier JM, Amrane M, Ward A, et al. Arterial complications of the thoracic outlet syndrome: fifty-five operative cases. J Vasc Surg 1989;9:778–87.

33. Marine L, Valdes F, Mertens R, et al. Arterial thoracic outlet syndrome: a 32-year experience. Ann Vasc Surg 2013;27:1007–13.

34. Longley DG, Yedlicka JW, Molina EJ, et al. Thoracic outlet syndrome: evaluation of the subclavian vessels by color duplex sonography. AJR Am J Roentgenol 1992;158:623–30.

35. Matsumura JS, Rilling WS, Pearce WH, et al. Helical computed tomography of the normal thoracic outlet. J Vasc Surg 1997;26:776–83.

36. Atasoy E. Thoracic outlet syndrome: anatomy. Hand Clin 2004;20:7–14.

37. Arnhjort T, Nordberg J, Delle M, et al. The importance of the costoclavicular space in upper limb primary deep vein thrombosis, a study with magnetic resonance imaging (MRI) technique enhanced by a blood pool agent. Eur J Intern Med 2014;25: 545–9.

38. Hunter DW, Mortazavi S. Imaging venous disease: pearls and pitfalls. Tech Vasc Interv Radiol 2014; 17:74–81.

39. Tanju S, Sancak T, Düşünceli E, et al. Direct contrast-enhanced 3D MR venography evaluation of upper extremity deep venous system. Diagn Interv Radiol 2006;12:74–9.

40. Sampson FC, Goodacre SW, Thomas SM, et al. The accuracy of MRI in diagnosis of suspected deep vein thrombosis: systematic review and meta-analysis. Eur Radiol 2007;17:175–81.

41. Rochlin DH, Orlando MS, Likes KC, et al. Bilateral first rib resection and scalenectomy is effective for treatment of thoracic outlet syndrome. J Vasc Surg 2014;60:185–90.

42. Brooke BS, Freischlag JA. Contemporary management of thoracic outlet syndrome. Curr Opin Cardiol 2010;25:535–40.

43. Molina JE, Hunter DW, Dietz CA. Paget-Schroetter syndrome treated with thrombolytics and immediate surgery. J Vasc Surg 2007;45:328–34.

44. Likes K, Dapash T, Rochlin DH, et al. Remaining or residual first ribs are the cause of recurrent thoracic outlet syndrome. Ann Vasc Surg 2014;28:939–45.

Pediatric Chest MR Imaging
Sedation, Techniques, and Extracardiac Vessels

Juan C. Baez, MD[a,b], Ravi T. Seethamraju, PhD[c], Robert Mulkern, PhD[b],
Pierluigi Ciet, MD, PhD[d,e], Edward Y. Lee, MD, MPH[b,*]

KEYWORDS

- MR imaging • MR imaging technique • Vascular anomalies and abnormalities • Pediatric patients

KEY POINTS

- Proper patient preparation is essential for thoracic MR imaging in pediatric patients.
- Sedation proves necessary to obtain diagnostic quality chest MR imaging in infants and young children.
- Various MR imaging techniques can visualize vascular anatomy both with and without the use of intravenous contrast.
- Evaluation of thoracic outlet syndrome is improved by dynamic MR imaging technique.

INTRODUCTION

Since its introduction to clinical practice, MR imaging has become a cornerstone of radiologic imaging. In recent years, advances in MR imaging technology including the use of 3T scanners and parallel imaging, have overcome many of the limitations that previously hindered the use of MR imaging for thoracic disorders. Particularly, the excellent soft tissue contrast and anatomic detail provided by MR imaging has encouraged its widespread adoption for thoracic vascular imaging. This review addresses practical strategies to improve thoracic MR image quality including overcoming motion artifacts and the necessity for sedation in many pediatric patients when performing thoracic

vascular MR imaging. With tailored pediatric protocols, one can accurately diagnose myriad conditions without exposing the patient to ionizing radiation. Selected examples of pathology that vascular thoracic MR imaging can diagnose in the pediatric population are also provided.

TECHNICAL ISSUES: MOTION

Motion in chest imaging is typically caused by cardiac and respiratory activities. Cardiac gating relies on the use of an electrocardiogram (ECG) for monitoring the cardiac cycle during the MR imaging examination, allowing for the acquisition of images during diastole, the most quiescent portion of the cardiac cycle.[1] Respiratory motion generally

Disclosures: no relevant disclosures (J.C. Baez, R. Mulkern, P. Ciet, and E.Y. Lee); Dr Seethamraju has stock ownership and an employment affiliation with Siemens AG.
[a] Mid-Atlantic Permanente Medical Group, 2101 East Jefferson Street, Rockville, MD 20852, USA; [b] Department of Radiology, Boston Children's Hospital, Harvard Medical School, 300 Longwood Avenue, Boston, MA 02115, USA; [c] Magnetic Resonance, Research and Development, Siemens Healthcare, 1620 Tremont St., Boston, MA 02120, USA; [d] Department of Radiology and Pediatric Pulmonology, Sophia Children's Hospital, Erasmus Medical Center, Wytemaweg 80, 3015 CN, Rotterdam, The Netherlands; [e] Department of Radiology, Beth Israel Deaconess Medical Center, Harvard Medical School, 330 Brookline Ave, Boston, MA 02215, USA
* Corresponding author. Department of Radiology, Boston Children's Hospital, Harvard Medical School, 300 Longwood Avenue, Boston, MA 02115.
E-mail address: Edward.Lee@childrens.harvard.edu

Magn Reson Imaging Clin N Am 23 (2015) 321–335
http://dx.doi.org/10.1016/j.mric.2015.01.010
1064-9689/15/$ – see front matter © 2015 Elsevier Inc. All rights reserved.

plays a much larger role in noncardiac thoracic imaging compared with cardiac motion. In an ideal setting, breath-hold imaging yields the highest quality images, as it can largely eliminate respiratory motion.[2] Because the ability to perform breath holding is limited in infants and young children (<5 years old), this technique is reserved for older (≥5 years) or intubated children and, of course, requires rapid pulse sequences.

Another way to manage respiratory motion involves acquiring signal over a longer period, but only during the same phase of respiration. One can perform respiratory gating with the use of a bellows or belt strapped to the patient that monitors the respiratory cycle. Such methods can be deployed to selectively acquire MR signals only during end expiration, the portion of the cycle at which the abdomen and chest remain motionless.[3] One can also monitor the phase of the respiratory cycle with the use a navigator echo. Navigator echoes allow either retrospective or prospective gating of signal by sampling a small area in the region of the diaphragm to assess diaphragmatic excursion.[4] Similar to the use of the bellows, only signals acquired during the

appropriate phase of the respiratory cycle are then used for final image reconstructions (**Fig. 1**).[5]

Children may have difficulty with extended breath holds or the concept of quiet breathing. In addition, the average resting respiratory rate increases with decreasing age. For this reason, multiple pulse sequences have been developed to optimize image quality.[6,7] A simplistic way of categorizing these sequences is to divide them into sequences that only acquire data while the lungs are not moving and those sequences that acquire signal throughout the respiratory cycle in quiet breathing. Other methods to perform non–breath hold imaging involve faster sequences that undersample k space or sample k space in a fashion that minimizes motion artifact such as periodically rotated overlapping parallel lines with enhanced reconstruction (PROPELLER/BLADE).[8]

PATIENT PREPARATION ISSUES: SEDATION

In the previous section, cardiac and respiratory motion were discussed as especially problematic to thoracic imaging. Even when optimizing the

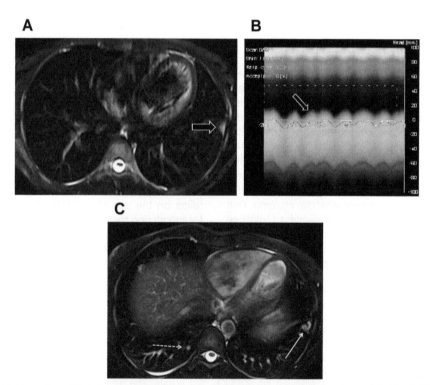

Fig. 1. Navigator gating. (*A*) Axial T2 HASTE MR image shows pleural thickening (*arrow*) in the left lower lobe, but motion artifact degrades image quality. (*B*) The use of navigator gating improves image quality by only accepting signal acquired during the same phase in the respiratory cycle, typically end expiration. The diaphragmatic excursion is plotted (*arrow*) on a time axis. (*C*) The use of navigator gating can improve image quality, although it increases overall imaging time. The previously noted pleural thickening (*solid arrow*) in the left lower lobe is better visualized. A right lower lobe pulmonary artery (*dashed arrow*) clearly seen on this gated sequence was not evident on the nongated sequence.

protocol using sequences such as PROPELLER that compensate for these two constant and implacable causes of motion, a moving patient can make a scan nondiagnostic. MR imaging relies on the acquisition of multiple series of images with the examinations taking anywhere between 15 minutes to more than an hour. Obtaining diagnostic MR imaging, therefore, requires either a cooperative or sedated patient.[9,10]

The age of a patient plays a central role in developing an individualized imaging plan for each MR imaging examination. Older patients (typically older than 5 years) who can follow commands may attempt to undergo MR imaging without sedation.[11] These pediatric patients, however, should undergo thorough preparation before the MR imaging examination is conducted either by the radiologist or medical staff familiar with the protocol to improve image acquisition. Children should be told what to expect with respect to the appearance of the magnet, the movement of the table, the loud noises they will hear, and the importance of laying still.[12] Some institutions provide coaching in a mock scanner environment to improve familiarization with the noisy MR imaging environment in an attempt to further improve examination quality and success.[13] Pediatric patients should also practice breathing instructions before the start of the examination. Although these steps result in additional time needed up front, they result in a high percentage of successful and diagnostic MR imaging examinations.[14,15]

Some children, as in the adult population, may require sedation for MR imaging because of claustrophobia or other anxiety.[12] Allowing the parent to stay in the room with the child, distraction methods such as goggles projecting a movie, or reassurance and coordination with ancillary staff accustomed to making children comfortable with imaging tests can often alleviate the need for sedation.[12,14] Neonates can often undergo MR imaging without sedation by using the "feed and wrap" method wherein the child is fed immediately preceding the examination and then placed in the scanner after being swaddled.[16] Although this technique works well in imaging of stationary body parts such as the brain, its application to chest imaging may prove limited given the sensitivity of MR imaging to respiratory motion and the high respiratory rates found in neonates, particularly those with underlying respiratory abnormalities.[17]

Children younger than 5 and older children with cognitive delay or inability to follow commands require a different approach. A diagnostic MR imaging examination in this patient population mandates the use of deeper sedation, often with endotracheal intubation performed in conjunction with anesthesiologists.[18] The risks of anesthesia should be weighed against the potential benefits of the imaging examination and should be explained to the parents of the patients. Recent studies in animal models have found that deep sedation in the early-developing brain may result in long-term sequelae.[19–21] These patients in particular may benefit from another examination not requiring sedation, such as computed tomography (CT), if the risks to brain development from anesthesia outweigh the radiation risk.

Sedation of children in the radiology department has traditionally been performed with chloral hydrate because of its well-established efficacy and safety profile.[22] Numerous other sedating agents have been used in children including fentanyl, midazolam, pentobarbital, propofol, chlorpromazine, and sevoflurane.[23–25] Dexmedetomidine is a newer agent with a short half-life (approximately 2 hours) that is highly selective for the $\alpha2$ adrenoceptor working at the level of the locus ceruleus in the central nervous system.[26–28] This agent provides both sedation and analgesia with minimal effect on respiration. A recent study evaluating this agent in 279 patients within a radiology department found no adverse respiratory effects, no pharmacologic therapy needed to treat hemodynamic variability, and rapid recovery after the examination.[27]

With the child sedated, the anesthesiologist can control patient respiration and potentially work in conjunction with the MR imaging technologist to time the acquisition of images. Hyperventilation, if properly timed, can recreate a breath hold type of state for those sequences requiring a breath hold. Alternatively, the anesthesiologist can hold respirations in a controlled environment with careful monitoring of the patient's vital signs including pulse oximetry to obtain the images. The radiologist should minimize the amount of time the patient is sedated by ensuring that the provided imaging is diagnostic and not performing superfluous pulse sequences. In addition, MR imaging should be performed as quickly as possible once the patient is intubated to minimize the development of atelectasis, which can obscure underlying abnormality and can be secondary to patient ventilation.[29–31] Once the examination is complete, the patient should be monitored in a controlled environment until the effects of anesthesia have worn off and the child is safe for discharge from the radiology department.

ANGIOGRAPHY TECHNIQUES

Traditional MR imaging has relied on the detection of precessing protons of the hydrogen atom in the body.[6,7] Most soft tissues contain an abundance of water molecules, which, in turn, are excellent sources of protons and hence provide abundant signal.[32–34] The vascular system also contains many circulating water molecules; however, their constant movement provides additional challenges and opportunities.

MR angiography provides a mechanism to evaluate the circulatory system in a less-invasive fashion than the traditional gold standard (ie, conventional angiography) and also provides unique advantages. Conventional angiography provides exquisite spatial and temporal resolution but can only image the patent lumen of the interrogated vessels. MR angiography, however, acquires images not only the lumen, but also the vessel wall, and surrounding structures. Although CT angiography provides much of the same data and is now considered standard of care for certain diagnoses such as pulmonary embolism, it requires exposing the patient to radiation and intravenous iodinated contrast.

One can perform MR angiography with and without contrast.[35] Contrast-enhanced MR relies on the use of gadolinium to shorten T1 times and thereby increase the signal of the blood relative to the remainder of the body (**Fig. 2**).[36] This robust technique is less prone to flow-related image artifacts than the unenhanced sequences and provides excellent vascular imaging. The advent of 3T imaging improved image quality by increasing signal-to-noise ratio with shortened scan times and also allowing the use of lower gadolinium doses without degrading image quality.[37] Depending on the timing of the image acquisition, traditional gadolinium contrast may be found primarily in the arterial system or venous system or diluted throughout both.[36] The use of newer intravascular gadolinium agents, such as gadofosveset, facilitates vascular studies by keeping the contrast within the blood vessels allowing exquisite vascular delineation for an extended period without significant signal loss.[38] If only a certain portion of the vasculature (ie, arterial system) is of interest, selective scanning early during the contrast injection cycle allows for delineation between the opacified signal-rich arteries and the signal-poor veins.

In some situations, current clinical guidelines preclude the use of gadolinium. Patients with a glomerular filtration rate of less than 30 mL/min are at risk of nephrogenic systemic fibrosis, a scleroderm alike condition.[39] Although certain formulations of gadolinium are considered low risk for development of nephrogenic systemic fibrosis because of improved stability between the chelate and gadolinium, a glomerular filtration rate less than 30 mL/min generally precludes the use of contrast in our institution.[39] Administering contrast in this situation would require a careful analysis of the risk-benefit ratio, informed consent from the

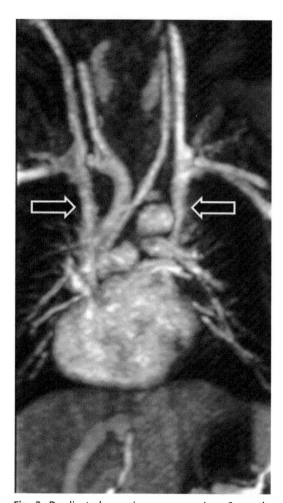

Fig. 2. Duplicated superior vena cava in a 6-month-old girl. Coronal maximum intensity projection image from an MR angiography shows 2 superior vena cavae (*arrows*). The left-sided superior vena cava drains into the coronary sinus.

parents, and nephrology consultation. The guidelines have also changed regarding the use gadolinium in children less than 1 year of age. In this population, gadolinium is contraindicated in neonates less than 4 weeks old and should be used cautiously in patients less than 1 year old.[39] In pregnant patients, the use of gadolinium is often generally avoided because of the theoretic, but unproven, risk to the fetus unless the benefits outweigh the potential risk.[40] In all these situations, non–contrast-enhanced MR angiography provides an excellent alternative. An added benefit of non–contrast-enhanced MR angiography is the ability to perform multiple sequential acquisitions should the initial images prove nondiagnostic.

Time-of-flight MR angiography relies on the use of either 2-dimensional or 3-dimensional gradient echo sequences in which the constant inflow of blood into the imaging slab results in a higher signal intensity within the vessel than the surrounding soft tissues saturated by repeated radiofrequency pulses.[41] These sequences are limited by long acquisition times and signal loss when blood flow is parallel to the imaging plane. Consequently, time-of-flight MR angiography can underestimate blood flow. Additional causes of signal loss include turbulent flow and susceptibility artifact associated with gradient-echo imaging.

Steady-state free precession images (SSFP), with a complicated T1 and T2 weighting, can provide anatomic information with good spatial and temporal resolution.[42,43] These properties have made SSFP one of the main sequences of cardiac imaging. Numerous studies have found that SSFP sequences accurately diagnose pathology in the aorta and smaller vessels.[43,44] SSFP sequences have high signal-to-noise ratio and are relatively independent of flow directionality; however, the sequences are susceptible to field inhomogeneities, especially at higher field strengths. The use of arterial spin labeling together with SSFP sequences has also been applied to angiographic imaging; however, discussion of this topic is beyond the scope of this article.

Double-inversion recovery imaging suppresses signal from flowing blood resulting in a black blood image. By eliminating signal from the flowing blood, one can better evaluate mural abnormalities. Black blood imaging requires ECG gating, resulting in long acquisition times. The use of different k space reconstruction algorithms (PROPELLER) is useful in decreasing motion artifact even in the absence of gating.[41]

ECG-gated fast spin echo MR angiography provides bright blood vascular imaging by subtracting systolic images from diastolic images.[45] In systole, the fast blood flow results in a signal void. During diastole, the more slowly flowing blood retains its signal. Consequently, the subtraction images eliminate the signal from the background tissues and only retain the fast flowing blood.[46] Limitations of this technique include the need for appropriate ECG triggering and sensitivity to motion, especially as subtraction of images is involved.

MR imaging is an excellent imaging modality for evaluation of thoracic vasculature. Routine MR imaging can often detect congenital aortic arch abnormalities such as a right-sided or double aortic arch.[47] A fundamental protocol would begin with a core number of T1-weighted and T2-weighted sequences. Additional angiographic pulse sequences as described above provide additional information about the blood vessels.[48] The use of contrast-enhanced MR angiography sequences with gadolinium increases the accuracy for detection of extracardiac mediastinal vascular abnormalities; however, the decision to administer contrast requires a careful weighing of both clinical necessity and risk factors. Newer blood pool contrast agents such as gadofosveset (Ablavar) continue to improve vascular imaging and may further increase diagnostic accuracy.[49]

EVALUATION OF EXTRACARDIAC MEDIASTINAL VASCULAR STRUCTURES
Vascular Rings and Slings

MR imaging can optimally illustrate congenital mediastinal vascular variants. Pediatric patients with unexplained dysphagia or respiratory symptoms often undergo evaluation for the presence of vascular rings, most commonly a double aortic arch or a right-sided aortic arch with an aberrant left subclavian artery. Although the diagnosis is often suggested by the impressions on the esophagus best seen on fluoroscopic contrast studies, confirmation and preoperative assessment typically rely on cross-sectional imaging (**Fig. 3**).[47] In

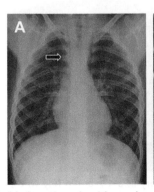
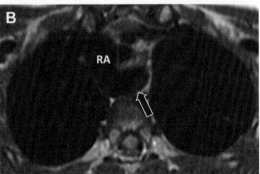

Fig. 3. Right-sided aortic arch with an aberrant left subclavian artery in an 8-year-old boy who presented with dysphagia. (A) Frontal chest radiograph shows a right-sided aortic arch (*arrow*) displacing the adjacent trachea to the left side. (B) Axial T1-weighted MR image shows the right-sided aortic arch (RA) with an aberrant left subclavian artery (*arrow*) arising from a diverticulum of Kommerell.

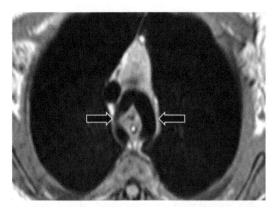

Fig. 4. Double aortic arch in a 29-day-old boy who presented with shortness of breath. Axial black blood sequence MR image shows 2 aortic arches (*arrows*) encircling trachea and esophagus.

the case of the double aortic arch, it is important for the surgeon to know which arch is dominant, as the contralateral arch is typically ligated, and such information affects the surgical approach (**Fig. 4**).[50] A left-sided aortic arch with an aberrant right subclavian is the most common arch anomaly, occurring in up to 2.5% of the general population; however, this congenital vascular anomaly does not represent a true vascular ring (**Fig. 5**). This variant is typically asymptomatic; however, in some cases it results in dysphagia lusoria or coughing.[51] Operative management, although controversial, has been used in symptomatic cases refractory to conservative management.[52]

Another mediastinal vascular variant that MR imaging can optimally illustrate is a pulmonary artery sling, in which the left pulmonary artery arises from the right pulmonary artery and passes posterior to the trachea and anterior to the

esophagus (**Fig. 6**). Although the characteristic impressions on the trachea and esophagus can be seen on a lateral radiograph or fluoroscopic study, MR imaging or CT permit direct visualization.[53]

Although it is not a true vascular ring or sling, the innominate artery sometimes compresses the trachea anteriorly, resulting in respiratory distress, which is best visualized on sagittal MR image (**Fig. 7**). It is thought that in some individuals, the innominate artery arises to the left of its normal location, requiring it to pass anterior to the trachea resulting in anterior tracheal compression. This origin is seen more frequently in young children and is often asymptomatic. As patients age, the origin of the innominate artery becomes progressively more rightward resulting in alleviation of symptoms.[54] Symptomatic patients may undergo aortopexy for definitive management.[55–57]

Aortic Anomalies

MR imaging evaluation of the aorta often takes place within the context of a dedicated cardiac MR imaging which is beyond the scope of this article. Nevertheless, aortic pathology can be seen on routine chest MR imaging requiring a familiarity with some of the more common manifestations.

Coarctation of aorta

Coarctation of the aorta is a condition in which the descending aorta is narrowed, commonly between the left subclavian artery and ductus arteriosus/ligamentum arteriosum.[58] A pressure gradient exists between the more proximal aorta and the aorta distal to the coarctation. This differentiates coarctation from the similar-appearing pseudocoarctation that does not have any hemodynamic

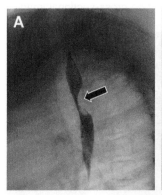
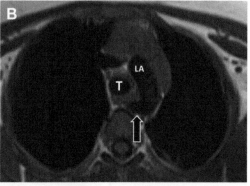

Fig. 5. Left-sided aortic arch with an aberrant right subclavian artery in a 4-year-old boy who presented with repeated vomiting after eating. (*A*) Lateral fluoroscopic image obtained during barium swallow study shows a posterior impression (*arrow*) of the esophagus caused by an underlying aberrant right subclavian artery. (*B*) Axial black blood sequence MR image shows a left-sided aortic arch (LA) with an aberrant right subclavian artery (*arrow*) coursing posterior to the esophagus. This is considered a normal variant, the lusory artery. T, Trachea.

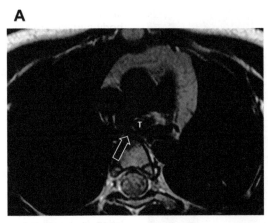

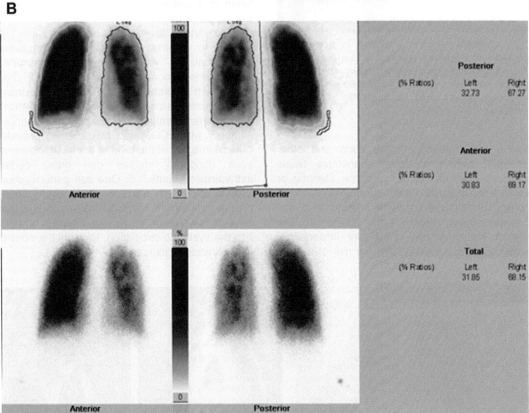

Fig. 6. Pulmonary artery sling in a 5-year-old girl who presented with respiratory distress. (*A*) Axial black blood sequence MR image shows the left pulmonary artery (*arrow*) arising from the right pulmonary artery and coursing posterior to the trachea (T). Also noted is compressed trachea (T). (*B*) Quantitative perfusion scan shows diffusely decreased radiotracer uptake in the left lung relative to the right.

significance. In the absence of dedicated flow analysis sequences, the presence of prominent collateral vessels point in the direction of a clinically significant coarctation (**Fig. 8**).[59,60] The presence of these collaterals gives rise to the classic rib notching sign seen on radiographs. Management of coarctation can be either surgical resection of the narrowed aortic segment or endovascular stent placement.

Aortic anomalies related to underlying connective tissue diseases

Pediatric patients with predisposing conditions including connective tissue diseases, such as Marfan's, Loeys-Dietz, and Ehler's Danlos, often undergo screening for aortic enlargement; however, these condition may go undiagnosed into adulthood. Arterial tortuosity syndrome is a rare connective tissue disorder that can result in

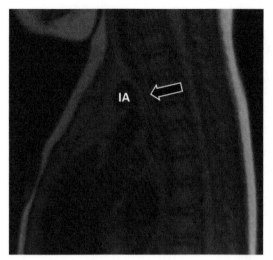

Fig. 7. Innominate artery syndrome in a 1-year-old girl with intermittent respiratory distress. Sagittal T1-weighted MR image best shows the marked tracheal narrowing (*arrow*) by the innominate artery (IA). The patient had symptomatic relief after aortopexy.

or dissection increases. Patient age, gender, and body surface area should be taken into account, because this demographic information can alter the risk of aneurysm rupture.[62] Mycotic aneurysms typically affect the aorta at the level of the arch and can be seen with several different causative agents. Timely recognition of these aneurysms is essential to help guide appropriate clinical management.

Partial Anomalous Pulmonary Venous Return

The role of MR imaging for evaluation of congenital and acquired heart disease in the pediatric population is a well-researched area that is beyond the scope of this report. Anomalies in pulmonary venous return, either total or partial, result in pulmonary to systemic shunts that are sometimes symptomatic.[63] Variations of this condition wherein one or more pulmonary veins fails to drain into the left atrium exist.[64] MR imaging illustrates the pulmonary veins and their drainage with excellent accuracy. Evaluation of the pulmonary venous anatomy with ECG-gated MR imaging provides optimal imaging at the level of the heart; however, even nongated studies can show certain extracardiac shunts.[63,65] One can perform shunt quantification with the use of velocity-encoded phase-contrast MR imaging.[66] When greater than 50% of the pulmonary venous blood is shunted into the systemic circulation, the shunt is considered clinically significant.

kinking and tortuosity of the aorta and other vessels.[61] Similar to other connective tissue disorders, the vessels can become stenotic or aneurysmal (**Fig. 9**). Other conditions such as bicuspid aortic valve and aortic stenosis also predispose to the development of the aneurysm. The size of the aneurysm is of key importance, because above a certain size, the risk of rupture

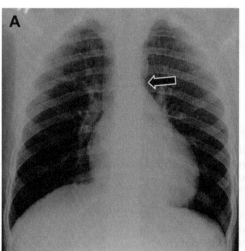
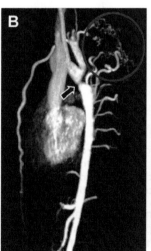
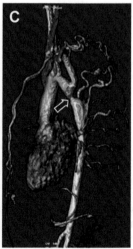

Fig. 8. Aortic coarctation in a 5-year-old boy who presented with upper extremity hypertension. (*A*) Frontal chest radiograph shows narrowing (*arrow*) of the proximal descending aorta resulting in the "3-sign." (*B*) Sagittal maximum intensity projection image from a contrast enhanced angiogram shows narrowing (*arrow*) of the proximal descending aorta just distal to the left subclavian artery takeoff. Also noted are prominent collateral arteries (*red circle*). (*C*) Three-dimensional volume-rendered image from a contrast-enhanced angiogram again shows the focal aortic narrowing (*arrow*) immediately distal to the origin of the left subclavian artery.

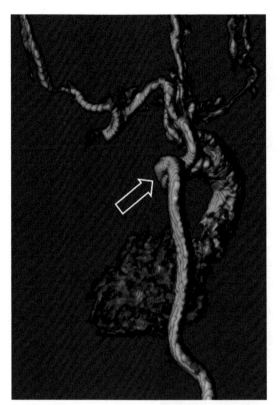

Fig. 9. Arterial tortuosity syndrome in a 6-month-old girl. Three-dimensional volume-rendered image of a contrast-enhanced MR angiogram shows marked tortuosity of the aortic arch and descending aorta (*arrow*). The great vessels arising from the aorta also have a tortuous appearance.

The most common form of partial anomalous venous return (PAPVR) involves anomalous right upper lobe venous drainage into the superior vena cava or the right atrium. This particular variant of example of PAPVR is often associated with a sinus venosus-type atrial septal defect.[67] The term *atrial septal defect* is actually a misnomer in this case, as the true atrial septum is not involved. Although the behavior of the lesion is similar to a large atrial septal defect, the abnormality is an extraseptal defect in the wall separating the superior vena cava/right atrial junction from the left atrium.[66] PAPVR involving the contralateral left upper lobe typically drains via a vertical vein, which is an anomalous vein to the left of the aorta that drains into the brachiocephalic vein.

A special case of aberrant pulmonary venous anatomy results in a characteristic appearance all radiologists should recognize. Scimitar syndrome is a process in which an aberrant right lung draining vein does not drain into to the left atrium but rather into the subdiaphragmatic inferior vena cava (most commonly) resulting in a left

to right shunt.[68] This vessel has a characteristic appearance, which is shaped like a Turkish sword thereby explaining its name (**Fig. 10**).[69]

Scimitar syndrome has other names including *hypogenetic lung syndrome* and *pulmonary venolobar syndrome*. Both of these names suggest that the abnormality is not limited to the pulmonary vasculature. The lung appears small because of hypoplasia with ipsilateral mediastinal shift. The contralateral lung often appears hyperlucent in comparison. Although the radiographic manifestations are suggestive, cross-sectional imaging is diagnostic.[70] MR imaging can show the aberrant vein and the feeding artery often supplied by the aorta (see **Fig. 10**). A significant percentage of patients with scimitar syndrome have other anomalies involving the cardiovascular, respiratory, genitourinary, and skeletal systems.[71]

Anomalous pulmonary venous drainage also occurs in the setting of extralobar pulmonary sequestration. These congenital lung abnormalities that do no communicate with the central trachea and bronchi drain their systemic arterial supply via the inferior vena cava, azygos vein, hemiazygous vein, or the portal veins.[72] Sequestration is further discussed in part II of this article.

Acquired Extracardiac Vascular Anomalies

Vasculitis

MR imaging has long been considered an excellent modality for initial detection and follow-up of vasculitis involving the thoracic vessels.[73] It permits excellent visualization of the thickened arterial wall well before significant luminal narrowing occurs.[74] The addition of contrast-enhanced phases shows vascular wall hyperenhancement in the affected portions of the vessel (**Fig. 11**).[75] Associated findings including stenosis and thrombi are also seen by MR imaging. Takayasu's arteritis is the prototypical vasculitis affecting large thoracic vessels in the pediatric population, most frequently in girls of Asian descent. Although the abdominal aorta is most frequently involved, the more proximal aorta and large branch vessels are often involved. Complications of Takayasu's arteritis caused by progressive destruction of the arterial media include aneurysm of the affected vessels and rupture.[76] MR imaging can be used to evaluate other vasculitides, including Kawasaki disease, whereby affected children are at risk for coronary artery aneurysms.[77]

Pulmonary Embolism

Detection of pulmonary embolism with MR imaging has been evaluated extensively in the literature. Although CT remains the gold standard, its use is

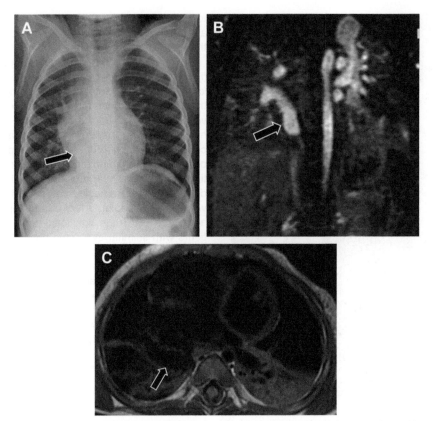

Fig. 10. Scimitar syndrome in a 3-year-old boy who underwent radiography for evaluation of possible pneumonia. (*A*) Frontal chest radiograph shows asymmetry in the lung volumes with the right lung appearing smaller than the left lung. There is a tubular and vertically oriented retrocardiac opacity to the right of the spine (*arrow*). (*B*) Coronal T1-weighted contrast-enhanced MR angiogram shows that the previously noted retrocardiac opacity represents an anomalous pulmonary vein (*arrow*). (*C*) Axial black blood MR image shows the anomalous pulmonary vein (*arrow*), which drains into the inferior vena cava (not shown). Atelectasis is noted posteriorly in bilateral lower lobes.

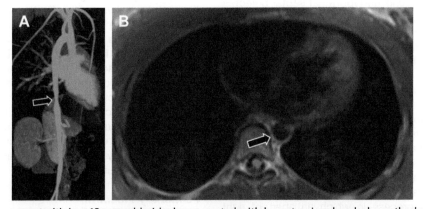

Fig. 11. Takayasu arteritis in a 13-year-old girl who presented with hypertension, headache, arthralgias, and erythema nodosum. (*A*) Oblique maximum intensity projection image from a contrast-enhanced MR angiogram shows focal narrowing (*arrow*) of the descending aorta. (*B*) Axial postcontrast MR image shows a hyper-enhancing and thickened aortic wall (*arrow*) corresponding to the site of luminal narrowing seen on the angiogram.

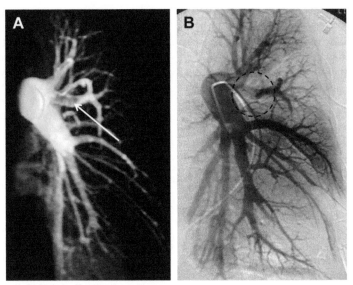

Fig. 12. Pulmonary embolism detected in an adolescent. (*A*) Three-dimensional MR pulmonary angiography with spoiled gradient recalled echo (SPGR) using short echo and repetition time. A filling defect (*arrow*) is seen in a left upper lobe segmental pulmonary artery. (*B*) Digital subtraction angiography of the pulmonary artery confirms the pulmonary embolism (*dotted circle*) seen on MR image. (*Courtesy of* Piotr Wielopolski, PhD, Rotterdam, Netherlands.)

sometimes contraindicated either by allergy or impaired renal function. In these cases, MR imaging may prove an attractive alternative to CT or scintigraphic imaging (ventilation/perfusion scan) without radiation exposure (**Fig. 12**).[78,79]

When evaluating pulmonary embolism with MR imaging, large central pulmonary embolism can be identified without contrast.[80] If the radiologist monitoring the examination detects the embolism on the initial sequences, contrast need not be administered, and the patient can receive appropriate therapy. If, however, pulmonary embolism is not detected on the initial images, the use of intravenous contrast increases sensitivity for

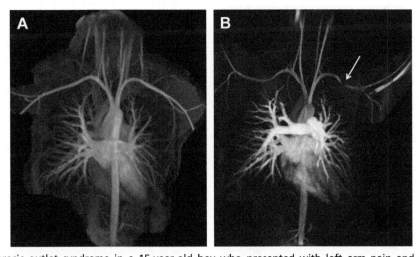

Fig. 13. Thoracic outlet syndrome in a 15-year-old boy who presented with left arm pain and swelling. (*A*) Coronal thick-slab maximum intensity projection image from a contrast-enhanced MR angiogram with the patient's arm adducted shows a normal appearance of upper extremity vessels including the subclavian arteries. (*B*) Coronal thick slab maximum intensity projection image from a contrast-enhanced MR angiogram with the patient's arms abducted now show focal narrowing (*arrow*) of the left subclavian artery as it courses inferior to the clavicle. This finding was confirmed on the source images.

detection of smaller pulmonary embolism.[81,82] Signs for pulmonary embolism are similar for CT and MR imaging. Filling defects within the pulmonary artery and sudden changes in vessel size are seen in MR imaging in case of pulmonary embolism.[81] Similar to CT, one can use the size of the pulmonary artery and the appearance of the right ventricle as an indicator of right strain caused by pulmonary hypertension. Wedge-shaped perfusion defects can also be seen on occasion. Pulmonary perfusion MR imaging provides additional functional data and increases the sensitivity for pulmonary embolism, especially when the embolus involves subsegmental branches.[83] Although the Prospective Investigation of Pulmonary Embolism Diagnosis (PIOPED III) study found that MR imaging had sensitivities and specificities greater than 90% for detection of pulmonary embolism, this finding only applied for patients who received technically adequate studies, which occurred approximately 50% of the time.[84] Consequently, evaluation of pulmonary embolism with MR imaging should only be used in centers with experience when other imaging studies are contraindicated.[85]

Thoracic Outlet Syndrome

Thoracic outlet syndrome occurs when the patient's subclavian artery or vein becomes compressed during arm abduction. The incidence of venous and arterial thoracic outlet syndrome is increased in the pediatric population compared with adults.[86] Symptoms can include loss of sensation, paresthesias, weakness, and pain.[87] Diagnosis depends on a corroborative clinical history, physical examination, and demonstration by imaging of vessel deformation with provocative maneuvers that is relieved by placing the arms in neutral position. Traditional imaging diagnosis has been performed with invasive angiography. Although CT can demonstrate the finding, it requires a 2-phase scan evaluating vessel patency with the arms in adduction and abduction.[88] MR imaging, however, can clearly show the abnormality and the surrounding structure causing the compression (**Fig. 13**).[89] Treatment of these patients is surgical.

SUMMARY

The performance of high-quality thoracic vascular MR imaging in the pediatric population requires close attention to patient selection, protocol optimization, appropriate sedation strategies, and an understanding of the basic physics principles of MR imaging as well as an appreciation for the appearance of varied pathologic entities. Although

the learning curve may seem steep, the potential rewards of added diagnostic information without the cost of radiation exposure to the child provide excellent motivation to incorporate thoracic vascular MR imaging into daily practice. Current applications have already proven its value, and future applications will only improve its importance and encourage widespread use.

REFERENCES

1. Ridgway JP. Cardiovascular magnetic resonance physics for clinicians: part I. J Cardiovasc Magn Reson 2010;12:71.
2. Wild JM, Marshall H, Bock M, et al. MRI of the lung (1/3): methods. Insights Imaging 2012;3(4):345–53.
3. Goo HW. Advanced functional thoracic imaging in children: from basic concepts to clinical applications. Pediatr Radiol 2013;43(3):262–8.
4. Oechsner M, Pracht ED, Staeb D, et al. Lung imaging under free-breathing conditions. Magn Reson Med 2009;61(3):723–7.
5. Morelli JN, Runge VM, Ai F, et al. An image-based approach to understanding the physics of MR artifacts. Radiographics 2011;31(3):849–66.
6. Bitar R, Leung G, Perng R, et al. MR pulse sequences: what every radiologist wants to know but is afraid to ask. Radiographics 2006;26(2):513–37.
7. Currie S, Hoggard N, Craven IJ, et al. Understanding MR: basic MR physics for physicians. Postgrad Med J 2013;89(1050):209–23.
8. Chavhan GB, Babyn PS, Vasanawala SS. Abdominal MR imaging in children: motion compensation, sequence optimization, and protocol organization. Radiographics 2013;33(3):703–19.
9. Boswinkel JP, Litman RS. Sedating patients for radiologic studies. Pediatr Ann 2005;34(8):650–4, 656.
10. Manson DE. MR imaging of the chest in children. Acta Radiol 2013;54(9):1075–85.
11. Liszewski MC, Hersman FW, Altes TA, et al. Magnetic resonance imaging of pediatric lung parenchyma, airways, vasculature, ventilation, and perfusion: state of the art. Radiol Clin North Am 2013;51(4):555–82.
12. Alexander M. Managing patient stress in pediatric radiology. Radiol Technol 2012;83(6):549–60.
13. De Bie HM, Boersma M, Wattjes MP, et al. Preparing children with a mock scanner training protocol results in high quality structural and functional MRI scans. Eur J Pediatr 2010;169(9):1079–85.
14. De Amorim e Silva CJ, Mackenzie A, Hallowell LM, et al. Practice MRI: reducing the need for sedation and general anaesthesia in children undergoing MRI. Australas Radiol 2006;50(4):319–23.
15. Hallowell LM, Stewart SE, de Amorim E Silva CT, et al. Reviewing the process of preparing children for MRI. Pediatr Radiol 2008;38(3):271–9.

16. Edwards AD, Arthurs OJ. Paediatric MRI under sedation: is it necessary? What is the evidence for the alternatives? Pediatr Radiol 2011;41(11):1353–64.

17. Olsen OE. MRI: how to perform a pediatric scan. Acta Radiol 2013;54(9):991–7.

18. Slovis TL. Sedation and anesthesia issues in pediatric imaging. Pediatr Radiol 2011;41(Suppl 2):514–6.

19. Murphy KL, Baxter MG. Long-term effects of neonatal single or multiple isoflurane exposures on spatial memory in rats. Front Neurol 2013;4:87.

20. Jevtovic-Todorovic V. Functional implications of an early exposure to general anesthesia: are we changing the behavior of our children? Mol Neurobiol 2013;48(2):288–93.

21. Yu D, Liu B. Developmental anesthetic neurotoxicity: from animals to humans? J Anesth 2013;27(5):750–6.

22. Bracken J, Heaslip I, Ryan S. Chloral hydrate sedation in radiology: retrospective audit of reduced dose. Pediatr Radiol 2012;42(3):349–54.

23. Griffiths MA, Kamat PP, McCracken CE, et al. Is procedural sedation with propofol acceptable for complex imaging? A comparison of short vs. prolonged sedations in children. Pediatr Radiol 2013;43(10): 1273–8.

24. Heng Vong C, Bajard A, Thiesse P, et al. Deep sedation in pediatric imaging: efficacy and safety of intravenous chlorpromazine. Pediatr Radiol 2012;42(5): 552–61.

25. Pedersen NA, Jensen AG, Kilmose L, et al. Propofol-remifentanil or sevoflurane for children undergoing magnetic resonance imaging? A randomised study. Acta Anaesthesiol Scand 2013;57(8):988–95.

26. Mason KP, Robinson F, Fontaine P, et al. Dexmedetomidine offers an option for safe and effective sedation for nuclear medicine imaging in children. Radiology 2013;267(3):911–7.

27. Mason KP, Fontaine PJ, Robinson F, et al. Pediatric sedation in a community hospital-based outpatient MRI center. AJR Am J Roentgenol 2012;198(2): 448–52.

28. Starkey E, Sammons HM. Sedation for radiological imaging. Arch Dis Child Educ Pract Ed 2011;96(3):101–6.

29. Tusman G, Böhm SH, Tempra A, et al. Effects of recruitment maneuver on atelectasis in anesthetized children. Anesthesiology 2003;98(1):14–22.

30. Blitman NM, Lee HK, Jain VR, et al. Pulmonary atelectasis in children anesthetized for cardiothoracic MR: evaluation of risk factors. J Comput Assist Tomogr 2007;31(5):789–94.

31. Lutterbey G, Wattjes MP, Doerr D, et al. Atelectasis in children undergoing either propofol infusion or positive pressure ventilation anesthesia for magnetic resonance imaging. Paediatr Anaesth 2007;17(2):121–5.

32. Jacobs MA, Ibrahim TS, Ouwerkerk R. AAPM/RSNA physics tutorials for residents: MR imaging: brief overview and emerging applications. Radiographics 2007;27(4):1213–29.

33. Barth MM, Smith MP, Pedrosa I, et al. Body MR imaging at 3.0 T: understanding the opportunities and challenges. Radiographics 2007;27(5):1445–62 [discussion: 1462–4].

34. Wehrli FW. Magnetic resonance of calcified tissues. J Magn Reson 2013;229:35–48.

35. Miyazaki M, Akahane M. Non-contrast enhanced MR angiography: established techniques. J Magn Reson Imaging 2012;35(1):1–19.

36. Vessie EL, Liu DM, Forster B, et al. A practical guide to magnetic resonance vascular imaging: techniques and applications. Ann Vasc Surg 2014; 28(4):1052–61.

37. Nael K, Krishnam M, Nael A, et al. Peripheral contrast-enhanced MR angiography at 3.0T, improved spatial resolution and low dose contrast: initial clinical experience. Eur Radiol 2008;18(12): 2893–900.

38. Lim RP, Bruno M, Rosenkrantz AB, et al. Comparison of blood pool and extracellular gadolinium chelate for functional MR evaluation of vascular thoracic outlet syndrome. Eur J Radiol 2014;83(7): 1209–15.

39. Daftari Besheli L, Aran S, Shaqdan K, et al. Current status of nephrogenic systemic fibrosis. Clin Radiol 2014;69(7):661–8.

40. Ciet P, Litmanovich DE. MR safety issues particular to women. Magn Reson Imaging Clin N Am 2015; 23(1):59–67.

41. Morita S, Masukawa A, Suzuki K, et al. Unenhanced MR angiography: techniques and clinical applications in patients with chronic kidney disease. Radiographics 2011;31(2):E13–33.

42. Scheffler K, Lehnhardt S. Principles and applications of balanced SSFP techniques. Eur Radiol 2003;13(11):2409–18.

43. Von Knobelsdorff-Brenkenhoff F, Gruettner H, Trauzeddel RF, et al. Comparison of native high-resolution 3D and contrast-enhanced MR angiography for assessing the thoracic aorta. Eur Heart J Cardiovasc Imaging 2014;15(6):651–8.

44. Tomasian A, Lohan DG, Laub G, et al. Noncontrast 3D steady state free precession magnetic resonance angiography of the thoracic central veins using nonselective radiofrequency excitation over a large field of view: initial experience. Invest Radiol 2008;43(5):306–13.

45. Miyazaki M, Sugiura S, Tateishi F, et al. Non-contrast-enhanced MR angiography using 3D ECG-synchronized half-Fourier fast spin echo. J Magn Reson Imaging 2000;12(5):776–83.

46. Mihai G, Simonetti OP, Thavendiranathan P. Noncontrast MRA for the diagnosis of vascular diseases. Cardiol Clin 2011;29(3):341–50.

47. Kir M, Saylam GS, Karadas U, et al. Vascular rings: presentation, imaging strategies, treatment, and outcome. Pediatr Cardiol 2012;33(4):607–17.

48. Wheaton AJ, Miyazaki M. Non-contrast enhanced MR angiography: physical principles. J Magn Reson Imaging 2012;36(2):286–304.

49. Lewis M, Yanny S, Malcolm PN. Advantages of blood pool contrast agents in MR angiography: a pictorial review. J Med Imaging Radiat Oncol 2012;56(2):187–91.

50. Cantinotti M, Hegde S, Bell A, et al. Diagnostic role of magnetic resonance imaging in identifying aortic arch anomalies. Congenit Heart Dis 2008;3(2):117–23.

51. Myers PO, Fasel JH, Kalangos A, et al. Arteria lusoria: developmental anatomy, clinical, radiological and surgical aspects. Ann Cardiol Angeiol (Paris) 2010;59(3):147–54.

52. Abraham V, Mathew A, Cherian V, et al. Aberrant subclavian artery: anatomical curiosity or clinical entity. Int J Surg 2009;7(2):106–9.

53. Eichhorn J, Fink C, Bock M, et al. Images in cardiovascular medicine. Time-resolved three-dimensional magnetic resonance angiography for assessing a pulmonary artery sling in a pediatric patient. Circulation 2002;106(14):e61–2.

54. Fawcett SL, Gomez AC, Hughes JA, et al. Anatomical variation in the position of the brachiocephalic trunk (innominate artery) with respect to the trachea: a computed tomography-based study and literature review of Innominate Artery Compression Syndrome. Clin Anat 2010;23(1):61–9.

55. Torre M, Carlucci M, Speggiorin S, et al. Aortopexy for the treatment of tracheomalacia in children: review of the literature. Ital J Pediatr 2012;38:62.

56. Wine TM, Colman KL, Mehta DK, et al. Aortopexy for innominate artery tracheal compression in children. Otolaryngol Head Neck 2013;149(1):151–5.

57. Gardella C, Girosi D, Rossi GA, et al. Tracheal compression by aberrant innominate artery: clinical presentations in infants and children, indications for surgical correction by aortopexy, and short- and long-term outcome. J Pediatr Surg 2010;45(3):564–73.

58. Holloway BJ, Rosewarne D, Jones RG. Imaging of thoracic aortic disease. Br J Radiol 2011;84(Spec No 3):S338–54.

59. Secchi F, Iozzelli A, Papini GD, et al. MR imaging of aortic coarctation. Radiol Med 2009;114(4):524–37.

60. Hom JJ, Ordovas K, Reddy GP. Velocity-encoded cine MR imaging in aortic coarctation: functional assessment of hemodynamic events. Radiographics 2008;28(2):407–16.

61. Ekici F, Uçar T, Fitöz S, et al. Cardiovascular findings in a boy with arterial tortuosity syndrome: case report and review of the literature. Turk J Pediatr 2011;53(1):104–7.

62. Davies RR, Gallo A, Coady MA, et al. Novel measurement of relative aortic size predicts rupture of thoracic aortic aneurysms. Ann Thorac Surg 2006;81(1):169–77.

63. Katre R, Burns SK, Murillo H, et al. Anomalous pulmonary venous connections. Semin Ultrasound CT MR 2012;33(6):485–99.

64. Dillman JR, Yarram SG, Hernandez RJ. Imaging of pulmonary venous developmental anomalies. AJR Am J Roentgenol 2009;192(5):1272–85.

65. Hellinger JC, Daubert M, Lee EY, et al. Congenital thoracic vascular anomalies: evaluation with state-of-the-art MR imaging and MDCT. Radiol Clin North Am 2011;49(5):969–96.

66. Vyas HV, Greenberg SB, Krishnamurthy R. MR imaging and CT evaluation of congenital pulmonary vein abnormalities in neonates and infants. Radiographics 2012;32(1):87–98.

67. Shariat M, Grosse-Wortmann L, Yoo SJ, et al. Normal drainage, abnormal connection: partial anomalous pulmonary venous connection and sinus venosus atrial septal defect with a net right-to-left shunt. World J Pediatr Congenit Heart Surg 2012;3(4):508–10.

68. Korkmaz AA, Yildiz CE, Onan B, et al. Scimitar syndrome: a complex form of anomalous pulmonary venous return. J Card Surg 2011;26(5):529–34.

69. Ferguson EC, Krishnamurthy R, Oldham SA. Classic imaging signs of congenital cardiovascular abnormalities. Radiographics 2007;27(5):1323–34.

70. Midyat L, Demir E, Aşkin M, et al. Eponym. Scimitar syndrome. Eur J Pediatr 2010;169(10):1171–7.

71. Wasilewska E, Lee EY, Eisenberg RL. Unilateral hyperlucent lung in children. AJR Am J Roentgenol 2012;198(5):W400–14.

72. Abbey P, Das CJ, Pangtey GS, et al. Imaging in bronchopulmonary sequestration. J Med Imaging Radiat Oncol 2009;53(1):22–31.

73. Matsunaga N, Hayashi K, Okada M, et al. Magnetic resonance imaging features of aortic diseases. Top Magn Reson Imaging 2003;14(3):253–66.

74. Schmidt WA. Imaging in vasculitis. Best Pract Res Clin Rheumatol 2013;27(1):107–18.

75. Restrepo CS, Ocazionez D, Suri R, et al. Aortitis: imaging spectrum of the infectious and inflammatory conditions of the aorta. Radiographics 2011;31(2):435–51.

76. Isobe M. Takayasu arteritis revisited: current diagnosis and treatment. Int J Cardiol 2013;168(1):3–10.

77. Mavrogeni S, Papadopoulos G, Hussain T, et al. The emerging role of cardiovascular magnetic resonance in the evaluation of Kawasaki disease. Int J Cardiovasc Imaging 2013;29(8):1787–98.

78. Zhang LJ, Luo S, Yeh BM, et al. Diagnostic accuracy of three-dimensional contrast-enhanced MR angiography at 3-T for acute pulmonary embolism detection: comparison with multidetector CT angiography. Int J Cardiol 2013;168(5):4775–83.

79. Schiebler ML, Nagle SK, François CJ, et al. Effectiveness of MR angiography for the primary diagnosis of acute pulmonary embolism: clinical outcomes at 3 months and 1 year. J Magn Reson Imaging 2013;38(4):914–25.

80. Herédia V, Altun E, Ramalho M, et al. MRI of pregnant patients for suspected pulmonary embolism: steady-state free precession vs postgadolinium 3D-GRE. Acta Med Port 2012;25(6):359–67.

81. Hochhegger B, Ley-Zaporozhan J, Marchiori E, et al. Magnetic resonance imaging findings in acute pulmonary embolism. Br J Radiol 2011;84(999):282–7.

82. Biederer J, Mirsadraee S, Beer M, et al. MRI of the lung (3/3)-current applications and future perspectives. Insights Imaging 2012;3(4):373–86.

83. Fink C, Ley S, Schoenberg SO, et al. Magnetic resonance imaging of acute pulmonary embolism. Eur Radiol 2007;17(10):2546–53.

84. Fink C, Henzler T, Shirinova A, et al. Thoracic magnetic resonance imaging: pulmonary thromboembolism. J Thorac Imaging 2013;28(3):171–7.

85. Stein PD, Chenevert TL, Fowler SE, et al. Gadolinium-enhanced magnetic resonance angiography for pulmonary embolism: a multicenter prospective study (PIOPED III). Ann Intern Med 2010;152(7):434–43, W142–3.

86. Chang K, Graf E, Davis K, et al. Spectrum of thoracic outlet syndrome presentation in adolescents. Arch Surg 2011;146(12):1383–7.

87. Ozoa G, Alves D, Fish DE. Thoracic outlet syndrome. Phys Med Rehabil Clin N Am 2011;22(3):473–83, viii–ix.

88. Ersoy H, Steigner ML, Coyner KB, et al. Vascular thoracic outlet syndrome: protocol design and diagnostic value of contrast-enhanced 3D MR angiography and equilibrium phase imaging on 1.5- and 3-T MRI scanners. AJR Am J Roentgenol 2012;198(5):1180–7.

89. Aralasmak A, Cevikol C, Karaali K, et al. MRI findings in thoracic outlet syndrome. Skeletal Radiol 2012;41(11):1365–74.

Pediatric Chest MR Imaging: Lung and Airways

Juan C. Baez, MD[a,b], Pierluigi Ciet, MD, PhD[c,d], Robert Mulkern, PhD[b],
Ravi T. Seethamraju, PhD[e], Edward Y. Lee, MD, MPH[b,*]

KEYWORDS

• MR imaging • Lungs • Airways • Pediatric patients

KEY POINTS

- Magnetic resonance (MR) imaging can reliably identify lung nodules larger than 5 mm in children.
- MR imaging can permit accurate and dynamic evaluation of large airways.
- MR imaging is a valuable imaging modality to assess the progression of chronic lung diseases such as cystic fibrosis.
- Future chest MR imaging techniques have a great promise for functional imaging of the lungs in pediatric patients.

INTRODUCTION

In recent years, MR imaging with advanced imaging techniques has been receiving a lot of attention mainly because of its ability to assess lungs and airways in the pediatric population. Although computed tomography (CT), which is regarded as the gold standard imaging modality, provides exquisite resolution of the anatomic structures of the lungs and airways, it exposes the pediatric patient to ionizing radiation. MR imaging has been advocated as an adjunctive tool, particularly in pediatric patients, for the evaluation of chest pathology. In the past, the proton-poor environment, rapid signal dephasing, and respiratory motion presented significant obstacles for widespread adoption and clinical use of MR imaging lung studies. Nevertheless, by optimizing protocols and tailoring them to the individual pediatric patient and with the clinical question at hand, MR imaging can now provide excellent visualization of the relevant anatomy and pertinent abnormalities. The future of chest MR imaging includes a greater emphasis on functional information. The use of hyperpolarized gases, where available, provides excellent imaging of lung ventilation. Upcoming technologies, such as Fourier decomposition, promise the ability to provide functional perfusion and ventilation data without the use of intravenous or inhaled contrast agents. The overarching goal of this article is to provide up-to-date information regarding MR imaging techniques for practical assessment of lungs and airways in the pediatric population. Furthermore, several pediatric thoracic disorders involving the lungs and airways that can be evaluated with advanced MR imaging techniques are highlighted.

Disclosures: no relevant disclosures (J.C. Baez, P. Ciet, R. Mulkern, and E.Y. Lee); Dr Seethamraju has stock ownership and an employment affiliation with Siemens AG.
a Mid-Atlantic Permanente Medical Group, 2101 East Jefferson Street, Rockville, MD 20852, USA; b Department of Radiology, Boston Children's Hospital, Harvard Medical School, 300 Longwood Avenue, Boston, MA 02115, USA; c Department of Radiology and Pediatric Pulmonology, Sophia Children's Hospital, Erasmus Medical Center, Wytemaweg 80, 3015 CN, Rotterdam, The Netherlands; d Department of Radiology, Beth Israel Deaconess Medical Center, Harvard Medical School, 330 Brookline Ave, Boston, MA 02215, USA; e Magnetic Resonance, Research and Development, Siemens Healthcare, 1620 Tremont St., Boston, MA 02120, USA
* Corresponding author. Department of Radiology, Boston Children's Hospital, Harvard Medical School, 300 Longwood Avenue, Boston, MA 02115.
E-mail address: Edward.Lee@childrens.harvard.edu

Magn Reson Imaging Clin N Am 23 (2015) 337–349
http://dx.doi.org/10.1016/j.mric.2015.01.011
1064-9689/15/$ – see front matter © 2015 Elsevier Inc. All rights reserved.

EVALUATION OF LUNG PARENCHYMAL ABNORMALITIES
MR Imaging Protocol

A fundamental MR imaging protocol evaluating the lung parenchyma includes a gradient recalled echo (GRE) multiplanar localizer, coronal T2 single-shot half Fourier turbo spin echo (HASTE), axial 3-dimensional (3D) GRE T1, coronal balanced steady-state free precession (true fast imaging with steady-state precession), and axial short tau inversion recovery.[1,2] One can complete this practical MR imaging examination in less than 25 minutes. If necessary, postcontrast imaging with a 3D GRE T1-weighted sequence with fat saturation can provide information regarding enhancement characteristics. Pediatric patients with difficulty after breathing instructions because of their young age or critical condition often benefit from a sequence that does not rely on breath holds such as an axial T2 periodically rotated overlapping parallel lines with enhanced reconstruction (PROPELLER/BLADE) performed with the patient free breathing.

Consolidation and Infection

Although CT remains the gold standard for evaluation of parenchymal lung abnormalities, the ability to characterize lung abnormality without exposing the child to ionizing radiation has propelled research into the use of alternative technology.[3] Several studies have shown that ultrasonography can diagnose peripherally located lung consolidation as well as or better than radiography.[4–6] However, chest ultrasonography becomes more difficult with increasing age because the acoustic windows become more limited with increasing ossification of the skeletal structures.[7]

Furthermore, deep parenchymal abnormalities surrounded by aerated lung go undetected by ultrasonography because of dissipation of the ultrasound beam by the air interface. For these reasons, the use of MR imaging to aid in the diagnosis of lung abnormalities has been evaluated by multiple investigators.[8,9] Although CT provides greater spatial resolution than MR imaging, the use of multiple sequences offers characterization of tissue beyond the limits of CT.[10]

Studies have shown that MR imaging can detect pneumonia and other consolidative processes in the lungs (**Figs. 1** and **2**). A prospective study comparing 1.5T MR imaging using fast T1 and T2 imaging sequences with radiography for the detection of pneumonia proved that the 2 modalities were comparable.[11] A comparison of different MR pulse sequences showed that HASTE was the best sequence for the detection of lung consolidation.[2] In addition to the consolidation, MR imaging can also detect complications of pneumonia such as necrosis/abscess and pneumonia.

Other studies have compared MR imaging with CT, the current gold standard, and shown that the former is a high-sensitivity examination for evaluation of lung abnormalities. In one recent prospective trial of 71 pediatric patients in which patients underwent both CT and MR imaging evaluation within 24 hours, diagnostic accuracy of MR imaging was 97% compared with that of CT. The only undiagnosed lung findings were a single case of mild bronchiectasis and another case with a pulmonary nodule measuring 3 mm that went undetected.[12] In addition, this study demonstrated excellent interobserver reliability between 2 readers, suggesting the robustness of this technique.

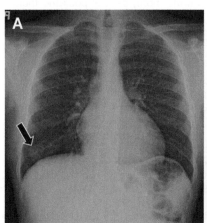 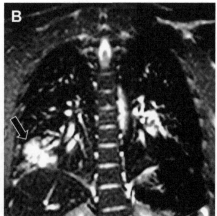

Fig. 1. Pneumonia. (*A*) Frontal chest radiograph demonstrates focal consolidative opacity (*arrow*) in the right lung base. (*B*) Coronal short tau inversion recovery MR image demonstrates a T2-hyperintense focus (*arrow*) in the right lower lobe corresponding to the consolidative opacity (see Fig. 1*A*) in this region.

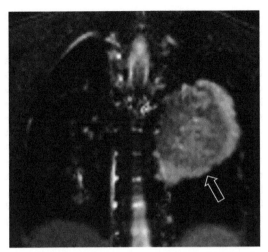

Fig. 2. Round pneumonia in an 8-year-old girl who presented with fever and cough. Coronal short tau inversion recovery MR image demonstrates a round consolidative opacity (*arrow*). Follow-up chest radiograph obtained after treatment demonstrated interval resolution.

Although MR imaging is unlikely to define the causative agent in infection, clues gleaned from the imaging may help narrow the differential diagnosis in cases in which additional imaging is performed for problem solving. Lung necrosis in tuberculosis, for example, can appear low in signal intensity on fluid-sensitive sequences likely because of the underlying caseating necrosis associated with *Mycobacterium*.[13] Iron deposition within foci of *Aspergillus* infection has also been associated with low signal on MR imaging.[14] Certain infections such as those caused by *Echinococcus* result in a characteristic appearance.

The resultant hydatid cysts present as cystic masses, often with smaller daughter cysts.[15] A T2-hypointense rim has been described in these cystic masses and should at least raise the possibility of this diagnosis (**Fig. 3**).[16]

Lung Masses

Congenital lung masses constitute a group of developmental disorders affecting lung parenchyma in vascular and airway development.[17] The diagnosis of congenital lung masses including sequestration and congenital pulmonary airway malformations (CPAMs) is increasingly being made prenatally with the use of fetal ultrasonography as a screening tool.[18] Also, fetal MR imaging can provide additional information in the evaluation of these abnormalities. In the neonatal period, thoracic MR imaging further aids in characterization of these masses and confirms prenatal diagnoses.[19,20] The use of T2-weighted sequences often permits reliable differentiation between normal and abnormal lung masses. In addition, T2-weighted imaging can help in identifying cystic components within these masses.[21] However, large air-filled cysts may go unrecognized on MR imaging because of the lack of signal.

MR imaging may also identify feeding vessels and draining veins associated with congenital lung malformation such as pulmonary sequestration.[22] Although one can identify flow voids on multiple MR sequences, MR angiography with postprocessed 3D images best illustrates feeding vessels, as in the case of a pulmonary sequestration wherein the anomalous arterial vessels arise from the aorta.[23] Recent research has suggested that bronchial atresia lies on the same spectrum

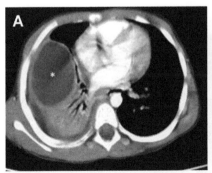
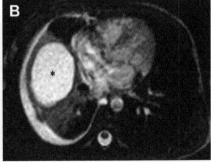

Fig. 3. (*A*) Hydatid cyst in a 15-year-old boy with known pulmonary hydatid infection who presented with fever, elevated white blood cell count, and opacity in the right lower lung on chest radiographs. Axial contrast-enhanced CT image shows large cystic lesion (*asterisk*) in the right lower lobe consistent with pulmonary hydatid infection. (*B*) Axial T2-weighted MR image shows large cystic lesion (*asterisk*) in the right lower lobe corresponding to the finding in Fig. 3A. (*From* Gorkem SB, Coskun A, Yikilmaz A, et al. Evaluation of pediatric thoracic disorders: comparison of unenhanced fast-imaging sequence 1.5T MRI and contrast enhanced MRI. AJR Am J Roentgenol 2013;200:1354; with permission.)

as these other types of congenital lung masses.[24,25] The atretic bronchus is a mucous-filled tubular structure, which is both T1 and T2 hyperintense. Other signs of bronchial atresia such as subtle air trapping, however, likely go unnoticed on MR imaging using standard protocols. The improved spatial resolution of CT compared with that of MR imaging and the ability to visualize air-filled structures and associated complications such as trapped air are a large part of the reason that CT remains the preferred modality for imaging diagnosis and surgical planning.[26] Nevertheless, the use of a proton-density-weighted GRE sequence with short repetition time(TR) and echo time (TE) and slice thickness between 5 to 8 mm can often allow detection of trapped air.

Primary lung neoplasms occur far less frequently in the pediatric population than in adults and are less common than metastatic disease.[27,28] A list of relatively rare diagnoses in this category includes entities such as papillomas, myofibromas, hemangiomas, and hamartomas. Mesenchymal hamartomas are masses that arise from the chest wall, but on presentation may seem as if they arise from the lung (**Fig. 4**). These masses constitute no risk of metastatic or recurrent disease and therefore require no treatment unless symptomatic.[29] Characteristic MR imaging features of the mesenchymal hamartomas include hemorrhagic fluid levels within secondary aneurysmal bone cysts and calcification seen as hypointense signal on MR imaging.

Pathologists often classify inflammatory myofibroblastic tumors as benign pulmonary neoplasms, although these lesions sometimes recur or act aggressively.[29] These masses often constitute a diagnostic and clinical dilemma because of their behavior. The other name for this lesion, inflammatory pseudotumor, also indicates that not all pathologists are convinced that these masses are neoplastic. MR imaging features of inflammatory myofibroblastic tumors include low signal on T1, high signal on T2, and homogeneous enhancement (**Fig. 5**).[30]

Malignant primary lung neoplasms also present in a variety of forms. Pleuropulmonary blastomas are uncommon malignancies with both mesenchymal and epithelial components that can present like CPAMs.[31,32] Numerous other pediatric primary lung malignancies can, although rarely, arise de novo, with a full discussion of these cancers lying beyond the scope of this article (**Figs. 6** and **7**).

Metastatic Pulmonary Nodules

Use of MR imaging for the detection of pulmonary nodules remains an alluring goal because many pediatric patients with cancer require routine surveillance for detection of lung recurrence or metastases. In these pediatric patients, the cumulative radiation dose of chest imaging may prove significant.[33,34] Furthermore, these patients may possess increased sensitivity to the damaging effects of radiation with predisposition to developing new malignancies because of prior therapy or congenital sensitivity, such as in pediatric patients with ataxia telangiectasia. Consequently, replacement of routine surveillance CT scans with MR imaging would allow continued evaluation without exposing the child to additional risks.

MR imaging can reliably detect lung nodules larger than 5 mm (**Fig. 8**).[12] Other studies suggest that MR imaging becomes less sensitive for

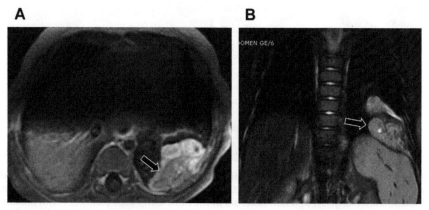

Fig. 4. Mesenchymal hamartoma. (*A*) Axial T1 postcontrast MR imaging demonstrates heterogeneous enhancement within this well-defined left lower chest wall mass (*arrow*) that proved a mesenchymal hamartoma on surgical excision. (*B*) Coronal T2-weighted MR image shows a left lower lobe heterogeneous mass (*arrow*) with internal foci of T2 prolongation and areas of susceptibility corresponding to known calcifications.

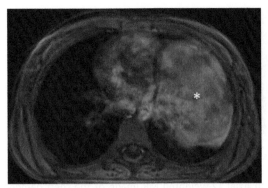

Fig. 5. Myofibroblastic tumor. Axial T1 postcontrast MR image shows homogeneous enhancement in the large lingular mass (*asterisk*).

detection of lung nodules smaller than 3 mm (sensitivity of 73%) (**Fig. 9**).[35] A known limitation in MR imaging evaluation concerns calcified lung nodules. Calcification results in susceptibility-related loss of MR imaging signal intensity. Consequently, calcified nodules, which would be easily identified on CT, become occult on MR imaging. The improved tissue contrast, however, may add additional information regarding the cause of the nodule not evident on other imaging. The use of diffusion-weighted MR imaging has been suggested to also aid in both detection and characterization of malignant nodules.[36,37]

Interstitial Lung Disease

The use of MR imaging for the evaluation of interstitial lung disease remains in an early stage of development. Few studies have compared it to the current radiological gold standard, high-resolution CT.[38–40] Nevertheless, T2-hyperintense areas that do not obscure the vascular markings correspond to ground glass opacity seen on CT.[41] Curvilinear bands and parenchymal distortion can also be visualized with MR imaging. The strength of MR imaging for interstitial lung disease, however, potentially resides in exploiting different signal characteristics of tissue to distinguish between active inflammation and fibrosis with inflamed tissue appearing T2 hyperintense. Rapid enhancement kinetics also seems to favor active inflammation.[42] Additional studies are necessary before MR imaging can play a pivotal role in evaluating interstitial lung disease.[39]

EVALUATION OF AIRWAYS

Appropriate evaluation of the airway depends on an assessment of the level of the problem. Either the large airways or the small airways can be involved, each with their own pathologic conditions and each requiring different approaches.

Small airways disease is radiologically defined by direct signs, such as bronchiectasis, bronchial wall thickening, and mucous plugging, as well as by indirect signs such as trapped air. Bronchiectasis, bronchial wall thickening, and mucous plugging can be assessed by T2-weighted sequences, either in breath hold (HASTE/single-shot fast spin echo) or in free breathing (PROPELLER/BLADE) methods. However, the diagnostic accuracy of these techniques for detecting bronchiectasis and mucous plugging at the periphery of the lung is currently lower compared with that of CT (**Fig. 10**). In fact, the level of the bronchi, bronchial diameter, wall thickness, and signal within the lumen all affect the ability of the radiologist to make the diagnosis.[43,44] Air trapping assessment with MR imaging is not as reliable as with CT.[1] The increased air content because of air trapping results in low-signal areas barely distinguishable from the surrounding normal lung parenchyma. One can partially improve detection of air trapping by using large voxel sizes and short TR/TE

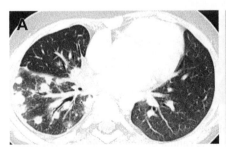
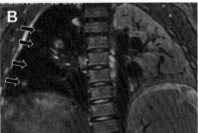

Fig. 6. (*A*) Pulmonary nodules in a 12-year-old girl with lymphoma. Axial noncontrast chest CT image demonstrates multiple right-sided pulmonary nodules. These pulmonary nodules were proved by biopsy to represent lymphoma. (*B*) Coronal T2-weighted MR image shows the pulmonary nodules (*arrows*). Extensive atelectasis of the left lung are noted posteriorly.

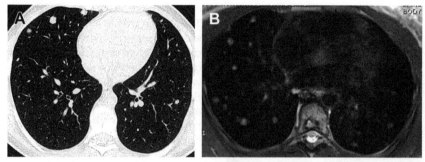

Fig. 7. (*A*) Epithelioid hemangioendothelioma in a 10-year-old boy. Axial noncontrast CT image demonstrates numerous bilateral pulmonary nodules of varying sizes. (*B*) Axial T2-weighted MR image of the chest demonstrates numerous bilateral pulmonary nodules correlating with the CT findings (see Fig. 7A).

(**Fig. 11**).[45] Finally, new techniques such as Fourier decomposition have recently shown promising results for improving the sensitivity of MR imaging for air trapping.[46]

Pathologic condition of the large airway can be subdivided into static and dynamic processes. Most large airway processes fall into the static category with tracheobronchial branching anomalies, bronchial atresia, tracheal stenosis, neoplasm, and infection residing in this category. MR imaging is well suited for the evaluation of these abnormalities and does not require radically new techniques. The air-filled large airways provide a natural contrast to the surrounding soft tissue because of the paucity of signal (**Fig. 12**). By tracing the black areas representing air in the

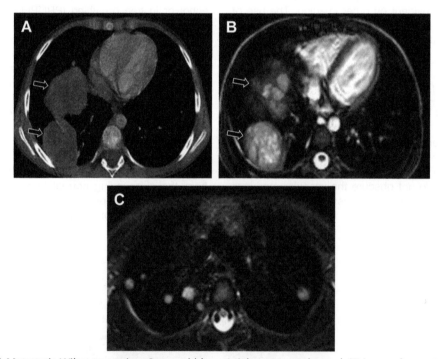

Fig. 8. (*A*) Metastatic Wilms tumor in a 2-year-old boy. Axial contrast-enhanced CT image demonstrates large masses (*arrows*) in the right lung representing "cannonball" metastases in Wilms tumor. (*B*) Axial short tau inversion recovery (STIR) MR image again demonstrates the large cannonball metastases (*arrows*) corresponding well with findings seen on CT image (see Fig. 8A). (*C*) Metastatic Wilms tumor in a 3-year-old girl. Axial STIR MR image shows bilateral smaller pulmonary nodules showing high signal intensity. (*From* Gorkem SB, Coskun A, Yikilmaz A, et al. Evaluation of pediatric thoracic disorders: comparison of unenhanced fast-imaging sequence 1.5T MRI and contrast enhanced MRI. AJR Am J Roentgenol 2013;200:1352–7; with permission.)

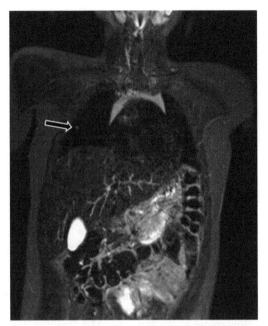

Fig. 9. Pulmonary nodule in a 6-year-old boy with Li-Fraumeni syndrome who underwent whole body MR imaging. Coronal T2-weighted MR image of the chest and abdomen demonstrates a 3-mm T2-hyperintense right lower lobe lung nodule (*arrow*).

airway, radiologists can reliably evaluate the airways to the proximal subsegmental branches assuming a high-quality examination without significant artifact.[22]

MR Imaging Protocol

Although the previously discussed fundamental lung protocol can also address many airway-related issues, additional sequences add useful information. A 3D spoiled gradient recalled echo (SPGR) sequence allows evaluation of lung anatomy and measurement of the airway. PD-weighted SPGR helps to depict the tracheal contours that are largely surrounded by mediastinal fat. Dedicated views of the large airways with improved spatial resolution may be obtained by using this sequence on a smaller field of view. Breathing maneuvers can be trained using an MR-imaging-compatible spirometer (**Fig. 13**).[47] The purpose of the training is to monitor and standardize breathing maneuvers and to reduce anxiety related to the MR imaging investigation, thereby increasing the probability of a successful MR imaging examination. Patients receive adequate training before the examination by a lung function technician who also triggers the image acquisition by closely interacting with the MR imaging technician during the scan.

Tracheobronchomalacia

Dynamic large airway pathology, by definition, changes over time and requires time-resolved imaging for diagnosis. Tracheobronchomalacia is the most common dynamic large airway process and occurs as a result of excessive narrowing or collapse of the airway during the respiratory cycle. Weakness in the airway walls and cartilage results in greater than 50% narrowing of the luminal area during expiration in affected pediatric patients.[48] Bronchoscopy can directly visualize the airway collapse; however, this is an invasive procedure.[49,50] Radiography with inspiratory and expiratory views as well as cine fluoroscopy can also attempt to visualize the abnormality; however,

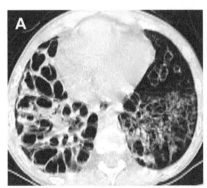
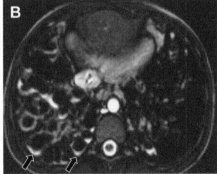

Fig. 10. (*A*) Cystic bronchiectasis in a 5-year-old girl. Axial CT image demonstrates cystic and cylindrical bronchiectasis, more prominent on the right. Fluid levels are noted in some of the ectatic airways. (*B*) Axial T2-weighted MR image of the chest demonstrates the same cystic and cylindrical bronchiectasis. The layering fluid (*arrows*) in the airways is again seen and better visualized on MR image. ([*A*] *Courtesy of* Dr Sureyya B. Gorkem, Kayseri, Turkey; and [*B*] *From* Yikilmaz A, Koc A, Coskun A, et al. Evaluation of pneumonia in children: comparison of MRI with fast imaging sequences at 1.5T with chest radiographs. Acta Radiologica 2011;52(8):914–9; with permission.)

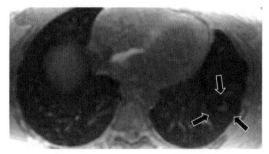

Fig. 11. Air trapping in a pediatric patient with asthma. Axial 3D spoiled gradient echo MR image obtained at expiration using a thick slice, low matrix, and short TR/TE shows air trapping (*arrows*) in the superior segment of the left lower lobe.

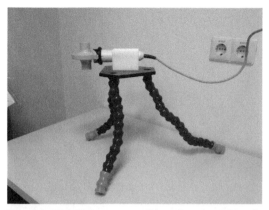

Fig. 13. MR-imaging-compatible spirometer. Mouthpiece of an MR-imaging-compatible spirometer is standing on a plastic tripod within the MR imaging suite.

they are limited in sensitivity compared with bronchoscopy.[51] Furthermore, radiography exposes the patient to ionizing radiations. CT, which remains the gold standard of noninvasive imaging of tracheobronchomalacia, allows excellent visualization of the affected anatomy, but it requires at least two phases (inspiratory and expiratory), thus exposing the patient to overall increased radiation.[52] In addition to exquisite visualization of the airway, CT demonstrates associated pulmonary findings such as air trapping.[53] The use of volumetric CT reduces the administered radiation dose while permitting dynamic CT evaluation, but it does not eliminate the radiation exposure.[54,55]

Spirometer-controlled cine MR imaging provides an alternative noninvasive imaging modality to evaluate for tracheobronchomalacia without exposing the pediatric patient to ionizing radiations.[47] Four-dimensional time-resolved imaging of the same field of view during specific breathing maneuvers, such as forced expiration, best elicits the collapse point in patients with tracheomalacia (**Figs. 14** and **15**).

Cystic Fibrosis

Despite the lower spatial resolution of MR imaging compared with that of CT, the improved tissue characterization provided by different MR imaging sequences suggests that it may play an increasingly important role in certain patient populations

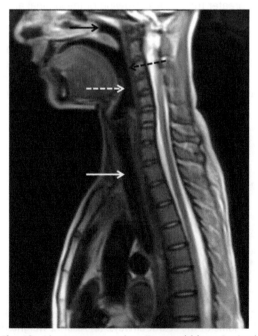

Fig. 12. Airway anatomy in a 5-year-old boy. Sagittal T2-weighted MR image shows the nasopharynx (*black solid arrow*), oropharynx (*black dotted arrow*), hypopharynx (*white dotted arrow*), and trachea (*white solid arrow*).

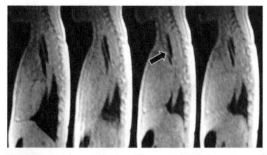

Fig. 14. Tracheomalacia. Time-resolved imaging of contrast kinetics/Time-resolved angiography With Intercalated Stochastic Trajectories (TRICKS/TWIST) in the sagittal plane demonstrates the dynamic appearance of the airway during forced expiration. A total of 48 frames are collected in 22 seconds for a temporal resolution of 500 milliseconds. Trachea completely collapses in the third image (*arrow*).

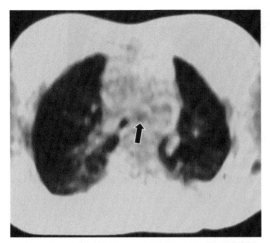

Fig. 15. Bronchomalacia. Axial PD-weighed MR image obtained during forced expiration demonstrates collapse (*arrow*) of the left main stem bronchus. Of note, patent right main stem bronchus is seen at this level.

such as those afflicted with cystic fibrosis.[56] Patients with cystic fibrosis undergo numerous imaging studies throughout their lives to better assess progression of their disease and determine management. In an effort to quantify disease progression and identify abnormalities before changes in pulmonary function tests, multiple scoring systems have been used, which rely on different imaging modalities including radiography, CT, and now MR imaging. Most of these scoring systems evaluate similar parameters including bronchiectasis, mucous plugging, lung

volumes, and parenchymal changes, with some investigators suggesting that bronchiectasis is the most important parameter.[57] Recent studies have attempted to validate MR imaging scoring systems by comparing with the CT equivalent and have shown that the results are comparable, suggesting that one may follow-up patients with cystic fibrosis less frequently with ionizing radiation examinations and perform MR imaging instead.[58]

In addition to simply proving comparable to CT, MR imaging can provide additional diagnostic data that are not available from CT. For example, although CT shows bronchial wall thickening well, it cannot characterize the underlying cause. The improved tissue contrast of MR imaging shows T2 hyperintensity within the bronchial wall if it is edematous and shows gadolinium enhancement in cases of active inflammation (**Figs. 16** and **17**).[22] The presence of air fluid levels within a dilated bronchus indicates contemporaneous infection. Although parenchymal changes such as consolidation and air bronchograms are seen just as well in MR imaging as in CT, the ability to directly assess lung function is unique to MR imaging. As cystic fibrosis destroys lung parenchyma and impairs ventilation, reflexive vasoconstriction occurs (Euler-Liljestrand reflex). Contrast-enhanced MR perfusion imaging demonstrates perfusion defects that correlate with diseased lung and precede the morphologic changes (**Fig. 18**).[56]

Direct visualization of small airways disease may ultimately be better performed with hyperpolarized

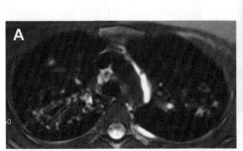
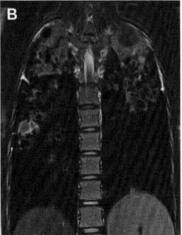

Fig. 16. Cystic fibrosis in a 17-year-old girl. (*A*) Axial T2-weighted MR image shows bilateral upper lobe bronchiectasis, right lung more severely affected than the left lung. Bronchial wall edema and mucous plugging is best seen in the right upper lobe. (*B*) Coronal T2-weighted MR image demonstrates bilateral upper-lobe-predominant bronchiectasis, mucous plugging, and consolidative opacities. (*Courtesy of* Goffredo Serra, MD, Rome, Italy.)

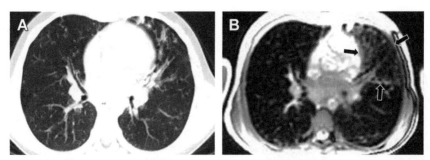

Fig. 17. Cystic fibrosis. (*A*) Axial noncontrast CT image demonstrates bronchiectasis and bronchial wall thickening, which is most evident in the lingula. (*B*) Axial T2-weighted MR image redemonstrates the bronchiectasis (*arrows*). The bronchial walls are thickened and edematous.

gas imaging or oxygen-enhanced imaging, 2 different investigational techniques that may eventually become part of the clinical evaluation of patients with small airways disease.[22,59]

FUTURE DIRECTIONS

Hyperpolarized gas is a tool currently in the research stage that allows radiologists to overcome the limitations of low ^{1}H MR imaging signals because of the low proton density in gas-filled lungs. Instead of obtaining MR signal from protons, the MR scanners operate at radiofrequencies sensitive to the resonant frequencies of either ^{129}Xe or ^{3}He nuclei, gases that are inhaled by the patient immediately preceding the scan. Both hyperpolarized gases (ie, ^{129}Xe and ^{3}He) produce excellent image quality, although the higher atomic weight of ^{129}Xe could make this agent more sensitive to airflow abnormalities. Furthermore, significant differences in the tissue permeability of ^{3}He (impermeable) and ^{129}Xe (very permeable) offer different and possibly complementary information regarding lung structure and function. The safety and efficacy of this technique suggest that it may soon enter into routine clinical practice particularly nowadays with advances in polarizer technology.[60]

Fourier decomposition is a new MR technique that provides perfusion and ventilation images without administration of intravenous or gaseous contrast agents. This technique uses a high-temporal-resolution steady-state free precession sequence to acquire thick slab coronal images in free breathing conditions. The images are first lined up using a nonrigid registration algorithm. Next, by computing voxelwise Fourier decomposition of the time series, the signal originating from the blood perfusion is separated (decomposed) from the signal related to the breathing cycle (**Fig. 19**). A recent study with Fourier decomposition has proved that this

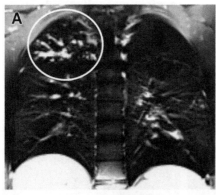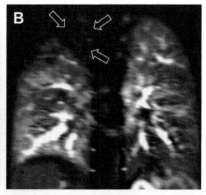

Fig. 18. Cystic fibrosis. (*A*) Coronal PROPELLER/BLADE proton-density-weighted MR image shows area of bronchiectasis and mucous impaction in the right upper lobe, which results in low parenchyma intensity because of air trapping (*white oval*). (*B*) Coronal TRICKS/TWIST, dynamic magnetic resonance angiography (MRA) with k-space manipulation image shows the same area of lung structural changes that is hypoperfused (*arrows*). (*Courtesy of Goffredo Serra, MD, Rome, Italy.*)

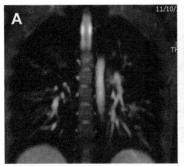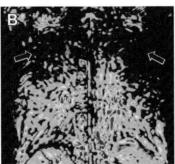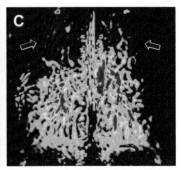

Fig. 19. (A) Air trapping detected in Fourier decomposition MR image. Coronal balanced steady-state free precession/true fast imaging with steady-state precession demonstrates bilateral upper-lobe-predominant bronchial wall thickening and bronchiectasis, which result in air trapping (low signal). (B) Ventilation defect detected in Fourier decomposition MR image. Ventilation map demonstrates decreased ventilation (*arrows*) in the lung apices compared with the lung bases. (C) Perfusion defect detected in Fourier decomposition MR image. Perfusion map shows that the bilateral lung apices are also hypoperfused (*arrows*). (*Courtesy of* Giovanni Morana, MD, PhD, Treviso, Italy.)

technique is feasible in pediatric populations and may represent an elegant alternative to intravenous contrast agents and hyperpolarized gases.[46]

SUMMARY

The performance of high-quality thoracic MR imaging in the pediatric population requires close attention to patient preparation, which includes patient selection, protocol optimization, and appropriate sedation strategies. In addition, it also requires a clear understanding of the basic physics principles as well as the appearance of varied pathologic entities. Although the learning curve may appear steep, the potential rewards of added diagnostic information without the cost of radiation exposure to the child provide excellent motivation to incorporate thoracic MR imaging into daily practice. Current applications have already proved its practical value, and future applications have a great potential to improve its importance and encourage its widespread use.

REFERENCES

1. Rajaram S, Swift AJ, Capener D, et al. Lung morphology assessment with balanced steady-state free precession MR imaging compared with CT. Radiology 2012;263(2):569–77.
2. Fink C, Puderbach M, Biederer J, et al. Lung MRI at 1.5 and 3 Tesla: observer preference study and lesion contrast using five different pulse sequences. Invest Radiol 2007;42(6):377–83.
3. Liu J. Lung ultrasonography for the diagnosis of neonatal lung disease. J Matern Fetal Neonatal Med 2014;27(8):856–61.
4. Darge K, Chen A. Point-of-care ultrasound in diagnosing pneumonia in children. J Pediatr 2013; 163(1):302–3.
5. Reissig A, Copetti R, Mathis G, et al. Lung ultrasound in the diagnosis and follow-up of community-acquired pneumonia: a prospective, multicenter, diagnostic accuracy study. Chest 2012;142(4):965–72.
6. Shah VP, Tunik MG, Tsung JW. Prospective evaluation of point-of-care ultrasonography for the diagnosis of pneumonia in children and young adults. JAMA Pediatr 2013;167(2):119–25.
7. Coley BD. Chest sonography in children: current indications, techniques, and imaging findings. Radiol Clin North Am 2011;49(5):825–46.
8. Biederer J, Beer M, Hirsch W, et al. MRI of the lung (2/3). Why … when … how? Insights Imaging 2012; 3(4):355–71.
9. Montella S, Maglione M, Bruzzese D, et al. Magnetic resonance imaging is an accurate and reliable method to evaluate non-cystic fibrosis paediatric lung disease. Respirology 2012;17(1):87–91.
10. Barreto MM, Rafful PP, Rodrigues RS, et al. Correlation between computed tomographic and magnetic resonance imaging findings of parenchymal lung diseases. Eur J Radiol 2013;82(9):e492–501.
11. Yikilmaz A, Koc A, Coskun A, et al. Evaluation of pneumonia in children: comparison of MRI with fast imaging sequences at 1.5T with chest radiographs. Acta Radiol 2011;52(8):914–9.
12. Gorkem SB, Coskun A, Yikilmaz A, et al. Evaluation of pediatric thoracic disorders: comparison of unenhanced fast-imaging-sequence 1.5-T MRI and contrast-enhanced MDCT. AJR Am J Roentgenol 2013;200(6):1352–7.
13. Peprah KO, Andronikou S, Goussard P. Characteristic magnetic resonance imaging low T2 signal intensity of necrotic lung parenchyma in children

with pulmonary tuberculosis. J Thorac Imaging 2012;27(3):171–4.

14. Hirsch W, Sorge I, Krohmer S, et al. MRI of the lungs in children. Eur J Radiol 2008;68(2):278–88.

15. Kantarci M, Bayraktutan U, Karabulut N, et al. Alveolar echinococcosis: spectrum of findings at cross-sectional imaging. Radiographics 2012;32(7):2053–70.

16. Pedrosa I, Saíz A, Arrazola J, et al. Hydatid disease: radiologic and pathologic features and complications. Radiographics 2000;20(3):795–817.

17. Lee EY, Dorkin H, Vargas SO. Congenital pulmonary malformations in pediatric patients: review and update on etiology, classification, and imaging findings. Radiol Clin North Am 2011;49(5):921–48.

18. Khalek N, Johnson MP. Management of prenatally diagnosed lung lesions. Semin Pediatr Surg 2013; 22(1):24–9.

19. Pacharn P, Kline-Fath B, Calvo-Garcia M, et al. Congenital lung lesions: prenatal MRI and postnatal findings. Pediatr Radiol 2013;43(9):1136–43.

20. Recio Rodríguez M, Martínez de Vega V, Cano Alonso R, et al. MR imaging of thoracic abnormalities in the fetus. Radiographics 2012;32(7):E305–21.

21. Naidich DP, Rumancik WM, Ettenger NA, et al. Congenital anomalies of the lungs in adults: MR diagnosis. AJR Am J Roentgenol 1988;151(1):13–9.

22. Liszewski MC, Hersman FW, Altes TA, et al. Magnetic resonance imaging of pediatric lung parenchyma, airways, vasculature, ventilation, and perfusion: state of the art. Radiol Clin North Am 2013;51(4):555–82.

23. Xu H, Jiang D, Kong X, et al. Pulmonary sequestration: three dimensional dynamic contrast-enhanced MR angiography and MRI. J Tongji Med Univ 2001;21(4):345–8.

24. Peranteau WH, Merchant AM, Hedrick HL, et al. Prenatal course and postnatal management of peripheral bronchial atresia: association with congenital cystic adenomatoid malformation of the lung. Fetal Diagn Ther 2008;24(3):190–6.

25. Griffin N, Devaraj A, Goldstraw P, et al. CT and histopathological correlation of congenital cystic pulmonary lesions: a common pathogenesis? Clin Radiol 2008;63(9):995–1005.

26. Yu H, Li HM, Liu SY, et al. Diagnosis of arterial sequestration using multidetector CT angiography. Eur J Radiol 2010;76(2):274–8.

27. Dishop MK, Kuruvilla S. Primary and metastatic lung tumors in the pediatric population: a review and 25-year experience at a large children's hospital. Arch Pathol Lab Med 2008;132(7):1079–103.

28. Weldon CB, Shamberger RC. Pediatric pulmonary tumors: primary and metastatic. Semin Pediatr Surg 2008;17(1):17–29.

29. Baez JC, Lee EY, Restrepo R, et al. Chest wall lesions in children. AJR Am J Roentgenol 2013; 200(5):W402–19.

30. Takayama Y, Yabuuchi H, Matsuo Y, et al. Computed tomographic and magnetic resonance features of inflammatory myofibroblastic tumor of the lung in children. Radiat Med 2008;26(10):613–7.

31. Demir HA, Yalcin B, Ciftci AO, et al. Primary pleuropulmonary neoplasms in childhood: fourteen cases from a single center. Asian Pac J Cancer Prev 2011;12(2):543–7.

32. Mut Pons R, Muro Velilla MD, Sangüesa Nebot C, et al. Pleuropulmonary blastoma in children: imaging findings and clinical patterns. Radiologia 2008; 50(6):489–94.

33. De Jong PA, Mayo JR, Golmohammadi K, et al. Estimation of cancer mortality associated with repetitive computed tomography scanning. Am J Respir Crit Care Med 2006;173(2):199–203.

34. Chawla SC, Federman N, Zhang D, et al. Estimated cumulative radiation dose from PET/CT in children with malignancies: a 5-year retrospective review. Pediatr Radiol 2010;40(5):681–6.

35. Biederer J, Hintze C, Fabel M. MRI of pulmonary nodules: technique and diagnostic value. Cancer Imaging 2008;8:125–30.

36. Wu LM, Xu JR, Hua J, et al. Can diffusion-weighted imaging be used as a reliable sequence in the detection of malignant pulmonary nodules and masses? Magn Reson Imaging 2013;31(2):235–46.

37. Regier M, Schwarz D, Henes FO, et al. Diffusion-weighted MR-imaging for the detection of pulmonary nodules at 1.5 Tesla: intraindividual comparison with multidetector computed tomography. J Med Imaging Radiat Oncol 2011;55(3):266–74.

38. Koyama H, Ohno Y, Seki S, et al. Magnetic resonance imaging for lung cancer. J Thorac Imaging 2013;28(3):138–50.

39. Lutterbey G, Gieseke J, von Falkenhausen M, et al. Lung MRI at 3.0 T: a comparison of helical CT and high-field MRI in the detection of diffuse lung disease. Eur Radiol 2005;15(2):324–8.

40. Lutterbey G, Grohé C, Gieseke J, et al. Initial experience with lung-MRI at 3.0 T: comparison with CT and clinical data in the evaluation of interstitial lung disease activity. Eur J Radiol 2007;61(2):256–61.

41. Müller NL, Mayo JR, Zwirewich CV. Value of MR imaging in the evaluation of chronic infiltrative lung diseases: comparison with CT. AJR Am J Roentgenol 1992;158(6):1205–9.

42. Yi CA, Lee KS, Han J, et al. 3-T MRI for differentiating inflammation- and fibrosis-predominant lesions of usual and nonspecific interstitial pneumonia: comparison study with pathologic correlation. AJR Am J Roentgenol 2008;190(4):878–85.

43. Eichinger M, Heussel CP, Kauczor HU, et al. Computed tomography and magnetic resonance imaging in cystic fibrosis lung disease. J Magn Reson Imaging 2010;32(6):1370–8.

44. Puderbach M, Hintze C, Ley S, et al. MR imaging of the chest: a practical approach at 1.5T. Eur J Radiol 2007;64(3):345–55.

45. Failo R, Wielopolski PA, Tiddens HA, et al. Lung morphology assessment using MRI: a robust ultra-short TR/TE 2D steady state free precession sequence used in cystic fibrosis patients. Magn Reson Med 2009;61(2):299–306.

46. Bauman G, Puderbach M, Heimann T, et al. Validation of Fourier decomposition MRI with dynamic contrast-enhanced MRI using visual and automated scoring of pulmonary perfusion in young cystic fibrosis patients. Eur J Radiol 2013;82(12):2371–7.

47. Ciet P, Wielopolski P, Manniesing R, et al. Spirometer controlled cine-magnetic resonance imaging to diagnose tracheobronchomalacia in pediatric patients. Eur Respir J 2014;43(1):115–24.

48. Tan JZ, Ditchfield M, Freezer N. Tracheobronchomalacia in children: review of diagnosis and definition. Pediatr Radiol 2012;42(8):906–15 [quiz: 1027–8].

49. Erdem E, Gokdemir Y, Unal F, et al. Flexible bronchoscopy as a valuable tool in the evaluation of infants with stridor. Eur Arch Otorhinolaryngol 2013;270(1):21–5.

50. Murgu S, Colt H. Tracheobronchomalacia and excessive dynamic airway collapse. Clin Chest Med 2013;34(3):527–55.

51. Sanchez MO, Greer MC, Masters IB, et al. A comparison of fluoroscopic airway screening with flexible bronchoscopy for diagnosing tracheomalacia. Pediatr Pulmonol 2012;47(1):63–7.

52. Lee EY, Strauss KJ, Tracy DA, et al. Comparison of standard-dose and reduced-dose expiratory MDCT techniques for assessment of tracheomalacia in children. Acad Radiol 2010;17(4):504–10.

53. Lee EY, Tracy DA, Bastos MD, et al. Expiratory volumetric MDCT evaluation of air trapping in pediatric patients with and without tracheomalacia. AJR Am J Roentgenol 2010;194(5):1210–5.

54. Tan JZ, Crossett M, Ditchfield M. Dynamic volumetric computed tomographic assessment of the young paediatric airway: initial experience of rapid, non-invasive, four-dimensional technique. J Med Imaging Radiat Oncol 2013;57(2):141–8.

55. Wagnetz U, Roberts HC, Chung T, et al. Dynamic airway evaluation with volume CT: initial experience. Can Assoc Radiol J 2010;61(2):90–7.

56. Wielpütz MO, Eichinger M, Puderbach M. Magnetic resonance imaging of cystic fibrosis lung disease. J Thorac Imaging 2013;28(3):151–9.

57. Tiddens HA, Rosenow T. What did we learn from two decades of chest computed tomography in cystic fibrosis? Pediatr Radiol 2014;44(12):1490–5.

58. Sileo C, Corvol H, Boelle PY, et al. HRCT and MRI of the lung in children with cystic fibrosis: comparison of different scoring systems. J Cyst Fibros 2014; 13(2):198–204.

59. Qing K, Ruppert K, Jiang Y, et al. Regional mapping of gas uptake by blood and tissue in the human lung using hyperpolarized xenon-129 MRI. J Magn Reson Imaging 2014;39(2):346–59.

60. Kirby M, Parraga G. Pulmonary functional imaging using hyperpolarized noble gas MRI: six years of start-up experience at a single site. Acad Radiol 2013;20(11):1344–56.

Index

Note: Page numbers of article titles are in **boldface** type.

Magn Reson Imaging Clin N Am 23 (2015) 351–354
http://dx.doi.org/10.1016/S1064-9689(15)00029-X
1064-9689/15/$ – see front matter © 2015 Elsevier Inc. All rights reserved.

mri.theclinics.com

Moving?

Make sure your subscription moves with you!

To notify us of your new address, find your **Clinics Account Number** (located on your mailing label above your name), and contact customer service at:

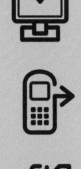

Email: journalscustomerservice-usa@elsevier.com

800-654-2452 (subscribers in the U.S. & Canada)
314-447-8871 (subscribers outside of the U.S. & Canada)

Fax number: 314-447-8029

Elsevier Health Sciences Division
Subscription Customer Service
3251 Riverport Lane
Maryland Heights, MO 63043